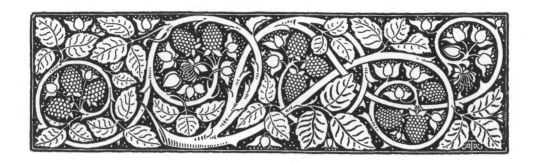

You can view this as a recipe book and use it as such, but I hope this book will inspire you to walk the path of the Hearth Witch, which is so much more. While you may begin to learn how to work with natural resources from books like this one, the true teaching only comes when you start listening to the land and its plants and animals.

When the sacred within you recognises the sacred that surrounds you everywhere, a deeper spiritual reality opens up in which all space becomes sacred space, all time becomes sacred time, and all acts become sacred acts.

This is the true path of the Hearth Witch. Walk it in beauty.

Anna Franklin

THE HEARTH Witch's COMPENDIUM

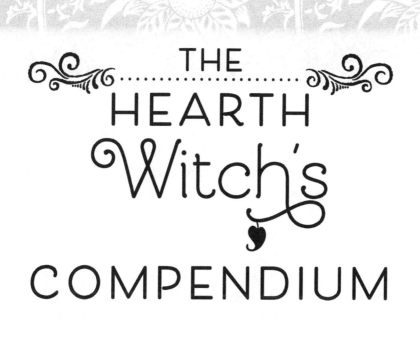

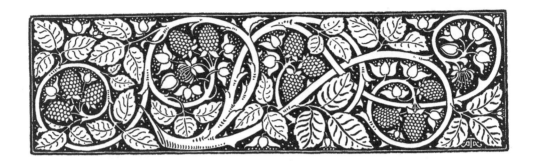

Anna Franklin is a third-degree witch and high priestess of the Hearth of Arianrhod, and she has been a practicing Pagan for more than forty years. She is the author of twenty-eight books and the creator of the *Sacred Circle Tarot*, *Fairy Ring Oracle*, and the *Pagan Ways Tarot* (Schiffer, 2015). Her books have been translated into nine languages.

Anna has contributed hundreds of articles to Pagan magazines and has appeared on radio and TV. She lives and works in a village in the English Midlands, where she grows her own herbs, fruit, and vegetables, and generally lives the Pagan life. Visit her online at www.AnnaFranklin.co.uk.

THE HEARTH Witch's

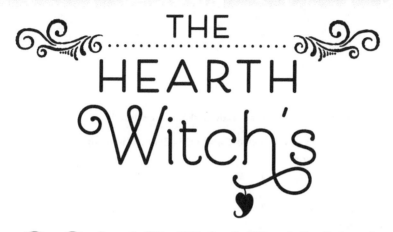

COMPENDIUM

MAGICAL AND NATURAL LIVING FOR EVERY DAY

ANNA FRANKLIN

Llewellyn Publications
woodbury, minnesota

FIRST EDITION
Ninth Printing, 2024

Book design by Rebecca Zins
Cover design by Ellen Lawson
Interior floral background © Dover Publications
Interior floral woodcut © *1167 Decorative Cuts* (New York: Dover Publications, 2007)

Llewellyn is a registered trademark of Llewellyn Worldwide Ltd.

Library of Congress Cataloging-In-Publication Data
Names: Franklin, Anna, author.
Title: The hearth witch's compendium : magical and natural living for every
    day / Anna Franklin.
Description: Woodbury : Llewellyn Worldwide, Ltd, 2017. | Includes
    bibliographical references and index.
Identifiers: LCCN 2016045983 (print) | LCCN 2016052034 (ebook) | ISBN
    9780738750460 (alk. paper) | ISBN 9780738751900 ()
Subjects: LCSH: Witchcraft. | Herbs—Miscellanea. | Plants—Miscellanea. |
    Formulas, recipes, etc.
Classification: LCC BF1566 .F694 2017 (print) | LCC BF1566 (ebook) | DDC
    133.4/3—dc23
LC record available at https://lccn.loc.gov/2016045983

Llewellyn Publications
A Division of Llewellyn Worldwide Ltd.
2143 Wooddale Drive
Woodbury MN 55125-2989

www.llewellyn.com
Printed in the United States of America

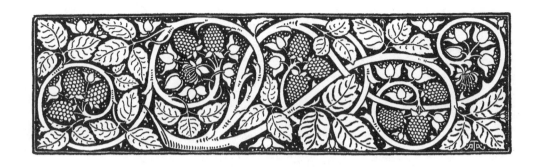

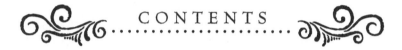

CONTENTS

CHAPTER 5
• • • • • • •

The Witch's Home   163

CHAPTER 11

Essential Oils   317

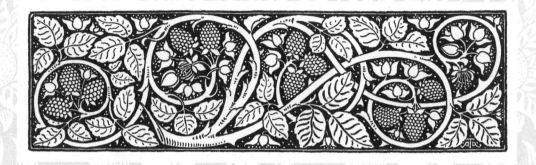

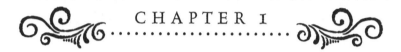

CHAPTER 1

Hearth Witchery

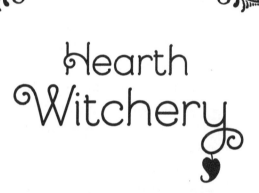

The garden is full of roses this week. They flop over the fences and scramble up the trellis, their soft, sensual blooms filling the air with a voluptuous perfume. It is easy to understand why they are sacred to so many gods and goddesses of love—Isis, Aphrodite, Venus, Eros, Cupid, Inanna, and Ishtar, to name just a few. I bless the plants and gather armfuls of flowers.

I take them into the house and lay them on the kitchen table and begin to separate the red flowers from the white. I'm reminded that in one Greek tale, when the goddess Aphrodite first arose from the ocean and stepped onto the shore, the sparkling sea foam fell from her body in the form of pale white roses and took root. Later, as she pursued the beautiful youth Adonis, she caught herself on a thorn and her blood dyed the roses crimson red, symbolising innocence turned to desire and maidenhood turned to womanhood.[1] For magical purposes, while my white roses stand for purity, perfection, innocence, virginity, and the moon, the red roses represent earthly passion and fertility. Wound together, they signify the union of opposites—symbolism we use at Beltane to celebrate the sacred marriage of the God and Goddess, an act which reconciles male and female, summer and winter, life and death, and flesh and spirit, and brings about all creation, driven by the most fundamental and powerful force in the universe: love.

However, Midsummer is tomorrow, and roses play a part in our solstice ritual since, like other flowers with rayed petals, they are an emblem of the sun. Like the sun, which dies each night and is reborn each day at sunrise, the rose is an emblem of renewal, resurrection, and eternal life, which is why the Celts, Egyptians, and Romans used them as funeral offerings. [2] [3] [4] I set aside some to make offerings for dead friends later, and others to make chaplets for Midsummer.

I'm still left with an abundance of blossoms. I take down two clean glass jars from my cupboard and pack both of them with the scented petals I carefully pull from the stems. One jar I top up with white vinegar and set it on the sunny kitchen windowsill. I will leave it there for two weeks before straining the liquid into a clean jar. My resulting rose vinegar can be used as a delicate salad dressing, an antiseptic wash for wiping down my kitchen surfaces, or be dabbed onto my forehead to relieve headaches. The second jar of rose petals I fill up with one part distilled water to three parts vodka. I label it and put it in a cool, dark place in my pantry, where it will stay for three weeks. When it is ready, I will strain the liquid into a clean jar—and lo and behold, I will have made my own rose hydrosol. I will use it as a skin toner just as it is, but I could chill it to make a compress for puffy eyes or use it as a final conditioning rinse for my hair. Next month I will incorporate some into skin lotions and creams.

The gorgeous fresh petals I have left could be baked into cakes and cookies, made into a delicate jam or a wine for next year's Midsummer solstice, or crystallised for cake decorations. Tonight I will drop some petals into my bath to make a relaxing soak after a hard day in the garden, and before I go to bed I will put a handful into the teapot and infuse them

---

1   Jennifer Peace Rhind, *Fragrance & Wellbeing: Plant Aromatics and Their Influence on the Psyche* (London: Singing Dragon, 2013).

2   Miranda Green, *Gods of the Celts* (Stroud: Sutton Publishing Ltd, 1986).

3   Roger Phillips and Martyn Rix, *The Ultimate Guide to Roses* (London: Macmillan, 2004).

4   Laurie Brink and Deborah Green, *Commemorating the Dead: Texts and Artifacts in Context; Studies of Roman, Jewish, and Christian Burials* (Berlin: de Gruyter, 2008).

in boiling water to make a subtle, fragrant tea that is mildly sedative and good for tension headaches.

I spread out more petals on a tray and put them to dry in the airing cupboard. These dried petals are not only good for rose tea later in the year and the usual potpourri, but can be employed in magical talismans, charm bags, and incense—red for love; yellow for Midsummer, renewal, and the sun; and white for moon rituals. So many virtues in just one plant, and I've only scratched the surface of what the rose has to offer. Each day Mother Nature has a different gift for me.

I've worked in this way for decades now. My kitchen is hung with drying plants, and my pantry contains jars of dried herbs to use for magic and healing tinctures and salves, as well as for brewing wines and making jars of jam. I am a hearth witch. Though there are many paths to magic, this is the term I invented some years ago to describe my own.[5] I consider my house to be a sacred place, a temple of the gods, where I live, work, and worship. As I make a fire in the hearth or light a candle, I honour the living goddess of the hearth fire (known as Brighid in Ireland, Hestia in Greece, and Vesta in Rome) and her presence in my home. On the shelves beside my hearth is a shrine to my household gods, and as I clean and tidy I think of it as honouring them. With intent, a physical cleansing can become a psychic cleansing, sweeping away negative energies.

I as prepare food, I try to do it with intent—to make my body healthy, to thank Mother Earth for her bounty, and to share it with love. Each ingredient is honoured for its individual life force and its inherent physical and spiritual properties. All the vegetable peelings and scraps go on to the compost heap, which will nourish my garden plants, and I think that recycling and composting are much more powerful ways of honouring Mother Earth than muttering a few words in a ritual now and again; the hearth witch not only believes that the earth is sacred, she treats it as such.

My garden teaches me more about the magic of nature than any book, as I try to understand how each plant grows and what it needs, and how to work with it so that it will give me food; ingredients for wine, dyes, and magical potions; or help me with my healing work. Season by season I collect its wealth, along with the wild bounty of the fields and hedgerows around my village.

In this way, the hearth witch sees the sacred within the physical, the magical in the mundane, and uses this knowledge to incorporate spiritual practice into everyday life. I suspect that most of us feel we should make a lot more time in our lives for spiritual practice,

---

5 Anna Franklin, *Hearth Witch* (Earl Shilton: Lear Books, 2004).

chiding ourselves that we really *must* put aside that thirty minutes for daily meditation or that evening for ritual, then struggling to fit it in and being left with feelings of guilt and failure. This approach is a reflection of a culture that sees the spiritual and physical as separate. Traditional Pagan societies have always recognised that the spiritual and the physical are indivisible and that one is a reflection of the other. When we bring our attention and intent into cooking a meal, lighting a candle, or just being aware of our feet meeting the earth as we walk, it becomes a spiritual practice and opens up a deeper reality, the great matrix of Nature connected in a unified, sacred whole. We recognise that the land beneath our feet is not merely dirt but a fountain of energy that sustains animals, plants, and people.[6] When this realisation dawns, all space becomes sacred space, all time becomes sacred time, and all acts become sacred acts.

Paganism is not a man-made religion created by a human prophet or guru but one that continually evolves out of a spiritual relationship with the natural world. As well as providing shelter, food, medicine, and all that is necessary for life, Mother Earth is the basis of our spiritual existence.[7] Paganism's many gods and goddesses represent the diversity of the natural world with indwelling divinity present in all things—from a blade of grass to a stream, from a mountain to a galaxy. When we open our souls to nature, we touch our gods; but when we turn our backs on it, we feel a sense of alienation, of spiritual and emotional loss, because we are cut off from our divine source.

In bygone ages, of course, most of us lived much closer to nature than we do now. Once every woman had to be something of an herbalist and healer, responsible for her household's health, since professional medical help was either unavailable or too expensive (and possibly dangerous to boot). Every home kept some drying herbs and flowers to make herbal infusions, powders, oils, and poultices; brewed wine and ale; preserved fruit; made jams and jellies, pickles and chutneys; and many also made inks, dyes, soaps, and household cleaners. A girl would be initiated into the secrets of these family formulas by her mother, who would also pass along her knowledge of folklore, stories, healing potions, minor surgery, gardening, brewing and wine making, spinning, weaving, dyeing, childcare, home management, animal husbandry, beekeeping, fortunetelling, and cookery know-how.

And then there were those in the community who knew a little bit more: the village wise woman or cunning man. When I joined my first coven, our high priestess, Julia, told us stories of the herb wives of the past, who cared for the bodies and spirits of those around

---

6   Aldo Leopold, A *Sand County Almanac* (New York: Oxford University Press, 1977).
7   Larissa Behrendt, "Aboriginal Urban Identity: Preserving the Spirit, Protecting the Traditional in Non-Traditional Settings," *Australian Feminist Law Journal* 4, no. 1 (1995): 55–61.

them, telling their fortunes, treating their bodily ailments with herbs, dowsing their lost property, and physicking their farm animals. She held them up to us as examples of powerful, magical women in an age when women otherwise had little influence. They were the midwives who brought new life into the world, she said, and who laid out the dead at the end of life.

Though such stories have often been wildly romanticised, folklore records and accounts do show that virtually every village seems to have had a wise woman or a cunning man of some sort. These village shamans had different names in different places, including handy-women, blessers, witches, conjurers, herb wives, wild herb men, snake doctors, fairy doctors, and currens.[8] In some parts of England they had the title Old Mother Redcap, since the red cap was a badge of office amongst wise women. There was often some oddity of dress among wise women and cunning men, such as odd socks or a garment worn inside out.[9] These practitioners didn't use athames and magic swords but everyday objects—stones, keys, shears, sieves, pitchforks, brooms, divining rods, wax, bottles, paper, and anything that came readily to hand from the kitchen or farm.

It wasn't only the poor that resorted to their services either. When the then-Prince of Wales bought Sandringham in 1863, he expelled "several wise women" who lived in a group of cottages there, which he had torn down and replaced by modern ones for his servants. Only one old wise woman was allowed to remain at Flitcham, for it was said that the prince's agent dared not remove her. She was endowed with a vast knowledge of herbal cures and was known to wander miles in search of a certain herb needed for a specific cure. When the prince was taken ill, he was advised to use the herbal remedies of the old wise woman, who made him drink mandrake wine for his cure.[10] [11]

Guided by some of my early teachers in the Craft, I began to study the ancient wisdom of the grandmothers, the wise women, once passed down from mother to daughter and crone to apprentice, and then improved by a lifetime of study and the daily observation of the patterns of nature. I certainly wasn't brought up in this way or taught any of those things as a child, and as an ardent feminist, for years I refused to do anything traditionally defined as "women's work." However, I gradually realised that such expertise had formed the pattern of women's lives for thousands of years and that women had developed highly

---

8   Nigel Pennick, *Secrets of East Anglian Magic* (Milverton: Capall Bann, 2004).

9   Ibid.

10 C. F. Tebbutt, *Huntingdonshire Folklore* (St. Ives, Huntingdon: The Friends of the Norris Museum, 1984).

11 Pennick.

skilful methods in all these areas, even though no contemporary historian wrote about them or accorded women due status for their invaluable work.

Indeed, any woman practicing fortunetelling, midwifery, or herbalism could be executed as a witch, while male doctors, astrologers, and alchemists were left unscathed. Following the fifteenth-century Council of Trent, the church specifically forbade women from having anything to do with medicine,[12] a profession they were not to be readmitted to until the late nineteenth century. While male university-trained doctors were sanctioned by the church, if any woman stood before a tribunal accused of practicing medicine or healing it was automatically assumed that she must have achieved any cure by witchcraft, and she was put to death.[13] According to the infamous *Malleus Maleficarum* ("Hammer of the Witches"), the inquisitor's handbook, "If a woman dare to cure without having studied than she is a witch and must die." Male doctors were trusted implicitly by the authors of the *Malleus Maleficarum*: "Although some of their remedies seem to be vain and superstitious cantrips and charms…everybody must be trusted in his profession."[14]

Women's knowledge has been derided and ignored for most of our history, and this is just as true today in Western culture, in which knowledge is "owned" by experts (mainly men) and can only be passed on through state-approved academic institutions, and where those seeking to follow traditional or alternative paths—such as herbalism—are dismissed as uneducated, naïve, or even dangerous.

But this is *our* knowledge, *our* heritage—as women and as witches, both male and female. Discovering it and practicing my Craft has been a marvellous adventure for me, and it never ceases to fill me with wonder and awe at the power of Mother Nature. It makes me aware of the magic that flows throughout the world in every uncurling oak leaf in spring, every blushing rose petal, every humming summer bee, every rutting stag, and every misty shore.[15] This is the reward of the path of the hearth witch, and this is what I want to share with you in this book.

12   Brian P. Levack (editor), *New Perspectives on Witchcraft, Magic and Demonology: Witchcraft, Healing and Popular Diseases*, Volume 5 (Routledge, 2002).

13   Heinrich Kramer and James Sprenger, trans. Montague Summers, *Malleus Maleficarum* (London: Bracken Books, 1996; first edition 1486).

14   Ibid.

15   Anna Franklin, *Pagan Ways Tarot* (Atglen: Schiffer Publishing Ltd, 2015).

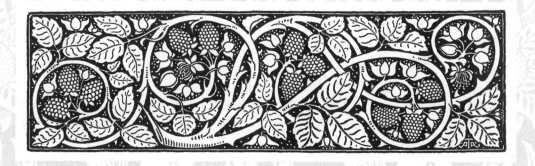

CHAPTER 2

The Witch's Kitchen

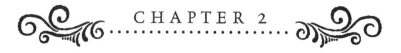

Food is one of the most basic necessities of life. Food is life, a gift of Mother Earth, and we acknowledge that gift only when we treat it with reverence. Preparing, cooking, and serving food is a day-to-day ritual of hospitality, love, and sharing that expresses the cycle of the year when fresh seasonal food is used.

Whether you are cooking for a sabbat or just for supper, treat it as a conscious act of magic and reflect that when you eat, you take in the life energy of the food you are consuming, not just its nutrition. Each ingredient possesses its own virtues and energies, and you can utilise these gifts to create culinary magic. Do you want to add sage for wisdom, rosemary for remembrance, lemon balm for joy? You can cook up a love feast, a meal for peace and healing, or a dish for abundance. All nuts are associated with fertility, all grains with abundance, and most fruits with love. The kitchen is a magical workshop and the oven an alchemical tool that transmutes raw ingredients into sustenance for body and spirit. Prepare your food with intent, stir your dishes sunwise to wind up the magic, eat consciously, and give thanks to Mother Earth for her gifts.

Food Ethics

Concerned Pagans have to consider the ethics of their food choices, which have an impact on health, the environment, and animal welfare. Most Pagans say that the code they live by is "an' it harm none, do what you will." It is difficult to make ethical choices in a world dominated by factory farming that treats animals as unfeeling "production units," that promotes genetically modified plants and processed foods full of strange chemicals, and that advocates the use of poisonous fertilizers and pesticides, wasteful packaging, overfishing, exploitative labour practices, and a global market that means many food miles are added to a product. Sometimes the tide of injustice and suffering seems overwhelming. So what are we to do?

I think the only answer is that we do as much as we can as best and as honestly as we can. For me that means being vegetarian, eating organic whole foods, and growing as much of my own food as possible. For some it means being vegan and buying only from local growers; for others it might mean buying high-welfare-standard meat or only using fair trade products.

Ritual Food

Foods have always played a key part in rituals and the worship of the gods. Without food we would not live at all, and its production was one of the central themes of ancient religions.

One of the most valuable of the ancient foods was grain, which could be made into flour and then bread. It is one of the most important symbols of the nurturing goddess, sometimes seen as her son, the vegetation god, who would awaken in the spring, grow through the summer, and mature in the autumn, only to be harvested and die. The shed seeds lay dormant in the cold winter earth, the belly of the Earth Mother, ready to shoot up again in the spring. This was a never-ending cycle of life, death, and rebirth, a cycle also promised to worshippers.

Eating bread and drinking wine were important parts of the rites of vegetation deities. An ear of corn was the central mystery of Eleusis in the worship of Demeter,[16] and bread

---

16 Harold R. Willoughby, *Pagan Regeneration: A Study of Mystery Initiations in the Graeco-Roman World* (Chicago: The University of Chicago Press, 1929).

was eaten in the rites of Artemis and Cybele, often baked in circles and marked with a cross,[17] probably representing the four solar festivals of the equinoxes and solstices. This is still seen today in our hot crossed buns that are eaten at Easter, which was once the spring-time observance of the vegetation god's resurrection.

For ancient Pagans, grain and wine were god essences. When we consecrate bread and wine in a ritual, we invoke that god essence—the spiritual core of the food—and through it we absorb the power of the gods. It nourishes us physically and spiritually.

Wine is one of the "god-containing" substances believed by the ancients to allow people to share in god consciousness. Whereas bread is viewed as the body of the sacrificed god, wine is his blood; sometimes it is seen in traditional British Craft as the blood of the earth goddess.[18] The taking of the two together signifies the union of opposites. The cup that contains the wine symbolises the cauldron or grail, which contains wisdom and inspiration.

The chalice of wine and the platter of bread are passed around the circle, with the words "blessed be," to be shared by all present with love and blessings. This intimate act creates a connection with every other person present as well as a communion with the gods. It comes at the end of the ritual and helps to ground the participants before the circle is broken.

MAKING THE WINE AND BREAD

The wine for ritual should be homemade. Country wines can be made with seasonal ingredients—strawberries at Midsummer, blackberries at the autumn equinox, hawthorn flowers at Beltane, and so on. Our favourite for Samhain is sloe gin, and for Yule we always have mulled mead. You can find recipes for all of these in this book.

The wine should be put to brew with a blessing such as:

> Let the wine be made ready in the name of the God and in the name of the Goddess. Let it be placed on the altar beneath the sign of the pentagram that the worshippers shall drink of it. Before the God and the Goddess we shall consume and be consumed by the wine of wisdom and blessing.

Festival bread is made especially for the ritual. It is made with due ceremony and intent; buying a machine-made loaf from the supermarket just isn't good enough as an offering to the gods. In many parts of the world different breads are made for different occasions,

---

17   John G. R. Forlong, *Encyclopedia of Religions* (Cosimo Classics, 2013).

18   Julia Isobel Reed, personal communication.

their shapes and varieties reflecting the festival and its symbolism. Traditional loaf shapes are based upon binding knots or in the shape of suns and moons, animals and humans.[19] It would be appropriate to have a sun-shaped loaf for Midsummer or one in the form of a sheaf of wheat for Lughnasa, and so on.

The bread is put to bake with a blessing, such as:

> Let the bread be baked in the name of the God and Goddess, for now is the time of the [insert name of sabbat] feast, when the secret worshippers meet once more. Before the God and Goddess we shall feast and rejoice.

THE BLESSING OF THE CAKES AND WINE

This is done in different ways by different Pagan groups and traditions. In some covens the consecration is done by a priest and priestess together. The priestess might hold the cup while the priest plunges his athame into it and one of them will speak the blessing. In those groups that believe polarity is reversed on the astral, the priest holds the cup (the feminine) and the priestess plunges her knife (the masculine) into it and utters the words of consecration. In other groups the priestess will bless the wine and the priest the bread or vice versa. We like to share this task out between coven members so that at each festival a different person is responsible for blessing both the cakes and wine. They are usually asked to write their own words, which makes them consider what the ceremony means, but you might like to use something like this:

> I conjure thee, O wine; the light of the sun and the light of the moon have ripened the swelling grape—the blood of the earth pressed smooth. I conjure thee, O wine, that as we drink of thee we drink of the power of the Goddess; we see more of the ancient ways and know the ancient laws.

> I conjure thee, O meal, who art indeed our body, since without thee we would not live. I conjure thee, O meal, that as we partake of thee we partake of the wisdom of the God: we learn more of the fields and the forests, the things that are wild and free.

---

19 Nigel Pennick, *Natural Magic* (Earl Shilton: Lear Books, 2005).

FOOD OFFERINGS AND LIBATIONS

If the food has been made with intent and consecration, it becomes more than ordinary food and thus makes a suitable offering to the gods and spirits. When we bless the bread and wine, before we take any for ourselves, we offer a portion to the gods. With the words "the first is always for the gods," bread is thrown onto the fire so that its essence might be released to them. A libation of wine is made in a similar manner. (A libation is a pouring of wine, milk, or other drink onto the ground or before an image as an offering to the gods.) We always leave more food behind in the woods for the local spirits after the feast. In reality, of course, it is the animals and birds that eat it, but we consider that first the spirits consume its essence.

· · · ·

LIBUM

This is the bread traditionally offered by the Romans to their household spirits, the Lar Familiaris, on special occasions.

1 EGG, BEATEN

SMALL POT OF CREAM CHEESE (SUCH AS RICOTTA)

PEPPER

4 OUNCES (1 CUP) SPELT FLOUR

4 FRESH BAY LEAVES

RUNNY HONEY

Beat the egg into the cheese and pepper, then add the sifted flour to form a soft dough. Place the bay leaves on a greased baking dish and cover with the dough. Bake at 220°C/425°F/gas mark 7 for 30–40 minutes or until golden brown. Cut the bread open and drizzle on the honey while it is still hot.

Food for the Sabbats

In addition to sharing the bread and wine in ritual, it is the custom to feast at the eight sabbats of the Pagan year.

In the past, people were acutely aware of the passing of the seasons and what each had to offer in terms of foods and herbs. Humankind was bound to the Wheel of the Year, which determined times for planting, times for weeding, times for gathering seeds, and times for harvest. During the summer and autumn a wide variety of food would be available, but during the winter there would only be stored produce. By the end of winter even that would have been consumed, and only the return of spring and the greening of the land could save the population from starvation. In a time when food is always available in the shops, we tend to forget the importance of the agricultural and pastoral cycle, which was everything to our ancestors—when different foods were available at different seasons and the various festivities and occasions of the year involved their own special dishes. The festivals of the Craft attempt to make us more aware of the natural cycles and our part in them. In our seasonal celebrations and feasts, we try to honour and reflect these magical connections of herbs and plants with the seasons.

Imbolc

Imbolc is the modern Pagan festival that marks the first signs that spring and life are returning after the darkness and death of winter. It is celebrated at the beginning of February in the northern hemisphere and the beginning of November in the southern hemisphere. It was one of the four pastoral festivals of the ancient Irish but was also recognised and celebrated in other parts of the world under different names. It was finally Christianised as Candlemas, and some Pagans call it by this name.

Light increases after Yule, and by Imbolc this escalation is very conspicuous. The earth responds to it and begins to stir back into action. Snowdrops and crocuses flower, and early trees begin to bud. Animals start to emerge from hibernation and lambing begins, an obvious sign of regeneration, renewal, and the purity of the new season.

For the ancient Irish, it was the feast of the goddess Brighid. Her name is variously interpreted as "Fiery Arrow" or "The Bright One." She is a goddess of transformation: the transformation of ore to metal objects, seed to birth, inspiration to poetry, and the passage from winter to spring. Finding that the worship of the Pagan goddess Brighid was too deeply ingrained to be eradicated, Christians turned her into a saint, St. Brigid, and gave her the role of the nursemaid of Jesus who distracted Herod's soldiers by dancing with two candles so that the holy family could escape. This is a direct appropriation of the role of the Pagan goddess nurturing the Child of Light, born at the winter solstice and growing stronger with each passing day.

In our feast we remember that although this is often the coldest month of the year, beneath the surface Mother Nature is renewing herself.

TRADITIONAL FOODS FOR IMBOLC

In the northern regions snow often covers the ground and there is little fresh food to be found. Our ancestors would have been using up their stored produce and root vegetables, so the recipes of Imbolc mostly reflect this, but they might have been lucky enough to find some early spring greens, and any young edible shoots are good at this time to remind us that the earth is about to bud. One of the most important themes of Imbolc is the birth of spring lambs—a promise of what is to come—and the consequent lactating of sheep, so if you can, and your diet allows it, include some dairy produce in your feast, especially sheep's milk and cheese.

Cauliflower and Bean Sprout Stir Fry

2 TABLESPOONS OIL

1 OUNCE (2 TABLESPOONS/30 GRAMS) BUTTER

1 CAULIFLOWER

8 OUNCES (2 CUPS/226 GRAMS) BEAN SPROUTS

2 OUNCES (½ CUP/60 GRAMS) ALMOND SLIVERS

1 TEASPOON CUMIN SEEDS

1 TEASPOON GARAM MASALA

SEASONING TO TASTE

Heat the oil and butter in a frying pan. Cut the cauliflower into very small florets and add to the pan with the bean sprouts, almonds, and spices. Stir over medium heat for 5 minutes. Season and serve.

Parsnip Soup

1 POUND (3 CUPS/450 GRAMS) PARSNIPS

2 PINTS (4¾ CUPS/1,136 MILLILITRES) STOCK

1 TEASPOON MIXED HERBS

Wash and chop the parsnips. Add to the stock with the herbs. Cook until tender. Remove from the heat and liquidise. Return to the pan, reheat, and serve.

Butter Bean Soup

½ POUND (1½ CUPS/227 GRAMS) BUTTER BEANS

2 LARGE ONIONS

1 CHOPPED TURNIP

2 PINTS (4¾ CUPS/1,136 MILLILITRES) STOCK

1 TEASPOON MIXED HERBS

SEASONING TO TASTE

Soak the beans overnight in cold water. Chop the vegetables. Add all the ingredients to the stock. Simmer until the beans are cooked. Remove from the heat and liquidise. Return to the saucepan, reheat, and serve.

Bean Sprouts

Bean sprouts are symbolic of the season. You can sprout alfalfa seeds, mung beans, soya beans, lentils, peas, and chickpeas.

Soak seeds for at least 12 hours. Drain and rinse at regular intervals. You can put the seeds in a glass jar with a muslin lid secured by an elastic band. Rinse the seeds in clean water 2–4 times a day. After 3–5 days they will have sprouted, and when the shoots are 2–3 inches long they can be eaten. Do not allow them to dry out during the process. Do not eat if the shoots become discoloured or mouldy.

Curd Cheese

Curd cheese can be rolled in herbs, ground black pepper, or crushed mustard seeds. Refrigerate and eat within 1 week.

1 PINT (2⅓ CUPS/568 MILLILITRES) FULL CREAM MILK

FEW DROPS VEGETARIAN RENNET OR LEMON JUICE

SEASONING

Heat the milk to 160°C. Add the rennet or lemon juice to curdle the mixture. Pour it all into a cheesecloth bag and suspend this over a large bowl. Leave to drain overnight. Take the remaining curd cheese from the bag, sprinkle with salt, and shape as required.

Elizabethan Curds

This was a delicate Elizabethan dessert.

8 OUNCES (1 CUP/230 GRAMS) CURD CHEESE

½ TEASPOON POWDERED CINNAMON

A PINCH OF GRATED NUTMEG

1 TABLESPOON ROSE WATER

2 TEASPOONS SUGAR

Beat the ingredients together and serve with cream.

Lentil Roast (Vegan)

1 POUND (2 CUPS/450 GRAMS) RED LENTILS

1 ONION, CHOPPED

1 POUND (3 CUPS/450 GRAMS) MASHED POTATOES

1 TEASPOON MIXED HERBS

1 OUNCE (⅓ CUP/30 GRAMS) BREADCRUMBS

Cook the lentils until soft. Mix with the rest of the ingredients and spoon into a greased bread tin. Bake for 30 minutes in a hot oven at 200°C/400°F/gas mark 6 until brown.

Leek Pie

1 POUND (3 CUPS/450 GRAMS) POTATOES, CHOPPED

2 POUNDS (6 CUPS/900 GRAMS) LEEKS, CHOPPED

4 OUNCES (1 CUP/115 GRAMS) GRATED RED CHEESE OR SHARP CHEDDAR

1 PINT (2⅓ CUPS/568 MILLILITRES) WHITE SAUCE

2 OUNCES (¼ CUP/60 GRAMS) BUTTER OR MARGARINE

WHITE PEPPER

A PINCH OF NUTMEG

Boil the potatoes in a pan and steam the leeks over them until both vegetables are soft. Remove from heat and drain the potatoes. Arrange the leeks in a greased pie dish and cover them with the white sauce. Mash the potatoes and combine with the butter, cheese, white pepper, and nutmeg. Spread this mixture over the top of the leeks and white sauce and bake in a hot oven at 200°C/400°F/gas mark 6 until top is golden.

TATTIE DROTTLE

1½ POUNDS (4½ CUPS/680 GRAMS) POTATOES

8 OUNCES (1½ CUPS/226 GRAMS) TURNIPS

8 OUNCES (1½ CUPS/226 GRAMS) SWEDE (RUTABAGA)

8 OUNCES (1½ CUPS/226 GRAMS) CARROTS

4 OUNCES (¾ CUP/115 GRAMS) ONIONS

2 PINTS (4¾ CUPS/1,130 MILLILITRES) STOCK

1 PINT (2½ CUPS/565 GRAMS) MILK

CHOPPED PARSLEY

SALT AND PEPPER

Peel and finely chop all vegetables. Put them in a large pan with the stock and season to taste. Cover and simmer for one hour. Remove from heat; cool slightly. Add the milk and blend until smooth. Return to the pan and bring to a boil. Serve sprinkled with a little fresh chopped parsley.

BRIGHID CAKES

1 POUND (3½ CUPS/450 GRAMS) ALL-PURPOSE FLOUR

A PINCH OF SALT

1 TEASPOON CREAM OF TARTAR

1 TEASPOON BICARBONATE OF SODA (BAKING SODA)

4 OUNCES (½ CUP/110 GRAMS) BUTTER OR MARGARINE

4 OUNCES (½ CUP/110 GRAMS) SUGAR

2 OUNCES (½ CUP/60 GRAMS) CHOPPED CANDIED PEEL

4 OUNCES (1 CUP/110 GRAMS) SULTANAS

¾ PINT (1¾ CUPS/425 MILLILITRES) MILK

Sieve the flour and salt, cream of tartar, and bicarbonate of soda into a bowl. Rub in the butter, then add the sugar, peel, and sultanas. Add the milk and knead into a dough. Place in a greased 7-inch tin and bake in a hot oven at 200°C/400°F/ gas mark 6 for 60 minutes. Turn the oven down to 180°C/350°F/gas mark 4 and bake for another 30 minutes. Turn out and cut into smaller pieces to serve.

Oatcakes

4 OUNCES (1 CUP/114 GRAMS) MEDIUM OATMEAL

½ TEASPOON BICARBONATE OF SODA (BAKING SODA)

½ TEASPOON SALT

1 TEASPOON MELTED BUTTER

HOT WATER

Mix the oatmeal, soda, and salt. Make a well in the centre and pour in the melted butter and enough hot water to make a soft dough. Turn onto a surface dusted with oatmeal and form into a smooth ball. Knead and roll out thinly. Cut into 8 pieces and put on a baking sheet. Bake at 180°C/350°F/gas mark 4 until the edges curl. The oatcakes should be toasted under the grill just prior to eating. Serve with butter, cheese, or jam.

Pottage (Vegan)

Pottage is a traditional meal that has been made by people in Britain for hundreds of years. It was a popular breakfast dish throughout the seventeenth century and was the main food given to the poor in workhouses—the gruel referred to in Dickens's Oliver Twist was probably pottage. The word pottage is probably derived from the Latin porrum, meaning "a leek," and this became "porray" in Middle English. Later the word became pottage, and its meaning was extended to any thick green broth.

1 TABLESPOON SPLIT PEAS

1 TABLESPOON LENTILS

1 TABLESPOON PEARL BARLEY

2 PINTS (4¾ CUPS/1130 MILLILITRES) WATER

1 LEEK

1 OUNCE (½ CUP/30 GRAMS) CHOPPED CABBAGE

3 TABLESPOONS CHOPPED MIXED FRESH HERBS
OF YOUR CHOICE

SALT AND PEPPER

Soak the pulses and barley overnight in some water. The next day, drain, add fresh water, and boil for 30 minutes. Discard this water. Add 2 pints of fresh water and simmer until tender. Meanwhile, finely chop the herbs and vegetables. Add them to the pulses with some pepper and salt. Cook until vegetables are tender.

. . . .
POTATO BREAD

8 OUNCES (1½ CUPS/226 GRAMS) POTATOES, BOILED AND SIEVED

½ PINT (1 CUP/280 MILLILITRES) WATER POTATOES WERE BOILED IN

2 TEASPOONS SUGAR

1 TABLESPOON BUTTER OR MARGARINE

1 OUNCE (30 GRAMS) FRESH YEAST OR ½ OUNCE (15 GRAMS) ACTIVE
    DRY YEAST OR ¼ OUNCE (7 GRAMS) INSTANT YEAST

1½ POUNDS (5½ CUPS/680 GRAMS) WHOLEMEAL (WHOLE WHEAT)
    FLOUR

3 TEASPOONS SALT

Mix the potatoes, potato water, sugar, and butter. Cool to lukewarm and crumble in the yeast. Leave in a warm place for 10 minutes. Add the flour and salt gradually, mixing with your hands. Knead until smooth and not sticky. Cover and leave in a warm place until doubled in size. Knead again and divide in two. Place in two oiled loaf tins, cover with a clean cloth, and leave in a warm place to rise again. Bake at 230°C/450°F/gas mark 8 for 15 minutes. Reduce the heat to 190°C/375°F/gas mark 5 for 35–45 minutes until brown and hollow-sounding when tapped.

. . . . .

DROP SCONES

To sour milk, add a few drops of vinegar to fresh milk.

4 OUNCES (1 CUP/110 GRAMS) SELF-RAISING FLOUR

A PINCH OF SALT

¼ TEASPOON BICARBONATE OF SODA (BAKING SODA)

3 TABLESPOONS SUGAR

¼ PINT (⅔ CUP/150 MILLILITRES) SOURED MILK

1 BEATEN EGG

2 TEASPOONS MELTED BUTTER

Sift the flour, salt, and bicarbonate of soda into a bowl. Add the sugar, milk, egg, and butter, and beat into a batter. Heat a greased heavy frying pan. Drop tablespoons of the batter into the pan and cook until the top bubbles and the bottom is golden brown. Turn over and cook the other side. Serve with butter, jam, and cream.

BAKEWELL PUDDING

8 OUNCES (225 GRAMS) SHORTCRUST PASTRY

1 EGG

1 TABLESPOON BROWN SUGAR

GROUND ALMONDS

STRAWBERRY OR RASPBERRY JAM

Line a shallow baking dish with pastry. Beat the egg and add sugar and enough ground almonds to make a thick paste. Spread the bottom of the tart with jam and cover with the almond mixture. Bake in a moderate oven at 180°C/350°F/ gas mark 4 for 30 minutes or until brown on top.

Ostara

Ostara celebrates the vernal equinox, when day and night stand at equal length (twelve hours each) but the light is gaining and the days are getting longer. We can really feel spring in the air and notice the ever-increasing warmth and the burgeoning of life. We experience a resurgence of vigour and hope as the energies of the natural world shift from the lethargy of winter to the lively expansion of spring. The flowering of the gorse, daffodils, primrose, and coltsfoot—sun-coloured spring flowers—celebrate and reflect the increasing strength of the sun. Animals and birds are nest building and mating. At Ostara the gods and goddesses of fertility return to the land, and we see new growth everywhere.

Two thousand years ago across the world there were a variety of Pagan religions with markedly similar themes of a god who dies and is reborn at this time. He represents the vegetative cycles of the year: the grain grows and is cut down, only to be reborn again; the trees lose their leaves and seem to die, only to bud once more. In Phrygia, for example, the spring equinox marked the resurrection of Attis, a vegetation god and lover of the goddess Cybele. In ancient Rome the ten-day festival in honour of Attis began on March 15. A pine tree, which represented Attis, was chopped down, wrapped in a linen shroud, decorated with violets, and placed in a sepulchre in the temple. On the Day of Blood, or Black Friday, the priests of the cult gashed themselves with knives as they danced ecstatically, sympathizing with Cybele in her grief and helping to restore Attis to life. Two days later a priest opened the sepulchre at dawn, revealing that it was empty and announcing that the god was saved. This day was known as Hilaria, or the Day of Joy, a time of feasting and merriment. This is a theme also explored in the Christian feast of Easter.

According to the seventh- to eighth-century English monk Bede, the Christian holiday of Easter was named after a Saxon goddess of spring, Eostre.[20] He wrote that Ēosturmōnaþ (Old English—"Month of Ēostre") was an English month corresponding to April, when feasts of Eostre were celebrated by Pagans. Building on this, Jacob Grimm, in his *Deutsche Mythologie*, described Eostre as the divinity of dawn, "of upspringing light, a spectacle that brings joy and blessing, whose meaning could be easily adapted into the resurrection-day of the Christian God."[21] Despite this—or perhaps because of it—there have been many scholarly efforts to discredit Bede's claims of the existence of such a goddess, disputing Grimm's

---

20 Bede, *De Tempore Ratione, The Reckoning of Time*, trans. Faith Wallis (Liverpool University Press, 1999).

21 Jacob Grimm, *Teutonic Mythology*, trans. James Stallybrass (New York: Dover, 1882).

· · · · ·

linguistic connections of Ostara, east, and dawn.[22] One suggestion is that the name of the month simply arises as a loan-translation of the Latin term *albae*, meaning both "white" and "dawn," since white robes were worn by churchmen at Easter.[23] There is certainly no evidence that Eostre was a pan-Germanic goddess of spring, as many modern Pagans often claim, but before we dismiss her existence completely, there is convincing etymological evidence (in the form of historical place and personal names) to suggest that she may have been a purely local goddess, worshipped in Kent.[24] If this is the case, Bede may simply have used the local name for the month, indeed named after a local goddess[25]—Anglo Saxon Christians were certainly happy to make use of Pagan names for days of the week.[26] Bede's book became one of the essential textbooks of the early Middle Ages, widely circulated in Europe, and it would be nice to think that in this manner he was perpetuating the feast of a local goddess.

TRADITIONAL FOODS FOR OSTARA

With Ostara comes the real arrival of spring. Fresh leaves green the trees, new vegetation covers the land, and flowers are abundant. The sacred foods of Ostara reflect the theme of the renewal of the sun and vegetation god and the beginning of the light half of the year. An essential Easter food was eggs, which were forbidden during Lent. At the equinox the old breeds of hens began to lay again, triggered by the increasing hours of daylight, and wild birds are mating and nest building. The egg is a symbol of new life. The ancient Egyptians and Romans gave each other presents of eggs at the spring equinox as a token of resurrection. Include some eggs in your feast, if your diet allows; if you are vegan, make a centrepiece of decorated papier-mâché eggs to reflect this theme.

---

22   Richard Sermon, "From Easter to Ostara: The Reinvention of a Pagan Goddess?" *Time and Mind: The Journal of Archaeology, Consciousness and Culture* 1 (November 2008).

23   Johann Knobloch, "Der Ursprung von nhd. Ostern, engl. Easter," *Die Sprache* 5:27–45.

24   Philip A. Shaw, *Pagan Goddesses in the Early Germanic World, Eostre, Hreda and the Cult of the Matrons* (London: Bristol Classical Press, Bloomsbury Academic, 2011).

25   Ibid.

26   Ibid.

. . . .

EGGS WITH SORREL

4 OUNCES (110 GRAMS) SORREL LEAVES

2 HEAPED TABLESPOONS CHOPPED ONIONS

4 TABLESPOONS WHITE WINE

3 EGG YOLKS

8 OUNCES (1 CUP/225 GRAMS) BUTTER OR MARGARINE

6 HARD-BOILED EGGS, SHELLED

Strip the sorrel leaves from the stems and cut them into strips. Boil the onions in the wine and 4 tablespoons of water, then put them into a food processor with the egg yolks and liquidise. Melt the butter and add half the sorrel leaves. Remove from the heat and pour on the yolk mixture. Add the rest of the sorrel and heat gently. Pour the sauce over the hard-boiled eggs and serve.

. . . .

CLIPPING PUDDING

This is another old recipe from the sheep-shearing time, when "clipping suppers" (referring to the clipping of the sheep) were held and were one of the highlights of the year for the workers and their children.

8 OUNCES (1 CUP/225 GRAMS) SHORT GRAIN RICE

1 PINT (2⅓ CUPS/568 MILLILITRES) MILK

½ TEASPOON POWDERED CINNAMON

3 TABLESPOONS SUGAR

1 EGG, BEATEN

4 OUNCES (1 CUP/110 GRAMS) CURRANTS

4 OUNCES (1 CUP/110 GRAMS) RAISINS OR SULTANAS

1 TABLESPOON BUTTER

GRATED NUTMEG

Wash rice in cold water, then put it in a pan with the milk, cinnamon, and sugar. Simmer gently until the rice is tender. Allow the rice mixture to cool before adding the egg. Fold in dried fruit and butter. Pour into an ovenproof dish and sprinkle with nutmeg to taste. Bake at 180°C/350°F/gas mark 4 for around 20 minutes or until a skin has formed on top.

. . . . .

LENTEN PIE

1 POUND (450 GRAMS) PUFF PASTRY

6 EGGS, HARD-BOILED AND CHOPPED

6 APPLES, PEELED AND CORED

4 OUNCES (1 CUP/110 GRAMS) RAISINS

1 OUNCE (¼ CUP/30 GRAMS) CANDIED PEEL

2 CLOVES, CRUSHED

A PINCH OF GINGER

A PINCH OF NUTMEG

A PINCH OF SALT

1 TABLESPOON BRANDY

1 TABLESPOON WHITE WINE

JUICE OF AN ORANGE

MILK TO GLAZE

Line a pie dish with half the pastry. Mix the eggs, apples, fruit, and spices, then add the brandy and wine. Spoon in the mixture over the pastry, pouring the orange juice over it. With the other half of the pastry, fit a pastry lid, brush with milk, and bake at 200°C/400°F/gas mark 6 for 50–60 minutes or until golden brown.

STUFFED EGGS

9 HARD-BOILED EGGS

1 BUNCH FINELY CHOPPED WATERCRESS

6 TABLESPOONS PLAIN YOGHURT

4 OUNCES (½ CUP/110 GRAMS) CREAM CHEESE

SALT AND PEPPER TO TASTE

Halve the eggs and remove the yolks. Mix yolks with the other ingredients and spoon or pipe the mixture back into the eggs.

. . . .

FIGGY PUDDING

This was traditionally served during Lent.

5 OUNCES (1¼ CUPS/140 GRAMS) ALL-PURPOSE FLOUR

3 OUNCES (½ CUP/90 GRAMS) VEGETABLE SUET

4 OUNCES (1 CUP/110 GRAMS) DRIED FIGS OR DATES

½ TEASPOON CINNAMON

½ TEASPOON GINGER

1 TEASPOON BICARBONATE OF SODA

A PINCH OF GRATED NUTMEG

2 TABLESPOONS GOLDEN SYRUP OR CORN SYRUP

1 LARGE EGG, BEATEN

4 TABLESPOONS CRÈME FRAICHE

Mix the dry ingredients. Warm the golden syrup and stir in the beaten egg and crème fraiche. Add this to the dry ingredients and stir. Spoon into a greased pudding basin (a heatproof ceramic or pyrex bowl) and cover with a circle of baking parchment, not too tight as the pudding will expand. Cover this with aluminium foil, but again, leave room on the top for expansion. Tie the pudding around the rim with string. Put a small trivet in a large, deep pan and place the pudding basin on top. Add enough just-boiled water to the pan to come halfway up the sides of the basin. Allow to steam over low heat for 2 hours, adding more water to the pan if necessary (do not allow it to boil dry). Remove from the heat and carefully lift out the pudding. Stand for 5 minutes and remove the foil and baking parchment. Serve in wedges with cream or custard.

Hot Cross Buns

These are traditionally eaten on Good Friday, but cakes marked this way are pre-Christian. For Pagans, the cross on the round bun may be seen as representing the quartered circle, the four directions, and solar increase. The hot cross buns eaten on Good Friday in the UK were thought to be very powerful, and some would be saved and kept tied in a bag hung from the kitchen rafters until the next Good Friday. It was thought that a portion of such a bun could cure any illness in man or beast. Eating buns marked with a cross was a traditional food at Pagan celebrations of the spring equinox in the ancient world and was adopted into Christian custom.[27] [28]

To make mixed spice, a common ingredient in the UK, blend 1 tablespoon ground allspice, 1 tablespoon ground cinnamon, 1 tablespoon ground nutmeg, 2 teaspoons ground mace, 1 teaspoon ground cloves, and 1 teaspoon ground ginger. Store in a sealed jar.

1½ POUNDS (5¼ CUPS/675 GRAMS) ALL-PURPOSE FLOUR

A PINCH OF SALT

2 TEASPOONS MIXED SPICE OR PUMPKIN PIE SPICE

2 OUNCES (¼ CUP/60 GRAMS) BUTTER

½ OUNCE (30 GRAMS) FRESH YEAST OR 1 SACHET DRIED YEAST

½ PINT (1 CUP/284 MILLILITRES) WARM WATER

1 OUNCE (1 TABLESPOON/30 GRAMS) CASTER (SUPERFINE) SUGAR

2 OUNCES (½ CUP/60 GRAMS) CURRANTS

2 OUNCES (½ CUP/60 GRAMS) MIXED CANDIED PEEL

1 EGG, BEATEN

To make the crosses:

3 OUNCES (⅓ CUP/90 GRAMS) ALL-PURPOSE FLOUR

4 TABLESPOONS WATER

For the glaze:

2 TABLESPOONS CASTER (SUPERFINE) SUGAR

1 TABLESPOON MILK

---

27 Encyclopaedia Brittanica, eleventh edition.
28 John G. R. Forlong, Encyclopedia of Religions (Cosimo Classics, 2013).

Sift the flour, salt, and spice into a bowl. Start the yeast in a cup with 1 teaspoon sugar and 1 tablespoon lukewarm water. Stir the started yeast into a well that has been made in the flour mixture. Add the dry ingredients and the egg. Knead well on a floured board. Return to the bowl, cover with a clean cloth, and leave in a warm place to rise for around an hour. Knead lightly again. Divide into 16 pieces and roll each piece into a ball. Flatten with your hand. Place on a baking tray, cover with a cloth, and leave to prove for 30 minutes.

To make the crosses, mix the flour and water to make a paste. Place in a piping bag and pipe a cross onto each of the risen buns. Bake the buns at 220°C/425°F/gas mark 7 for 15–20 minutes. Meanwhile, make the glaze by dissolving sugar in milk; bring to a boil and remove from heat. Brush the buns with the glaze as soon as they come out of the oven.

Nettle Pudding

1 POUND (450 GRAMS) YOUNG NETTLE TOPS

1 ONION

4 OUNCES (½ CUP/110 GRAMS) PEARL BARLEY

1 EGG

SALT AND PEPPER TO TASTE

BUTTER

Chop the greens and onion. Add the salt and barley and place in a pudding bag. Boil for 2 hours. Beat the resulting mixture with the egg and seasoning. Make into burger shapes and fry in butter.

. . . .

DAWN'S SHEARING CAKE

Typically, sheep shearing is carried out in March. In the past it was a social as well as a working occasion, and this traditional cake was served to the workers and their families.

1 POUND (3½ CUPS/450 GRAMS) ALL-PURPOSE FLOUR

1 TEASPOON BAKING POWDER

A PINCH OF SALT

9 OUNCES (1 CUP/240 GRAMS) BUTTER

13 OUNCES (1¾ CUPS/360 GRAMS) CASTER (SUPERFINE) SUGAR

2 EGGS

½ PINT (1 CUP/300 MILLILITRES) MILK

A PINCH OF FRESHLY GRATED NUTMEG

3 TEASPOONS CARAWAY SEEDS, LIGHTLY CRUSHED

FRESHLY GRATED ZEST OF 1 LEMON

Sift the flour, baking powder and salt into a bowl. Add the butter, rubbing it in with your fingers until the mixture resembles fine breadcrumbs, and then add sugar. Beat the eggs in a separate bowl along with the milk, then add to the flour mixture. Finally add the nutmeg, caraway seeds, and lemon zest, and stir to combine. Spoon the batter into a springform cake tin that's been well buttered and lined with greaseproof paper. Place in an oven preheated to 180°C/350°F/gas mark 4 and bake for about 30 minutes or until the top is golden brown and a skewer inserted into the centre of the cake emerges cleanly. Allow to cool for 10 minutes in the tin, then tip out and place on a wire rack to cool completely.

. . . .

SIMNEL CAKE

This is a traditional Easter cake. The thirteen decorations represent Jesus and the twelve apostles but are equally applicable to the thirteen lunar months of the year.

4 OUNCES (½ CUP/110 GRAMS) BUTTER

4 OUNCES (½ CUP/110 GRAMS) BROWN SUGAR

3 EGGS, BEATEN

5 OUNCES (⅛ CUP/140 GRAMS) ALL-PURPOSE FLOUR

1 OUNCE (¼ CUP/30 GRAMS) GROUND ALMONDS

½ TEASPOON MIXED SPICE (SEE PAGE 26)

½ TEASPOON BAKING POWDER

GRATED RIND AND JUICE OF ½ A LEMON

6 OUNCES (1 CUP/170 GRAMS) CURRANTS

4 OUNCES (1 CUP/110 GRAMS) RAISINS

6 OUNCES (¾ CUP/170 GRAMS) MARZIPAN (ALMOND PASTE)

Cream the butter and sugar and gradually add the beaten eggs. Fold in the flour, almonds, spice and baking powder. Stir in the lemon juice and rind, and the dried fruits. Grease and line an 8-inch cake tin and spoon in half the mixture. Reserving an ounce of marzipan for the decoration, roll out the remaining 5 ounces of marzipan and put in a layer. Add the rest of the cake mixture and bake at 180°C/350°F/gas mark 4 for 2 hours. Decorate the top with 13 marzipan balls.

EIGHTEENTH-CENTURY PANCAKES

In England the traditional pancake accompaniment is a generous sprinkling of lemon juice and sugar, but if you like you could serve the pancakes with cooked fruit, fresh or dried fruit, and cream.

4 OUNCES (1 CUP/110 GRAMS) ALL-PURPOSE FLOUR

A PINCH OF SALT

2 EGGS

7 TABLESPOONS MILK

3 TABLESPOONS CREAM

1 TEASPOON SUGAR

A PINCH OF NUTMEG

1 TABLESPOON BRANDY

OIL FOR COOKING

Sift together the flour and salt. Make a well in the centre and break the eggs into it. Combine the milk and cream. Add half of this into the well with the eggs. Beat together until smooth. In a separate bowl, combine the remaining milk and cream with the sugar, nutmeg, and brandy. Beat until smooth. Combine the two mixtures, once again beating until smooth. Cover the bowl and allow the mixture to rest for 30 minutes. Put just enough oil in the pan to coat thinly and heat until very hot. Drop in spoonfuls of the mixture and fry until cooked, turning once (this takes only around 30 seconds a side).

Beltane

Beltane marks the return of summer with all its warmth and promise of plenty. The blossoming of the fruit trees marks the coming of the summer goddess, while the hedgerows blaze with the flowering of the hawthorn, which is said to carry the scent of female sexuality as the Goddess prepares to mate with the God.

In medieval England the first of May was celebrated by going out into the greenwood "a-maying" to collect greenery and hawthorn blossoms. Love chases were customary, and the fertility of the land would be ensured by sympathetic magic. In many areas a May Queen was crowned with flowers, and her male counterpart was Jack-in-the-Green, or the Green Man. She is covered in blossoms; he is covered in ivy, holly, birch, poplar, fir, and other greenery. Once they may have been appointed by the village as representations of the Goddess and the God, and in some places they are still called "the bride and groom."

The maypole is a phallic symbol with obvious connotations of fertility and revelry. Throughout Europe there are long traditions of a stripped tree of birch erected in the village square or sacred site, decorated with ribbons and greenery. The dance around the maypole with some dancers circling sunwise, some widdershins, suggests a dance of death and rebirth.

TRADITIONAL FOODS FOR BELTANE

By now there is a greater choice of fresh foods from the garden, such as spring cabbage, rhubarb, herbs, broad beans, early lettuce, spring onions, radishes, and early new potatoes. The special ritual foods of Beltane include flowers, such as primrose, hawthorn, violet, and cowslip, plus fresh green herbs and leaves, such as dandelion, dill, hawthorn, sorrel, chickweed, and nettle.

· · · · · · · · ·

SORREL SOUP

*Sorrel (*Rumex acetosa*) honours the goddess of love and evokes the lusty currents of Beltane and its fertility aspects.*

2 MEDIUM ONIONS, CHOPPED

1 OUNCE BUTTER

12 OUNCES (2 CUPS/340 GRAMS) RED LENTILS, WASHED

2½ PINTS (6 CUPS/1,420 MILLILITRES) VEGETABLE STOCK

BOUQUET GARNI

8 OUNCES (225 GRAMS) FRESH SORREL

¼ PINT (⅔ CUP/150 MILLILITRES) PLAIN YOGHURT

Simmer together the onion, butter, lentils, stock, and bouquet garni in a large covered pan until lentils are soft, around 1–1½ hours, adding more liquid as required. Meanwhile, wash the sorrel and discard the stalks. Chop coarsely and add to the pan once the lentils are cooked. Cook uncovered until the leaves soften slightly. Put in a blender and liquidise. Just before serving, return to the heat and stir in the yoghurt.

· · · · · · · · · · · · · ·

CRYSTALLISED FLOWERS

Primrose is associated with the lusty currents of the season, growing life, and fertility. Violets are associated with twilight, a magical "time between times" when the otherworld is closer and it is easier to slip into, especially the turning of the wheel at Beltane.

DRIED EDIBLE FLOWER BLOSSOMS, SEPARATED FROM THE STEM (PRIMROSE, APPLE, ROSE, OR VIOLET)

1 LARGE EGG WHITE

A FEW DROPS OF WATER

CASTER (SUPERFINE) SUGAR

Combine the egg white with the water and beat lightly. Dip a paint brush into the egg white and paint the flower. Sprinkle sugar evenly all over on both sides. Place the flower or petal on greaseproof paper to dry. Allow to dry for 12–36 hours. Store in an airtight container. Use for cake decorations.

· · · · ·

SPRING CABBAGE CASSEROLE (VEGAN)

1 SPRING CABBAGE

2 LARGE ONIONS

2 LARGE POTATOES, ABOUT 1 POUND (3 CUPS/450 GRAMS)

4 TOMATOES

2 TABLESPOONS OIL

SALT AND PAPRIKA

¾ PINT (1¾ CUPS/426 MILLILITRES) VEGETABLE STOCK

Wash and chop the cabbage. Peel and slice the onions, potatoes, and tomatoes. Fry onions in oil until soft. In a lightly greased casserole dish, arrange layers of cabbage, fried onions, potatoes, and tomatoes, beginning and finishing with cabbage. Season each layer with the salt and paprika. Pour on the stock until it reaches the top layer of cabbage. Cover the dish and bake in the oven for 1½ hours or until done.

MAI BOWL

May wine is a German drink flavoured with fresh sweet woodruff (Galium oderatum/ Aspererula oderata), an herb which should be used only in May when the new leaves are tender (make sure you have the right herb, as there is a garden variety which is not suitable). Woodruff marks the turning of the wheel to summer. It is added to the Beltane cup and may be employed in garlands and posies during the festivities.

12 SPRIGS YOUNG SWEET WOODRUFF, CHOPPED

5 OUNCES (1¼ CUPS/140 GRAMS) POWDERED (ICING) SUGAR

2 BOTTLES (750 MILLILITRES EACH) DRY WHITE WINE

2 PINTS SPARKLING WINE

CHOPPED STRAWBERRIES

Place all the ingredients except the sparkling wine and strawberries in a bowl. Cover for 30 minutes. Strain out the herbs and reserve the wine, then add the sparkling wine and strawberries.

Note: Avoid woodruff if pregnant or breastfeeding.

NETTLE SOUP

Nettle is an herb of transformation; used at this time, it marks the leaving behind of the winter and past painful experiences, and embracing the warmth of the coming summer. Nettles are also full of vitamins and minerals, and they make an excellent tonic at this time of year.

2 ONIONS

1 CLOVE GARLIC

2 POTATOES

OIL FOR FRYING

LEAVES STRIPPED FROM 10 NETTLE STEMS

1½ PINTS (3½ CUPS/850 MILLILITRES) VEGETABLE STOCK

½ PINT (1 CUP/284 MILLILITRES) MILK OR SOYA MILK

SALT AND PEPPER TO TASTE

FRESH PARSLEY TO GARNISH

Peel and chop the onion, garlic, and potatoes, fry gently in some oil until soft. Add the nettle leaves and the stock. Boil for 20 minutes. Liquidise, then return to the pan, add the seasoning and the milk, and reheat. Garnish with parsley to serve.

Midsummer

Midsummer is the celebration of the summer solstice, when the sun is at its peak. Now is the time of brightness, long days, and warmth. Foliage and flowering are at their fullest just before fruiting begins. The earth is pregnant with goodness made fertile by the light of the sun. The Sun God is in his glory as the strong, virile husband and lover of the Goddess. The power of the sun on this day is protective, healing, empowering, revitalizing, and inspiring. It imbues a powerful magical charge into spells, crystals, and herbs. This makes it the ideal time to gather herbs, part of the bounty of the sun god, who is always a patron of healing and medicine.

But we must remember that after this day the sun starts to decline. It was therefore natural for people to want to protect themselves and their crops and animals from the looming powers of decay and winter that are an inevitable consequence of the decrease of the sun's warmth and vigour. Fire, the little brother of the sun, naturally gains greater power when the force of the sun is at its strongest. Bonfires once blazed all across Europe and North Africa at the solstice, and people leaped the fires to cleanse themselves.

TRADITIONAL FOODS FOR MIDSUMMER

By this time of year food is plentiful, with salad vegetables, soft fruits, and herbs in peak condition. This is the best time for picking most herbs; they obtain potent virtues for magic on the solstice and should be included in the feast.

· · · · · · · · · · · · · · ·

ELDERFLOWER FRITTERS

4 OUNCES (1 CUP/110 GRAMS) CORNFLOUR (CORNSTARCH)

WATER

2 EGG WHITES

SUGAR

6 ELDERFLOWER HEADS

Mix the cornflour with a little cold water to form a thin paste. In a separate bowl, whisk the egg whites until fairly stiff. Add a little sugar and continue to whisk for a further minute. Carefully fold the egg whites into the cornflour paste to make a light, frothy batter. Dip the elderflower heads into this batter and fry them until golden brown. Whilst still hot, roll the fritters in sugar and serve immediately.

· · · · ·

Watercress Soup

1 OUNCE (2 TABLESPOONS/30 GRAMS) BUTTER

1 HEAD OF LETTUCE SUCH AS COS OR BUTTERHEAD

BUNCH OF WATERCRESS

8 SPRING ONIONS

2 PINTS (5 CUPS/1,136 MILLILITRES) VEGETABLE STOCK

3 TEASPOONS CORNFLOUR (CORNSTARCH)

WATER TO BIND

SEASONING TO TASTE

½ PINT (1 CUP/284 MILLILITRES) PLAIN YOGHURT

Melt the butter in a pan. Add the chopped vegetables and fry for 5 minutes. Add the stock and simmer for 10–15 minutes or until the vegetables are tender. Blend the cornflour with a little water, stir into the soup, and boil to thicken. Season to taste and liquidise in a blender. Chill in the fridge until ready to serve and swirl in the yoghurt.

Sage and Potatoes

1 OUNCE (2 TABLESPOONS/30 GRAMS) BUTTER

1 ONION, FINELY CHOPPED

1 TEASPOON SAGE, FINELY CHOPPED

1 PINT (2½ CUPS/568 MILLILITRES) VEGETABLE STOCK

SALT AND PEPPER

2 POUNDS (6 CUPS/900 GRAMS) NEW POTATOES,
    PEELED AND BOILED

Melt the butter in a pan and add the onion. Cook without browning until the onion is transparent. Add the sage, stock, and seasoning, and boil until the liquid is reduced to just under half its volume. Slice the potatoes, add them to the pan, and cook until the potatoes are thoroughly heated.

. . . .
Herb Tart

For the pastry:

> 4 OUNCES (1 CUP/110 GRAMS) ALL-PURPOSE FLOUR
>
> A PINCH OF SALT
>
> 2 OUNCES (¼ CUP/60 GRAMS) BUTTER OR MARGARINE
>
> WATER

For the filling:

> 1 TABLESPOON OLIVE OIL
>
> 1 SMALL ONION, CHOPPED
>
> 2 TABLESPOONS CHOPPED PARSLEY
>
> 3 TABLESPOONS MIXED FRESH HERBS
>   (WHATEVER YOU HAVE AVAILABLE)
>
> 3 EGGS
>
> ½ PINT (1 CUP/284 MILLILITRES) CREAM
>
> A PINCH OF NUTMEG
>
> SALT AND PEPPER

Sift the flour and salt into a bowl. With your fingertips, lightly rub in the butter or margarine until the mixture resembles fine breadcrumbs. Add just enough cold water to bind the ingredients together. Cover and refrigerate for 20 minutes, then roll out the pastry and line a quiche dish. Prick all over with a fork to keep the pastry flat whilst cooking. Bake blind at 190°C/375°F/gas mark 5 for 15 minutes.

Meanwhile, heat the oil and fry the chopped onion until transparent. Add the herbs and remove from the heat. In a bowl beat the eggs, cream, nutmeg, salt and pepper together. Add the onion and herbs and mix together thoroughly. Pour this mixture into the hot tart pastry case and bake until the filling is set (around 30 minutes) at 180°C/350°F/gas mark 4.

. . . .
GOOSEBERRY FOOL

14 OUNCES (4 CUPS/400 GRAMS) GOOSEBERRIES

2 OUNCES (¼ CUP/60 GRAMS) BUTTER

SUGAR TO TASTE

½ PINT (1 CUP/284 MILLILITRES) SINGLE (LIGHT) CREAM

3 EGG YOLKS

Wash the gooseberries and top and tail them (remove the stalks and base). Put them in a pan with the butter and cook over low heat until soft. Crush the gooseberries with a wooden spoon and sweeten to taste. In another pan boil the cream. Remove the pan from the heat and whisk in the egg yolks. Set the pan over a larger one of hot water and stir briskly until the mixture thickens. Cool and add the gooseberries, spoon into individual serving glasses, and chill to set.

. . . .
CHERVIL SOUP

3 CARROTS, SCRUBBED

½ POUND (1½ CUPS/225 GRAMS) POTATOES, PEELED

2 STICKS CELERY

¼ POUND (¾ CUP/110 GRAMS) SHALLOTS,
    PEELED AND SLICED INTO RINGS

2 PINTS (5 CUPS/1,136 MILLILITRES) VEGETABLE STOCK

1 TEASPOON SUGAR

SALT AND PEPPER

BUNCH OF FRESH CHERVIL

4 TABLESPOONS PLAIN YOGHURT

Finely dice the carrots, potatoes, and celery. Put them in a pan with the shallots and the stock, reserving a few slices of shallot for garnish. Bring to a boil and then reduce heat. Simmer gently for 10 minutes or until the vegetables are tender. Add the sugar and season to taste. Rinse the chervil with boiling water, drain immediately, and chop it very finely, reserving a little for garnish.

Add this to the soup, stir in the yoghurt, and continue heating for a further 2 minutes. Do not allow the soup to boil. Serve garnished with one or two shallot rings and a sprinkling of chervil.

VEGAN PÂTÉ

Turn out the pâté just before serving and garnish with a little fresh herb and a twist of lemon.

14 OUNCES (2 CUPS/400 GRAMS) DRIED CHICKPEAS

1 LEVEL TEASPOON WHOLE MUSTARD SEEDS

1 LEVEL TEASPOON BLACK PEPPERCORNS

1 SMALL ONION, CHOPPED

2 CLOVES GARLIC, CHOPPED

½ TEASPOON ROSEMARY

¼ TEASPOON DILL

½ TEASPOON THYME

½ TEASPOON MARJORAM

JUICE OF 1 LEMON

OLIVE OIL

Boil the chickpeas in unseasoned water until soft, adding water as required. Drain them and put them in a food processor. Process the chickpeas until they are well chopped and resemble biscuit crumbs. Add the mustard seeds, peppercorns, onion, garlic and herbs. Process until the mixture begins to resemble dry pâté. Add the lemon juice and enough oil to bind to the desired consistency. Press the pâté into a lightly oiled mould and chill it well.

Lughnasa

Lughnasa is named for the pan-Celtic god Lugh, who is said to have founded annual funeral games on this date to commemorate Tailtu, his foster mother. The festival is also called Lammas, from the Anglo-Saxon *hlaef-mass* (meaning "loaf-mass"), and the Anglo-Saxon Chronicle of 921 CE mentions it as "the feast of first fruits."

Lughnasa is a harvest festival, marking the end of the period of summer growth and the beginning of the autumn harvest. Lughnasa celebrates the fruition of the year's work with the weaning of calves and lambs, the ripening of the corn, and the first apples, pears, bilberries, blackberries, and grapes. An old custom was to pick the first apples and make them into a drink called Lammas Wool (see page 45).

At this point in the Wheel of the Year the Goddess becomes the mother who gives birth to the fruits of the land. She is Mother Nature, from whom all life emerges, who sustains all life. She is the earth itself which bears fruit.

In an age when crops can be imported all year round, we tend to forget just how important this time was to our ancestors; the failure of the harvest meant starvation and death. This is just as true today in many parts of the world, as heartbreaking pictures of hungry children show us. It would be as well to remember these as we thank the gods for their bounty and offer a prayer for the less fortunate or dedicate the celebration to them.

TRADITIONAL FOODS FOR LUGHNASA

This is the time of summer ripeness, with an abundance of fresh produce including tomatoes, cucumbers, onions, baby carrots, broccoli, cabbage, beetroot, cauliflowers, fresh salad, courgettes/zucchini, beans, and peppers. Lughnasa is also the start of the apple and grape harvest, and there are ripe fruits such as peaches, apricots, gooseberries, and plums. The special ritual foods of Lughnasa are apples, basil, borage, chicory, fenugreek, fennel, honeysuckle, poppy seeds, grapes, vine leaves, and nasturtium flowers, as well as new potatoes, bilberries and other soft fruit, wine, beer, and bread.

WHITE CURRANT SOUP

1 POUND (4 CUPS/450 GRAMS) WHITE CURRANTS ON STALKS

¼ PINT (⅔ CUP/150 MILLILITRES) WATER

1½ TABLESPOONS CORNFLOUR (CORNSTARCH)

WATER

SUGAR TO TASTE

SPRIG OF MINT TO GARNISH

Rinse the currants. Drain them well and place in a pan with the water. Heat gently to the boiling point and simmer until the berries burst. Strain through a jelly bag, which will take about two hours. Make the liquid up to 2 pints with more water. Return to the pan and boil. Mix the cornflour with a little cold water and blend it into the soup to thicken. Simmer to cook the flour and allow the soup to thicken as desired. Add sugar to taste. Serve with a sprig of mint.

SUMMER SOUP

½ CUCUMBER

2 POUNDS (8 CUPS/900 GRAMS) TOMATOES

1 GREEN PEPPER

1 ONION

2 CLOVES GARLIC

2 SLICES BREAD

1 TABLESPOON OLIVE OIL

2 PINTS (5 CUPS/1,136 MILLILITRES) WATER

½ TEASPOON CHILI POWDER

A PINCH OF BLACK PEPPER

Blanch and skin the tomatoes. Put everything into a blender and liquidise. Heat through.

. . . .

Floral Salad

A HANDFUL OF BABY SPINACH LEAVES

1 BABY COS (ROMAINE) LETTUCE

1 SMALL CUCUMBER, CUBED

1 CARROT, CUBED

A FEW APPLE MINT OR GINGER MINT LEAVES

NASTURTIUM FLOWERS

VIOLETS

BORAGE FLOWERS

3 TABLESPOONS OIL

JUICE AND GRATED RIND OF ½ A LEMON

1 GARLIC CLOVE, CRUSHED

Break up the lettuce and arrange it with the spinach, cucumber, carrots, mint leaves, and flowers in a salad bowl. In a sealable container, mix together the oil, lemon, and garlic. Shake well and pour it over the salad just before serving.

. . . .

Basil and Tomato Crumble

1 POUND (4 CUPS/450 GRAMS) GREEN TOMATOES, SLICED

BLACK PEPPER AND SALT TO TASTE

1 TABLESPOON BASIL, CHOPPED

1 BUNCH SPRING ONIONS (SCALLIONS), FINELY CHOPPED

3 OUNCES (90 GRAMS) BREAD CRUMBS (ABOUT 3 SLICES)

1 OUNCE (¼ CUP/30 GRAMS) GRATED CHEESE

In an ovenproof dish arrange a layer of the tomato slices and sprinkle with salt and pepper. Mix the basil and the onions together and sprinkle a layer of this mixture over the tomatoes. Repeat these layers, using up all the tomatoes, onions, and basil. Cover the layers with a thick topping of bread crumbs. Sprinkle with the cheese and bake at 180°C/350°F/gas mark 4 for 3–4 hours or until golden brown.

. . . . .

SUMMER PUDDING

8-10 SLICES DAY-OLD WHITE BREAD

4-6 OUNCES (¾ CUP/140 GRAMS) CASTER (SUPERFINE) SUGAR

2-3 TABLESPOONS WATER

2 POUNDS (8 CUPS/900 GRAMS) MIXED SOFT FRUIT (ANY SUMMER
SOFT FRUIT AVAILABLE SUCH AS RASPBERRIES, REDCURRANTS,
BLACKCURRANTS, ETC.)

Rinse a 2-pound pudding basin in cold water. Trim the crusts from the bread and line the damp basin with the slices, pressing the bread down firmly and leaving no gaps. Reserve enough bread to cover the top. Over low heat, dissolve the sugar in the water; add the fruit and simmer for a few minutes. Strain off about ¼ pint of the liquid and put it to one side. Put the fruit in the basin and cover with the remaining bread. Stand the basin on a plate and cover it with a saucer. Press the saucer down and place a weight on top. Leave it like this overnight. To turn out the pudding, remove the saucer and invert the basin onto a plate. Remove the basin and pour the remaining liquid over the top.

GAELIC HERB POTATOES

This is based on a traditional Irish dish called "champ."

2 POUNDS (6 CUPS/900 GRAMS) POTATOES, PEELED AND SLICED

1 TABLESPOON FRESH MIXED HERBS, CHOPPED

SEASONING

WATER TO COVER

3 TABLESPOONS MILK

3 OUNCES (⅓ CUP/90 GRAMS) BUTTER

Boil the potatoes with the herbs, adding seasoning to taste and enough water to cover the potatoes. Simmer until the water has fully evaporated. Stir in the milk and butter and continue to cook until they have been fully absorbed and the potatoes are soft and fluffy. Mix well with a wooden spoon and serve.

PLAITED LUGHNASA LOAF

½ OUNCE (15 GRAMS) YEAST

1 TEASPOON PLUS 1½ TABLESPOONS SUGAR

6 FLUID OUNCES (¾ CUP/180 MILLILITRES) MILK

1 POUND (4 CUPS/450 GRAMS) PLAIN STRONG (BREAD) FLOUR

A PINCH OF SALT

3 EGGS, BEATEN

For glaze:

1 EGG, BEATEN

POPPY SEEDS

Start the yeast with a teaspoon of sugar and slightly warmed milk. Sift the flour and salt into a bowl. When the yeast is frothy, add it to the bowl with the eggs and 1½ tablespoons sugar. Mix to a smooth dough. Cover and leave in a warm place for an hour to double in size. Punch down, remove from bowl, and turn out on a lightly floured surface. Knead until smooth, divide into three strands, and plait together. Place on a baking tray, cover, and leave to prove for another 40 minutes. Brush with egg and sprinkle on the poppy seeds. Bake at 220°C/425°F/gas mark 7 for 15 minutes. Reduce the temperature to 190°C/375°F/gas mark 5 and bake for another 25 minutes.

SODA BREAD

2 POUNDS (8 CUPS/900 GRAMS) PLAIN STRONG (BREAD) FLOUR

2 TEASPOONS BICARBONATE OF SODA (BAKING SODA)

1 TEASPOON SALT

12 FLUID OUNCES (1½ CUPS/370 MILLILITRES) BUTTERMILK OR MILK

Sift the flour, bicarbonate, and salt into a bowl. Add the buttermilk and mix to a smooth dough. Shape into a large flat pancake and mark the centre with a cross. Bake for 35 minutes at 220°C/425°F/gas mark 7.

LAMMAS WOOL

4 LARGE COOKING APPLES

HONEY

NUTMEG

4 PINTS (9½ CUPS/2,273 MILLILITRES) ALE

Core the apples, place them upright in a deep baking tin, and fill the centres with honey. Sprinkle with nutmeg and bake in the oven for 40 minutes. Remove from the oven and pour the ale over the apples. Heat gently on the hob for a few minutes, spooning the ale over the apples. Strain off the liquid and serve warm. The apples can be served separately.

Autumn Equinox

At the autumn equinox, light and darkness stand in balance once more, with equal hours of night and day, but the darkness is gaining. Day by day, we move towards winter. It is a dual festival of light and darkness, joy and sorrow. It is a time of abundance when the bounty of the earth must be gathered in and safely stored against the bleak times ahead because the vegetation god dies and winter is coming.

The expansive, active part of the year is over; it is time to turn inwards. The sun's power is waning, but, being deprived of the external light, we encounter inner illumination.

TRADITIONAL FOODS FOR THE AUTUMN EQUINOX

This is a time of plenty, with a profusion of foods available including main crop potatoes, mature root vegetables such as carrots, swedes, turnips, and beetroot, as well as cauliflowers, broccoli, beans, and the last of the fresh salads, tomatoes, wild nuts, and mushrooms. This is a busy time, when the harvest must be gathered in before the first frosts and food must be prepared, stored, and preserved for the dead time of winter to come. The special ritual foods of the occasion include apples, acorns, basil, beans, blackberries, corn, chicory, rose hips, parsley, poppy seeds, hazel and other nuts, and hawthorn berries. Traditionally the harvest loaf is plaited or shaped to resemble wheat sheafs. We put a representation of John Barleycorn on top of the loaf, tear up the bread, and throw pieces to each member of the group. Whoever gets John Barleycorn's "special bit" becomes lord or lady of the feast and can order stories, entertainment, and food from the others.

. . . .

HERFEST CAKES

6 OUNCES (1½ CUPS/170 GRAMS) GROUND HAZELNUTS

4 FLUID OUNCES (½ CUP/120 MILLILITRES) HONEY

1 OUNCE (¼ CUP/30 GRAMS) ALL-PURPOSE FLOUR

1 TABLESPOON GRATED LEMON PEEL

1 EGG, BEATEN

1 TABLESPOON LEMON JUICE

Blend the ground nuts and honey into a paste. Mix in the flour and lemon peel. Blend the lemon juice and egg together and add to the mixture. Drop small amounts onto a greased baking tray and bake at 180°C/350°F/gas mark 4 for 20 minutes.

. . . . .

HARVEST LOAF

3 POUNDS (10½ CUPS/1350 GRAMS) WHOLEMEAL
(WHOLE WHEAT) FLOUR

1 TEASPOON SALT

5 TABLESPOONS BUTTER

1 OUNCE (30 GRAMS) FRESH YEAST

1½ PINTS (3½ CUPS/850 MILLILITRES) WARM WATER

Mix together the flour and salt and rub in the butter. Start the yeast by putting it into a cup with a teaspoon of sugar and a tablespoon of lukewarm water. Add to the flour mixture and stir in the water to make a dough. Knead well and return to the bowl. Cover with a clean cloth, leave in a warm place for 2 hours, then turn out onto a lightly floured surface and knead again. Divide into 4 pieces and place in greased 1-pound loaf tins. Cover again and prove for 30 minutes. Bake at 220°C/425°F/gas mark 7 for 30–40 minutes.

CARROT SOUP

2 POUNDS (6 CUPS/900 GRAMS) CARROTS, CHOPPED

1 ONION, CHOPPED

2 PINTS (5 CUPS/1,136 MILLILITRES) VEGETABLE STOCK

A PINCH OF MARJORAM

SEASONING TO TASTE

1 TABLESPOON CORNFLOUR (CORNSTARCH)

WATER TO BIND

A DASH OF SHERRY

1 TABLESPOON CHOPPED FRESH PARSLEY

Boil the carrots and onion in the stock with the marjoram. Simmer for 20 minutes. Liquidise. Mix the cornflour in a little water. Stir into the soup and boil to thicken. Add the sherry and the parsley.

. . . .
Stuffed Marrow

Marrows are big vegetables (about a foot long) that are basically overgrown zucchinis. For this recipe, you could stuff several large zucchinis instead.

1 MARROW

3 ONIONS

2 OUNCES (½ CUP/60 GRAMS) CHOPPED NUTS

2 OUNCES (½ CUP/60 GRAMS) PINE KERNELS, CHOPPED

4 OUNCES (1 CUP/110 GRAMS) BREAD CRUMBS

2 OUNCES (¼ CUP/60 GRAMS) BUTTER

1 TEASPOON MIXED HERBS

1 TEASPOON MARMITE, VEGEMITE, OR MISO

1 EGG

SALT AND PEPPER

Peel the marrow and chop in half. Scoop out the centre and discard. Fry the chopped onions in the butter and add the other ingredients. Fill the centre of the marrow with the mixture and bake, covered, in a hot oven at 200°C/400°F/ gas mark 6 for 60 minutes.

. . . .
Hazelnut Tart

The hazel or cobnut (Corylus avellana) is Coll, one of the seven chieftain trees of Ogham. Nuts are a Celtic symbol of concentrated wisdom, the sweetness of knowledge contained within a hard shell. The hazel has many connections with the festival of the autumn equinox, the harvest festival celebrated in the ninth month of the year, when the tree produces nuts. It represents the fruition of what has gone before and the culmination of the work.

8 OUNCES (225 GRAMS) WHOLEMEAL PASTRY

1 ONION, FINELY CHOPPED

1 OUNCE (2 TABLESPOONS/30 GRAMS) BUTTER OR MARGARINE

3 OUNCES (¾ CUP/90 GRAMS) GROUND HAZELNUTS

2 EGGS, BEATEN

¼ PINT (⅔ CUP/150 MILLILITRES) STOCK

1 TEASPOON MARMITE, VEGEMITE, OR MISO

1 TABLESPOON FRESH SAGE, CHOPPED

SALT AND PEPPER TO TASTE

Line a flan dish with the pastry. Cook the finely chopped onion in the butter and add the other ingredients. Pour into the pastry case and bake in a moderate oven at 180°C/350°F/gas mark 4 for 40 minutes.

. . . .

APPLE PUDDING

The apple represents immortality. Legendary isles of apples are common and always lie in the west. The western point of the circle marks the festival of Herfest, the setting of the sun at the autumn equinox, when the Lord dies and the dark days of winter begin.

12 OUNCES (3 CUPS/340 GRAMS) SELF-RAISING FLOUR

6 OUNCES (¾ CUP/170 GRAMS) BUTTER

5 OUNCES (¾ CUP/140 GRAMS) SUGAR

MILK TO BIND

1 POUND (4 CUPS/450 GRAMS) COOKING APPLES,
    PEELED, SLICED, AND CORED

Rub the flour and butter together. Add 4 ounces of sugar and mix in enough milk to form a soft dough. Lightly roll out to slightly more than ½-inch thick in a circular shape. Place on a greased baking tray. Pile the apples in the centre and sprinkle the remaining sugar over them, then bring up the sides of the dough and seal the edges together with a little water. Bake in a moderate oven at 180°C/350°F/gas mark 4 until risen and golden brown, about 30 minutes. Can be eaten hot or cold.

DAWN'S MUSHROOM AND WALNUT QUICHE

You can make spinach and walnut quiche as below but use 1 pound of fresh wilted spinach instead of mushrooms and add 2 crushed garlic cloves as you fry the onion.

1 COOKED PASTRY CASE

2 OUNCES (¼ CUP/30 GRAMS) BUTTER OR MARGARINE

1 WHITE ONION, CHOPPED

12 OUNCES (3 CUPS/340 GRAMS) MIXED MUSHROOMS, SLICED

SALT AND PEPPER

2 OUNCES (½ CUP/30 GRAMS) WALNUTS, ROUGHLY CHOPPED

3 OUNCES (¾ CUP/90 GRAMS) CHEDDAR CHEESE, GRATED

3 EGGS, BEATEN

7 FLUID OUNCES (¾ CUP/210 MILLILITRES) DOUBLE (HEAVY) CREAM

Preheat the oven to 180°C/350°F/gas mark 4. Use the butter to fry the onion and mushrooms until golden. Add the seasoning and walnuts. Sprinkle the cheese in the pastry case, then cover with mushroom mix. Beat the eggs into the cream, then pour over. Bake for approximately 15–20 minutes.

APPLE AND BLACKBERRY FOOL

The blackberry (Rubus fructicosus) was a sacred plant of the Celts and was thought to belong to the fairy folk. In Scotland, the bramble—along with the rowan and the yew—constituted the sacred fire.

1 POUND (4 CUPS/450 GRAMS) APPLES, PEELED, CORED, AND SLICED

10 OUNCES (2½ CUPS/280 GRAMS) BLACKBERRIES

2 OUNCES (¼ CUP/60 GRAMS) CASTER (SUPERFINE) SUGAR

½ PINT (1 CUP/284 MILLILITRES) FRESH DOUBLE (HEAVY) CREAM

Cook the apples and blackberries with the sugar in very little water until very soft. Liquidise. Whip the cream until fairly stiff and put a little to one side for topping. Fold the fruit puree into the cream. Spoon into individual glasses. Chill. Before serving, top with a little of the cream and decorate with pieces of fruit as desired.

MUSHROOM PÂTÉ

This pâté will store in the fridge for up to a month. Serve with toast.

1 ONION, CHOPPED

8 OUNCES (1 CUP) BUTTER

1 POUND (4 CUPS/450 GRAMS) MUSHROOMS

A PINCH EACH OF SALT, BLACK PEPPER, AND CAYENNE PEPPER

1 TEASPOON WORCESTER SAUCE

1 EGG, BEATEN

Cook the onion with 6 ounces butter until soft. Wash and chop the mushrooms; add to the pan with the seasonings. Cook slowly for 30 minutes, stirring now and then; afterwards boil fast to reduce the excess liquid. Transfer to a blender and liquidise, adding the beaten egg. Return to the pan and cook slowly, stirring, until the mixture becomes thick. Do not boil.

Pour the mixture into a pâté dish. Melt the remaining butter and pour over the surface to seal. Leave to cool. Keep chilled.

WARDEN PIE

4 HARD PEARS

WINE

2 SHORTCRUST PASTRIES

3½ OUNCES (½ CUP/100 GRAMS) SUGAR

½ TEASPOON CINNAMON

⅙ TEASPOON GROUND CLOVES

¼ TEASPOON GINGER

Peel and core the pears. Cover the pears in wine and parboil about 5 minutes. Drain and lay in the pastry shell, sprinkle with sugar and spices, and cover with a second pastry crust. Bake 45 minutes at 180°C/350°F/gas mark 4.

Samhain

Samhain is the modern Pagan festival that marks the start of winter, around the beginning of November. In the modern world it is known as Halloween. Several ancient cultures, such as the Celts, recognised a twofold division of the year: summer and winter. When the sun is stronger in summer and the days are longer, we have light, warmth, and plentiful food as animals produce young and plants grow. In the winter the power of the sun declines and we have darkness and cold; vegetation dies back. Nature is in decline; hunger and death may come to many.

By Samhain the grain harvest has long been gathered in and the root crops, nuts, berries, and apples have been stored against the hungry winter. Animals were brought down from their summer pastures to more sheltered winter quarters, to be fed on stored hay. Any surplus animals were culled and the meat preserved. Some of the animals would have been ritually sacrificed to propitiate the powers of winter.

With the death of vegetation and the decline of the sun, the spirits of winter, decline, and death are released from the otherworld to stalk the land. It is the beginning of the time of chaos that rules until Yule and the return of the sun. The social order is reversed, and guisers play tricks and demand food.

TRADITIONAL FOODS FOR SAMHAIN

By Samhain we usually have had the first winter frosts, and tender plants have been damaged or killed. The fresh salad season is over, but root vegetables are still viable in the ground. Ritual foods for Samhain include apples, parsley, sloes, pumpkin, hops, juniper, and rowan. Closely associated with Halloween is the hollowed-out pumpkin or turnip carved with a frightening face and lit with a candle inside. It is intended to frighten away the spirits that roam the land at this dangerous time.

. . . .

MASH O'NINE SORTS

It is traditional to put a gold ring into the mash, and whoever finds it in their portion will be lucky for the coming year. Don't forget to warn people about this if you do it!

2 POUNDS (6 CUPS/900 GRAMS) POTATOES, PEELED AND DICED

2 CARROTS, PEELED AND DICED

1 SMALL TURNIP, PEELED AND DICED

1 LARGE PARSNIP, PEELED AND DICED

. . . . .

SALT AND PEPPER TO TASTE

2 LEEKS, CLEANED AND CHOPPED THINLY

2 TABLESPOONS SINGLE (LIGHT) CREAM

8 OUNCES (2 CUPS/225 GRAMS) HARD OR SEMI-HARD CHEESES SUCH AS
MATURE CHEDDAR, DOUBLE GLOUCESTER, OR WENSLEYDALE, GRATED

Preheat the oven to 180°C/350°F/gas mark 4. Boil the potatoes, carrots, turnip, and parsnip together until soft. Mash them thoroughly and season with salt and pepper. Simmer the leeks in water until tender but firm. Add them to the root vegetable mix and stir in the cream and grated cheese (and a gold ring if you like). Transfer to an ovenproof dish, sprinkle grated cheese on top, and bake for 40 minutes.

PUMPKIN BREAD

1½ POUNDS (5¼ CUPS/675 GRAMS) ALL-PURPOSE FLOUR

¼ OUNCE (7 GRAMS) DRIED YEAST

¾ PINT (1¾ CUPS/425 MILLILITRES) WATER

¾ PINT (1¾ CUPS/425 MILLILITRES) MILK

A PINCH OF SALT

3 OUNCES (6 TABLESPOONS/90 GRAMS) BUTTER, MELTED

12 OUNCES (2½ CUPS/340 GRAMS) WHOLEMEAL (WHOLE WHEAT) FLOUR

1 POUND (5⅓ CUPS/450 GRAMS) ROLLED OATS

5 OUNCES (1 CUP/140 GRAMS) CHOPPED PUMPKIN SEEDS

Put the white flour into a bowl with the dried yeast. Boil the water and add to the milk, which should make the combined liquids lukewarm. Stir together the flour with the yeast mixture and knead it well. Cover the dough with a cloth and put it in a warm place for 1 hour. When the dough is risen, knead in the salt, melted butter, wholemeal flour, oats, and pumpkin seeds. Knead for a few minutes, cover with a cloth, and leave to rise in a warm place for 40 minutes. Shape into two loaves and place on greased baking trays. Cover and leave in a warm place to prove for about an hour. The loaves should double in size. Bake at 220°C/425°F/gas mark 7 for 1 hour.

. . . .

APPLE SPIRAL FLAN

At Samhain the apple represents the journey through the underworld, contact with the otherworlds, divination, and intuition. Apples and cider are sometimes used at Samhain in place of the cakes and wine. A libation of cider is made before the closing of the circle. Leave a couple of apples on the ground to keep wandering spirits happy.

6 OUNCES (¾ CUP/170 GRAMS) BUTTER, CHILLED,
    CUT INTO SMALL PIECES

8 OUNCES (1½ CUPS/225 GRAMS) PLAIN ALL-PURPOSE FLOUR

2 OUNCES (5 TABLESPOONS/50 GRAMS) SUGAR, DIVIDED

WATER TO BIND

1 EGG, BEATEN

3 COOKING APPLES

3 RED EATING APPLES

GINGER JAM

APRICOT JAM FOR GLAZE

Rub two-thirds of the butter into the flour and then mix in 1 ounce sugar. Add a little water to bind and roll out to ¼-inch thick. Line a shallow flan case with the pastry and prick over the surface with a fork. Cover with a layer of foil, pressing carefully into the corners of the tin, and weight this down with dried peas to prevent the pastry rising. Bake blind at 190°C/375°F/gas mark 5 until just beginning to turn light brown. Remove the peas and foil. Brush the beaten egg over inside of flan case and bake for a further 10 minutes to seal the pastry. Cool.

Meanwhile, cook the cooking apples over low heat with a tiny amount of water so the apples simmer in their own juices; cool and drain. Neatly cut the eating apples into narrow wedges without peeling and fry gently with the remaining butter and 1 ounce sugar until brown, turning once. Spread a layer of ginger jam over the pastry and cover this with the cooking apples. Arrange the slices of eating apples over the top in a spiral, starting around the outside and overlapping the slices, leaving the red skin visible. Ensure that the whole flan is completely covered by the spiral of apple slices, and return to the oven for a further 15 minutes to finish cooking. Warm a little apricot jam or more ginger jam and brush over the top of the flan to glaze whilst still hot.

. . . . .

PUMPKIN PIE

9-INCH (23-CENTIMETRE) PREBAKED WHOLE WHEAT PASTRY CASE

12 FLUID OUNCES (1½ CUPS/350 MILLILITRES) COOKED, DRAINED PUMPKIN

12 FLUID OUNCES (1½ CUPS/350 MILLILITRES) DOUBLE (HEAVY) CREAM

2 OUNCES (6 TABLESPOONS/50 GRAMS) BROWN SUGAR

A PINCH OF SALT

1 TEASPOON CINNAMON POWDER

1½ TEASPOONS GROUND GINGER

⅛ TEASPOON GROUND CLOVES

3 EGGS, LIGHTLY BEATEN

3 FLUID OUNCES (⅓ CUP/95 MILLILITRES) WARM GOLDEN SYRUP
    OR CORN SYRUP

1 TEASPOON VANILLA EXTRACT

Into a saucepan place the pumpkin, cream, sugar, salt, spices, eggs, and syrup. Mix well and cook over a low heat for a few minutes, stirring constantly. Allow to cool slightly and then stir in the vanilla essence. Pour the mixture into the pastry case, leveling the top if necessary. Cool completely before serving.

SUGAR-FREE OATEN FRUIT CRUMBLE

Oats are a traditional food at Samhain, utilized in a variety of sweet and savory dishes, blood puddings, and drinks. They are considered a warming food that helps build up a resistance to cold. Serve this crumble hot or cold with cream or custard.

2 COOKING APPLES

3 MEDIUM PEARS

2 TABLESPOONS WHITE GRAPE JUICE

6 OUNCES (2 CUPS/170 GRAMS) OATS

3 OUNCES (6 TABLESPOONS/90 GRAMS) BUTTER

Prepare and slice the apples and pears. Place both in the bottom of an ovenproof dish and pour the grape juice over the fruit. Rub together the oats and butter to make a crumble and spread over the fruit. Press down firmly. Bake in a moderate oven at 190°C/375°F/gas mark 5 until golden brown, about 40 minutes.

LANCASHIRE PARKIN

This is a traditional spiced oatmeal cake served at Halloween in the north of England. Make it a few days in advance and store in an airtight tin. The cake will become soft and stickily delicious.

8 OUNCES (1½ CUPS/250 GRAMS) ALL-PURPOSE FLOUR

8 OUNCES (2½ CUPS/250 GRAMS) MEDIUM OATMEAL (LIGHTLY GROUND ROLLED OATS)

4 TEASPOONS (20 MILLILITRES) GROUND GINGER

4 OUNCES (½ CUP/125 GRAMS) BUTTER

8 OUNCES (⅔ CUP/250 GRAMS) BLACKSTRAP MOLASSES (BLACK TREACLE)

4 OUNCES (⅓ CUP/125 GRAMS) HONEY

4 OUNCES (¾ CUP/125 GRAMS) SOFT BROWN SUGAR

4 TABLESPOONS (60 MILLILITRES) MILK

2 TEASPOONS (10 MILLILITRES) BICARBONATE OF SODA (BAKING SODA)

Grease an 11 x 7-inch (28 x 18 cm) cake tin. Preheat oven to 160°C/325°F/gas mark 3. Blend together the flour, oats, and ginger in a mixing bowl. Gently heat the butter, treacle, and honey in a pan until melted and add to the flour mixture. Gently heat the milk until lukewarm and stir in the baking soda. Add to the oatmeal mixture and beat well. Pour the mixture into the prepared cake tin. Bake in the preheated oven for 1½ hours. Cool in the tin for about 15 minutes, then finish cooling on a wire rack.

THOR CAKES OR THARF CAKES

These are traditional Derbyshire oatmeal and black treacle biscuits associated with Halloween and Bonfire Night. Several English villages celebrated "Tharf Cake Joinings" on Bonfire Night, 5 November. It is not known whether the name really has anything to do with the god Thor, but it may derive from the Old English theorf, meaning "unleavened," and has been recorded as Tharf-kyek, Thor Cake, and Tharfy.

8 OUNCES (2¾ CUPS/230 GRAMS) OATMEAL

8 OUNCES (2 CUPS/230 GRAMS) SELF-RAISING FLOUR

6 OUNCES (¾ CUP/170 GRAMS) BUTTER

8 OUNCES (1 CUP/230 GRAMS) SUGAR

1 TEASPOON BAKING POWDER

A PINCH OF GROUND GINGER

A PINCH OF SALT

1 TEASPOON CORIANDER SEEDS

1 OUNCE (¼ CUP/30 GRAMS) CANDIED PEEL

6 OUNCES (½ CUP/170 GRAMS) BLACK TREACLE (MOLASSES), WARMED

Grease a baking tray. Combine the oatmeal and flour and rub in the butter. Add the sugar, spices, and candied peel, then add the warmed treacle. Knead lightly before rolling out and cutting into thin rounds. Bake for about 10 minutes at 190°C/375°F/gas mark 5.

IRISH BARM BRACK

Brack is a Celtic word for bread, and barm means yeast. Found in Ireland, Wales, and Brittany, these fruit breads are traditionally served at Halloween.

1 POUND (3¾ CUPS/450 GRAMS) MIXED DRIED FRUIT

½ PINT (1¼ CUPS/280 MILLILITRES) COLD BLACK TEA

12 OUNCES (2½ CUPS/340 GRAMS) SELF-RAISING FLOUR

6 OUNCES (1¼ CUPS/170 GRAMS) BROWN SUGAR

½ TEASPOON MIXED SPICE (SEE PAGE 26)

2 EGGS, BEATEN

Soak the fruit overnight in the tea. Sieve the flour into a bowl. Stir the sugar and spice into the tea and fruit. Gradually add the beaten eggs, stirring well to mix. Turn into a well-greased loaf tin and bake in a moderate oven at 180°C/350°F/gas mark 4 for 1–1½ hours.

SAINT CATHERINE CAKES

St. Catherine's Day is celebrated in November. She was reputed to have been martyred on a wheel, but many Pagans believe that she was originally a spinning goddess whose wheel represents both creation and the turning of the year. These cakes are eaten in Devon, in southern England, on the saint's feast day of November 24.

4 OUNCES (½ CUP/125 GRAMS) BUTTER

4 OUNCES (½ CUP/125 GRAMS) SUPERFINE (CASTOR) SUGAR

1 LARGE EGG

8 OUNCES (1½ CUPS/250 GRAMS) SELF-RAISING FLOUR

½ LEVEL TEASPOON GROUND MIXED SPICE (SEE PAGE 26)

4 LEVEL TABLESPOONS GROUND ALMONDS

2 OUNCES (⅓ CUP/60 GRAMS) SULTANAS

Cream the butter and sugar together. Gradually beat in the egg with a spoonful of the flour to prevent curdling. Sift in the rest of the flour and spice, then add the almonds and sultanas. Mix well until the dough binds together. Knead lightly and roll out on a floured board to ¼ inch (½ cm) thick by 8 inches (20 cm) wide. Cut into ½-inch (1 cm) strips and twist round to make about 30 flattened spiral shapes, or Catherine wheels. Bake 10–15 minutes at 200°C/400°F/gas mark 6.

Yule

The winter solstice was celebrated on every continent of the earth—by the ancient Egyptians, Babylonians, Jews, and Persians, throughout Europe by the Greeks, Roman, Norse, Celtic, Germanic, and Slavic peoples, as well as the inhabitants of North and South America, the Far and Near East, and Africa.

The sun hangs low and weak in the sky during the brief daylight hours, casting long shadows. It is the shortest day and longest night, but from this time forward the sun gradually strengthens, thus it is the death of the old solar year and the start of the new. Ancient man would have realised that we depend on the sun for life: in the summer the long hours of daylight and warmth make the crops grow. In the winter days of darkness and cold, the crops shrivel and die; humans and animals struggle to find food and survive. Each day up to the winter solstice, the sun grows weaker and weaker. If it does not regenerate, then life must end. Then, on the shortest day, in the time of darkness, the light is reborn—and, with it, hope. For the Romans, *Deis Natalis Invicti Solis*, "the Birthday of the Unconquered Sun," celebrated the birth of Sol (the sun) on 25 December. Roman women would parade in the streets and cry, "Unto us a child is born!"

TRADITIONAL FOODS FOR YULE

In the past, little fresh food was available at this time, but Yule was a time of great feasting and merrymaking, when special, carefully hoarded and stored foods such as sweets, costly spices, liqueurs, and spirits were brought out to celebrate the rebirth of the sun and impart a little cheer in the depths of winter.

. . . .

CREME DE MARRONS

¼ PINT (⅔ CUP/150 MILLILITRES) DOUBLE (HEAVY) CREAM

8 OUNCES (225 GRAMS) CHESTNUT CREAM
(SWEETENED CHESTNUT PUREE), BEATEN

1 TABLESPOON BRANDY

Whip the double cream. Fold it into the beaten chestnut cream and add the brandy. Chill for an hour before serving.

. . . .

Chestnut Soup

1 POUND (4 CUPS/450 GRAMS) CHESTNUTS

1 PINT (2½ CUPS/568 MILLILITRES) VEGETABLE STOCK

2 OUNCES (¼ CUP/60 GRAMS) BUTTER

½ PINT (1 CUP/284 MILLILITRES) MILK

SALT

CAYENNE PEPPER

Split open the chestnuts and cook in just enough water to cover for 12–15 minutes. Drain and discard the chestnut cooking water. Remove from heat and peel them before they cool. Return to the pan and top up with the vegetable stock. Cook gently for 40 minutes or until tender. Liquidise and return to the pan with the butter, milk, and seasoning. Heat without boiling.

. . . .

German Yule Tiles

In Germany these biscuits are traditionally cut into tile shapes for tree ornaments. Before baking, extra dough can be cut out or piped onto the biscuits to make raised patterns, and a hole for hanging can be made with a clean drinking straw. After cooling, the biscuits can be iced with royal icing and painted with food colourings, threaded on ribbons, and hung on the tree.

3 OUNCES (⅜ CUP/90 GRAMS) BUTTER

4 OUNCES (½ CUP/110 GRAMS) MARGARINE

2 OUNCES (1¾ CUP/60 GRAMS) POWDERED (ICING) SUGAR

5 OUNCES (1¼ CUP/140 GRAMS) ALL-PURPOSE FLOUR

4 OUNCES (1 CUP/110 GRAMS) SELF-RAISING FLOUR

1 TABLESPOON CORNFLOUR (CORNSTARCH)

Cream together the butter and margarine, then fold in the icing sugar. Add the flours and cornflour. Knead lightly to make a smooth dough. Wrap in cling film and chill in the fridge for half an hour. Roll out the dough on a floured board to ¼-inch (½ cm) thick. Bake at 180°C/350°F/gas mark 4 for 15 minutes. Transfer to a cooling rack.

. . . . .

Chocolate Yule Log

3 EGGS

3 OUNCES (½ CUP/90 GRAMS) SUGAR

2½ OUNCES (½ CUP/75 GRAMS) SELF-RAISING FLOUR

½ OUNCE (2 TABLESPOONS/15 GRAMS) COCOA POWDER

¼ PINT (⅔ CUP/150 MILLILITRES) DOUBLE (HEAVY) CREAM

1 TABLESPOON OF YOUR FAVOURITE LIQUEUR

Place the eggs in a bowl and stand this in hand-hot water. Whisk the eggs for two minutes. Add the sugar and continue to whisk until the eggs have doubled their volume (around ten minutes). Remove the bowl from the water and continue whisking until the mixture is cool. Carefully fold in the flour and cocoa powder. Turn the batter into a greased and lightly floured Swiss roll tin lined with greaseproof paper and bake at 200°C/400°F/gas mark 6 for 10 minutes or until well risen and firm to the touch.

Whilst the cake is still hot, place a clean tea towel on your work surface and a sheet of greaseproof paper over it. Turn out the cake onto this and cut away the hard edges. Roll up the cake loosely and cover it with a damp tea towel. Allow it to go completely cold. Meanwhile, whisk the cream until it forms peaks. Stir in the liqueur. Carefully unroll the cake and remove the paper from the underside. Fill with the cream and re-roll. Hold in position for a minute or so to set. Decorate as liked.

Rum Truffles

8 OUNCES (225 GRAMS) DARK CHOCOLATE

2 TABLESPOONS POWDERED (ICING) SUGAR

1½ TEASPOONS RUM ESSENCE

2 OUNCES (60 GRAMS) CHOCOLATE SPRINKLES

Melt the chocolate in a bowl over a pan of hot water or in the microwave. Combine with the sugar and rum essence, stirring with a wooden spoon until well blended. Cool for 15 minutes, then shape into small balls with your hands. Roll them in chocolate sprinkles or cocoa powder.

. . . .

BRANDY SNAPS

3 OUNCES (⅜ CUP/90 GRAMS) BUTTER

2 OUNCES (¼ CUP/60 GRAMS) SUGAR

3 FLUID OUNCES (⅓ CUP/80 MILLILITRES) GOLDEN SYRUP

2 OUNCES (½ CUP/60 GRAMS) ALL-PURPOSE FLOUR

1 TEASPOON GROUND GINGER

JUICE OF ½ A LEMON (ABOUT 1 TABLESPOON)

6 FLUID OUNCES (¾ CUP/180 MILLILITRES) DOUBLE (HEAVY) CREAM

2 TABLESPOONS BRANDY

Heat the oven to 180°C/350°F/gas mark 4. Grease a baking sheet. In a pan melt the butter, sugar, and golden syrup over low heat. Remove from the heat and add the flour, ginger, and lemon juice. Beat until the mixture is smooth. Drop spoonfuls onto a baking sheet and bake for 10 minutes. Turn off the oven and leave the biscuits in there to keep warm; if they cool, they won't be malleable. One by one, remove them from the baking sheet with a palette knife and curl them round the handle of a greased wooden spoon. Ease them off and put them on a cooling rack. When you are ready to serve them, beat up the cream until thick and add the brandy. Whisk up again until stiff and pipe into the brandy snaps.

. . . . . .

WASSAIL

The wassail cup is a traditional Yuletide drink. Formerly it was mulled mead to which whole fruits and seasonings were added. The exotic spices are a more modern addition.

2¼ PINTS (5⅓ CUPS/1,278 MILLILITRES) ALCOHOLIC CIDER

3 APPLES, GRATED

2 OUNCES (¼ CUP/60 GRAMS) BROWN SUGAR

½ TEASPOON GROUND GINGER

GRATED NUTMEG

Put a ¼ pint (½ cup) of cider in a pan and add the grated apples. Cook until the apple is soft, and add the brown sugar, ginger, and the remaining 2 pints of cider. Heat through but do not allow to boil. Add some grated nutmeg and pour into a large cup or bowl. This is passed from one person to another with the blessing *waes haelinch* ("good health").

. . . .
MULLED WINE

½ POUND (1 CUP/225 GRAMS) BROWN SUGAR

½ PINT (1 CUP/284 MILLILITRES) WATER

1 LEMON

1 ORANGE

12 CLOVES

CINNAMON STICK

½ TEASPOON GINGER POWDER

2 OUNCES (½ CUP/60 GRAMS) RAISINS

2 BOTTLES RED WINE

To *decorate:*

ORANGE AND LEMON SLICES

Put the sugar and water in a pan and heat slowly to dissolve; add the juice of the lemon and orange and their grated rinds and the spices. Boil for five minutes and leave to infuse for an hour. Strain into a large pan, add the raisins, and bring to a boil. Add the wine, but do not allow it to boil (all the alcohol disappears), just warm it through. Serve hot in glasses decorated with orange and lemon slices.

. . . .
TWELFTH NIGHT CAKE

Twelfth Night celebrations brought the Yuletide season to a close and traditionally involved feasting and mischief. A special cake, the forerunner of all today's Christmas cakes, was the centrepiece of the party, and a piece was given to everyone present. Traditionally, it contained a dried bean and a dried pea. Whoever found the bean was elected king for the night, and whoever found the pea was queen, and they ruled the rest of the evening. By the nineteenth century the cake had become highly decorated with icing and figures made of sugar paste.

2¼ POUNDS (9 CUPS/1010 GRAMS) MIXED DRIED SULTANAS, RAISINS, AND CURRANTS

2 OUNCES (½ CUP/60 GRAMS) MIXED CANDIED PEEL

¼ PINT (⅔ CUP/150 MILLILITRES) WHISKEY

¼ PINT (⅔ CUP/150 MILLILITRES) MILK

12 OUNCES (1½ CUPS/340 GRAMS) BUTTER

12 OUNCES (1½ CUPS/340 GRAMS) MUSCAVADO SUGAR

4 EGGS, BEATEN

1 POUND 4 OUNCES (5 CUPS/560 GRAMS) ALL-PURPOSE FLOUR

1 LEVEL TABLESPOON BAKING POWDER

2 LEVEL TEASPOONS MIXED SPICE (SEE PAGE 26)

2 OUNCES (½ CUP/60 GRAMS) GLACÉ CHERRIES

2 OUNCES (½ CUP/60 GRAMS) CHOPPED WALNUTS

Place the dried fruit and peel in a bowl. Stir in the whiskey and milk, cover, and leave overnight. Heat the oven to 140°C/275°F/gas mark 1. Oil a large tin (approximately 12 x 10 inches) and line the base and sides with greaseproof paper. Brush the paper with oil. Cream the butter and sugar, then add the beaten eggs a little at a time. If the mixture curdles, add a little flour. Sift the flour, baking powder, and spice, and fold into the creamed mixture. Add the fruit, nuts, and whiskey. Stir well. Turn into the tin. Bake in the centre of the oven for 2¼–2½ hours. Leave to cool in the tin. Turn out and remove the paper. If you really must, you can sprinkle more whiskey. The cake can be iced and decorated with stars, ribbons, wheat ears, nuts, and glacé fruit.

. . . .
YULE PUDDING

Plum pudding or Christmas pudding is the crowning glory of every Christmas dinner in Britain. In the seventeenth century the word "plum" was used to refer to any dried fruit. Plum pudding was originally a soup made by boiling beef with dried fruit, wines, and spices. Christmas was the time to use all the rare and costly ingredients such as spices that were otherwise carefully rationed.

1½ POUNDS (6 CUPS/675 GRAMS) MIXED DRIED FRUIT

3 FLUID OUNCES (⅓ CUP/80 MILLILITRES) DARK ALE

JUICE AND RIND OF 1 LEMON

6 OUNCES (¾ CUP/170 GRAMS) BUTTER

8 OUNCES (1 CUP/225 GRAMS) DEMERARA SUGAR

4 EGGS, BEATEN

8 OUNCES (4 CUPS/225 GRAMS) FRESH BREADCRUMBS

4 OUNCES (1 CUP/110 GRAMS) CHOPPED MIXED CANDIED PEEL

1 OUNCE (¼ CUP/30 GRAMS) ALMONDS, PEELED AND CHOPPED

1 TEASPOON GROUND MIXED SPICE (SEE PAGE 26) OR PUMPKIN SPICE

¼ TEASPOON CINNAMON

1 TEASPOON GRATED NUTMEG

2 OUNCES (½ CUP/60 GRAMS) SLOES FROM SLOE GIN, STONED (OPTIONAL)

SMALL SILVER COIN OR FAVOUR

Combine the fruit, ale, and lemon; cover and stand overnight. In a bowl cream together the butter and sugar. Beat in the eggs. Add all the other ingredients, including the coin or favour, and mix well. Everyone who helps to stir the pudding can have a wish, so share this chore with as many as possible. Grease a large pudding bowl and press the mixture in, tying a cloth or greaseproof paper over the top and making a pleat in the middle to allow for expansion. Stand the bowl in a large pan of hot water and boil for 4 hours, topping up the water as necessary. Turn out whilst still hot, pour over 1 or 2 tablespoons whiskey, and light the pudding in the traditional way. Don't forget to warn everyone to check their dish for the coin or favour!

. . . . .

JÓLAGRAUTUR (YULE PORRIDGE)

This is the traditional Christmas breakfast in Finland. Whoever finds the almond will be very lucky for the coming year. They can also make a wish but must not reveal it to anyone.

- ½ PINT (1 CUP/250 MILLILITRES) WATER
- 3 PINTS (7 CUPS/1,700 MILLILITRES) MILK
- 6 OUNCES (1 CUP/170 GRAMS) RICE
- A PINCH OF SALT
- 2½ OUNCES (¾ CUP/70 GRAMS) RAISINS
- 1 ALMOND
- MILK TO TASTE
- CINNAMON AND SUGAR TO TASTE

Boil the water, stir in the rice, and cook for 10 minutes. Add the milk and cook over a low heat for 1 hour. Put the raisins in for the last 10 minutes along with a pinch of salt. Stir in the almond at the last minute and divide the mix into bowls. Add extra milk if liked, and sprinkle on sugar and cinnamon to taste.

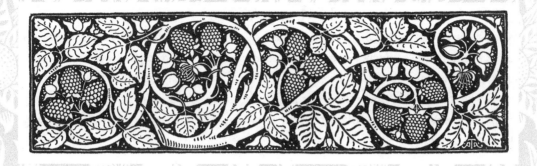

CHAPTER 3

Wine, Cider & Beer

I've been brewing for many years now. I started by making wine from the fruits and flowers I foraged from the local hedgerows and woodlands, but now that I have a large garden, brewing is a great way to use up a glut of fruits or vegetables. As I write, I have a whole shelf in the pantry filled with gooseberry jam. I can't get any more fruit in the freezer, so I've turned the rest of the gooseberries into wine and mead. Next Midsummer we will be drinking a bottle or two during our solstice vigil.

Homemade wine is important for the hearth witch, as we can make our own ritual brews organic, chemical free, and with honour for the plant that supplies the fruit and love for Mother Earth who supports it. Wine is usually ready to drink one year after it is made, linking one cycle to the next, part of the ever-evolving pattern of the Wheel of the Year.

Making Wine

Making wine is actually a very simple process. Wine can be made out of anything that is edible, from turnips and oak leaves to hawthorn blossoms and rose petals. Just add water, sugar, and yeast, and then the clever yeast eats up all the sugar and turns it into alcohol. It really is that easy! Wine making requires little specialist equipment. Though looking around brewing shops you might think it requires a large investment in materials and chemicals, it doesn't.

BASIC EQUIPMENT

You will need some basic equipment, as follows:

- A large plastic bucket or brewing bin for fermenting the pulp. You can buy purpose-made bins that have tightly fitting lids, but a plastic bucket well sealed with cling film (plastic wrap) will serve exactly the same purpose.

- A demijohn or glass fermentation jar. The wine is left in this until fermentation has finished. Demijohns can be obtained relatively cheaply from a number of outlets or online.

- An airlock. This is partially filled with water and fitted on top of the demijohn to allow the gasses produced from the fermentation process to escape from the jar and prevent bacteria entering. For several years I made wine without using airlocks; I just sealed the top of the jar with a plug of cotton wool. While it is possible to do this, the use of an airlock is advisable since they are inexpensive.

- A muslin bag or material to strain the vegetable matter. Muslin is closely woven and strains all the fibres from any pulp, though in the past I have used the knotted sleeve from an old shirt.

- A siphon tube is a necessity; it allows you to remove your wine from the jar without disturbing any sediment. If you just try to pour wine from one large vessel to another, you might spill some—and we don't want that kind of wastage, do we?

- You will also need bottles and corks for the finished product. Glass bottles are no problem; you will probably have several lying around ready to go to the bottle bank. Make a habit out of washing and saving them. Unless your bottles have screw tops, you will need to buy new corks, as old ones cannot be reused. With a bit of effort and squashing, corks can be inserted without the need for a bottling machine, or you can do as I do and only save screw-cap bottles. Be sure to sterilize them before use.

In addition, you can buy a large variety of equipment including thermometers, filtering kits, hydrometers, bottle corking machines, and so on. Personally, I have never found any of them necessary, but if your wine making turns into a serious hobby, you might want to invest in them.

THE BASIC STEPS OF WINEMAKING

1. The ingredients (fruit, vegetables, flowers, etc.) are gathered and washed.

2. The equipment is thoroughly sterilised.

3. The fruit or flowers are placed in a brewing bin with water and some of the sugar.

4. After a day or two, the yeast is added and allowed to ferment on the pulp for a few days.

5. The liquor is strained into a fermentation jar, any remaining sugar is added, and an airlock is fitted. The jar is put in a warm place to encourage fermentation.

6. When fermentation has finished after a few weeks (or sometimes months), the wine is "racked off," which means it is siphoned into a clean jar. (I often omit this stage.)

7. The wine is left to clear. This can take a few weeks, depending on the variety.

8. The wine is then siphoned off into bottles. Depending on the variety, wines must be left to mature for several months at least before drinking, and a year or two is better.

THE YEAST

You can buy a variety of yeasts developed for particular types of wines and beers. These will definitely give you a better result, though it is possible to use fresh or dried bread yeast. The main thing to remember about yeast is that it is a living ingredient and you need to keep it that way. It will not be active at low temperatures and will be killed by high temperatures. It is generally activated before being added to the other ingredients at around 20°C, which is just lukewarm. This method is employed in some of the recipes in this book.

YEAST NUTRIENT

A nutrient is generally added at the same time as the yeast. This helps to keep the yeast working and makes sure it converts more of the sugar to alcohol. You can make wine without it, but for a better fermentation and a stronger brew, it is best to use one. Old recipes call for the yeast to be floated on a piece of toast, which presumably served the same purpose. Some brewing yeasts already come with nutrients added.

THE SUGAR

Refined white sugar is generally used for wine making, but if you prefer you can use brown sugar, though this will alter the taste of the wine. If you use honey instead, this makes the finished product a mead.

CHEMICALS—TO USE OR NOT TO USE

A large variety of chemicals are available for use with wine and beer making. I try to avoid them wherever possible or use a natural alternative—after all, people have been making alcoholic beverages for millennia without them.

Acids

Wine needs a little acid to work. If none is present in the raw ingredients, it is necessary to add some, usually in one of two forms, citric acid or tannin. Sometimes recipes call for tannin. This is present in the skins of some fruits and in black tea, which means a cup of cold black tea can be added rather than a tannin powder. It also helps the wine to keep. Citric acid is present in all citrus fruits, so instead of adding a teaspoon of citric acid, add the fresh juice of a lemon. It helps fermentation and improves the bouquet.

Pectic Enzyme

This is usually used in combination with fruits that contain a lot of pectin. If you make jam, you will know that pectin causes things to jellify. Pectic enzyme helps to break down the pectin and get all the juice out of the fruit. Sometimes you might also have a wine that won't clear because of the high pectin content of the fruit, and pectic enzyme can be added to clarify the wine. The only wine I use it for is plum.

Sterilising Tablets and Solutions

One of the most important things in wine and beer making is the cleanliness and thorough sterilisation of the equipment. Bacteria can cause your must (the mass of skins, pulp, and seeds, etc.) to go mouldy, spoil the wine, or turn it to vinegar. In former times sulphur fumes were used to sterilise the equipment and ingredients. These days sterilisers generally come in the form of sodium metabisulphate/sodium metabisulfite, which gives off sulphur dioxide when combined with water. This can be used to clean equipment. In the form of Campden tablets it is added to the fruit pulp, etc., at the rate of one tablet per gallon. Be sure to wait twenty-four hours before adding the wine yeast or the Campden tablets may kill the yeast. Though I rarely bother, I occasionally find the addition of a Campden tablet to some wines is necessary to kill off bacteria and prevent mould forming. Some recommend the use of a Campden tablet each time the wine is transferred to a new vessel.

Wine from Fruit

THE BASIC METHOD

Use good-quality fruit and cut off any bad parts before washing thoroughly. If you have large fruits, such as apples or pears, you will need to roughly chop them. Put the fruit in a plastic bin and pour boiling water over it. Stir, cover, and cool to lukewarm. Crush the fruit (using a wooden spoon or a potato masher) and add half of the sugar, stirring to dissolve. Add the yeast and nutrient, following the manufacturer's instructions. Cover with the lid or cling film (plastic wrap) and stand in a warm place for three days, stirring daily. Strain the liquor off the pulp into a demijohn, add the rest of the sugar, and fit an airlock.

. . . .

BLACKBERRY WINE

The fruit of the blackberry changes from green to red and finally black. Representing the cycle of the harvest and its completion, this rich, fruity wine is perfect for the autumn equinox ritual and feast, when the vegetation god enters the underworld to dwell in the land of the dead until he returns with the spring. Blackberries are also sacred to the sidhe, the fairy folk, and the wine is employed in rituals to contact them or is poured out onto the ground as an offering to them.

4 POUNDS BLACKBERRIES

2 POUNDS SUGAR

JUICE OF 1 LEMON

YEAST

Wash the fruit, place in a brewing bin, and pour 6 pints of boiling water over it. Leave it for 3 days, stirring regularly. Strain the juice, dissolve the sugar in 2 pints of hot water, and add to the mixture, together with the lemon juice. Cool to lukewarm (20°C) and add the yeast. Transfer the must to a demijohn and fit an airlock.

APPLE WINE

Apple wine is one of the most versatile ritual drinks. Apples are associated with sun gods and sun goddesses as the red, rosy shape of the apples is symbolic of the sun, which makes apple wine suitable for use at the solstices and equinoxes. Apples are harvested between Lughnasa and Samhain, so the wine is also apropos for any harvest rituals and celebrations. Associated with initiation and knowledge, apples are also considered fruits of the otherworld and are used for making contact with it.

4 POUNDS APPLES

3 POUNDS SUGAR

YEAST

Chop the apples and place in a brewing bin. Pour 6 pints boiling water over them. Cover and leave for 4 days, stirring daily. Strain into a demijohn, add the sugar and yeast, and fit an airlock.

ELDERBERRY WINE

Elderberries are sacred to the Crone Goddess of winter, and the wine is suitable for the Samhain ritual cup. If you can find any berries in December, these are a rare and potent gift of the Goddess; any wine made from them will be a mighty sabbat brew. Use sparingly as an aid to clairvoyance.

5 POUNDS ELDERBERRIES

JUICE AND GRATED RIND OF 1 LEMON

3 POUNDS SUGAR

YEAST

Strip the berries from the stalks with a fork. Put into a brewing bin and pour 6 pints of boiling water over them, mash down, and stir in the lemon juice and peel. Cover and leave for 3 days, stirring daily, then strain into a demijohn. Dissolve the sugar in 3 pints of water and add this to the demijohn. Cool to lukewarm (20°C) and add the yeast. Fit an airlock and leave to ferment out. This wine needs to be kept at least a year before drinking, and two is better.

ROWAN WINE

Rowan's associations are with witchcraft, protection, divination, and the dead. The berries are marked at their base with the sign of the pentagram, a sign of protection, magic, and the calling and banishing of spirits; rowan wine may be used in these rituals. Rowan is also sacred to the goddess Brighid, and we sometimes use rowan wine at Imbolc; its folk name is the quicken tree, and Imbolc is the quickening of the year.

2 POUNDS ROWAN BERRIES, STALKS REMOVED

3 POUNDS SUGAR

2 ORANGES

2 TEASPOONS DRIED YEAST

Wash the berries and place them in a brewing bin. Pour ½ gallon boiling water over them and leave for 3 days, stirring daily. Put a further 1½ pints of water in a pan and bring to a boil. Dissolve sugar in it, then add to the brewing bin along with the juice and rind of the oranges. Stir thoroughly and strain into a demijohn. When cooled to lukewarm, add the yeast and top up with lukewarm water to the gallon mark. Fit an airlock.

WHITE GRAPE WINE

Grape wine is suitable for most occasions when you have nothing else ready, but in particular it celebrates the vegetation god and wine god in aspects such as Dionysus and Bacchus.

4 POUNDS GRAPES

YEAST

3 POUNDS SUGAR

Crush the grapes and put them in a brewing bin. Add 1 gallon of water and yeast. Cover and leave for 3 days, stirring daily. Strain off the juice, stir in the sugar, and pour into a demijohn. Fit an airlock.

HEDGEROW WINE

This wine is a real celebration of the wild bounty of the earth in the autumn. This wine will never taste the same twice, as the quantities of the different berries will vary each time.

4 POUNDS HEDGEROW BERRIES (ANY COMBINATION OF HAWS, ELDERBERRIES, BLACKBERRIES, AND ROSEHIPS)

1 LEMON

2 POUNDS SUGAR

YEAST AND NUTRIENT

Wash the berries well and place in a fermenting bin. Cover with 1 gallon of boiling water and stir in the lemon and sugar. Cool to lukewarm (20°C) and add the yeast and nutrient. Cover closely and stand in a warm place for 3 days. Strain into a demijohn and fit an airlock.

HAWTHORN BERRY WINE

This golden wine makes a suitable offering and ritual drink at the autumn equinox, representing the fruits of the sacred marriage of the God and the Goddess.

4 POUNDS BERRIES

2 POUNDS SUGAR

1 LEMON

YEAST

Place berries in a brewing bin, cover with boiling water, cover, and leave for a week, stirring daily. Strain. Melt the sugar in about 2 pints of warm water and add the lemon juice, then mix with the fruit juice. Start the yeast with a tablespoon of lukewarm water and a teaspoon of sugar, and leave until it goes frothy. Add yeast, transfer to a demijohn, and fit an airlock.

ROSEHIP WINE

The rose is sacred to the goddess of love, and the rosehip is sacred to the Mother Goddess and the fruits of love. This pale, delicate wine is a suitable drink for the rituals and feast of the autumn equinox.

> 2 POUNDS ROSEHIPS
>
> 2 POUNDS SUGAR
>
> 1 LEMON
>
> YEAST AND NUTRIENT

Wash and crush the berries. Put the sugar in a brewing bin with the hips and cover with 1 gallon boiling water. Stir well and cool to lukewarm (20°C). Add the yeast, lemon juice, and nutrient. Cover and leave for 14 days, stirring daily. Strain well, transfer to a demijohn, and fit an airlock.

GINGER AND LEMON WINE

This is a spicy winter warmer made with shop-bought ingredients when the earth is fallow.

> 1 OUNCE GINGER ROOT, BRUISED
>
> 4 LEMONS, SLICED
>
> 3 POUNDS RAISINS, CHOPPED
>
> 3 POUNDS SUGAR
>
> YEAST

Put the ginger, lemons, and raisins into a brewing bin and pour 1 gallon of boiling water over them. Add the sugar, stirring to dissolve. Cool to lukewarm (20°C). Add the yeast. Keep in a warm place for 10 days, stirring daily. Strain into a demijohn, fit an airlock, and leave to ferment out.

ORANGE WINE

If you live in northern climes, orange wine is good to make in the winter with shop-bought fruit when no fresh fruit is available in the garden. It brings the promise of the sun, and its scent makes us think of warmer days. It is suitable for use at the solstices and equinoxes.

14 ORANGES

3 POUNDS SUGAR

YEAST AND NUTRIENT

Peel 7 of the oranges, making sure to remove all the white pith. Pour 2 pints of water over them and let stand for 24 hours. Strain into a brewing bin. Add the rest of the water and sugar. Squeeze the juice from all the remaining oranges. Add the yeast and nutrient. Cover and keep in a warm place for 3 days. Strain into a demijohn, fit an airlock, and leave to ferment out.

STRAWBERRY WINE

Strawberry wine is taken at Midsummer to facilitate contact with the fairy wildfolk. Strawberries are sacred to the Mother Goddess, who nurtures all living things, as well as to the goddess of love.

1 GALLON STRAWBERRIES

3½ POUNDS SUGAR

½ POUND RAISINS

YEAST

Mash the strawberries and add 1 gallon of water. Let stand for 24 hours, strain off the liquid, and add the sugar and raisins. Return to the brewing bin. Stir in the sugar until it has dissolved and add the yeast. Cover and let stand for 2 days, stirring daily. Transfer to a demijohn and fit an airlock. This wine should be ready to bottle in 6 months.

RASPBERRY WINE

The juicy red raspberries of late summer make a delicious drink for Lughnasa celebrations.

1½ POUNDS RASPBERRIES

2 ORANGES

2 POUNDS SUGAR

YEAST

Wash the raspberries and pour 5 pints boiling water over them. Mash up with a wooden spoon. Leave 2 days and strain off the liquid. Add the juice of the 2 oranges. Boil 3 pints of water with the sugar and add to the fruit juice. Cool to lukewarm (20°C) and add the yeast. Ferment in a brewing bin for 3 days, pour into a demijohn, and fit an airlock.

PLUM WINE

All fruits are sacred to the goddess of the harvest and the Mother Goddess, and this full-bodied, fruity wine is a suitable drink in her rituals.

7 POUNDS PLUMS

3½ POUNDS SUGAR

PECTIC ENZYME

YEAST AND NUTRIENT

Cut up the plums and squash them. Place in a brewing bin. Boil 4 pints of water and pour it over the fruit. Leave for 5 hours. Add 4 pints of cold water and pectic enzyme. Cover and leave for 2 days, then strain off the juice into a large pan. Bring to boil, turn off the heat, and add the sugar, stirring until it dissolves. Cool to lukewarm (20°C). Add the yeast and nutrient. Pour into a demijohn and fit an airlock. You may need to use additional pectin enzyme to clear this wine.

Wine from Flowers

THE BASIC METHOD

Pick your flowers on a dry day and use them as quickly as possible. Take off any green parts and wash them gently but thoroughly. Flowers need the addition of acids (such as lemon juice) and nutrients, as well as something like chopped raisins or grape juice to give the resulting wine body. Start off the yeast and put it to ferment on the grape juice with the sugar in a brewing bin. When it is fermenting add the flower heads and acids, cover, and stand for seven days, stirring daily, pressing the flowers against the sides of the bin. Strain into a demijohn and fit an airlock. You can put the flowers in a muslin bag so that they can be removed easily.

. . . .

HAWTHORN BLOSSOM WINE

Hawthorn flowers are considered so potently magical that they may not be brought indoors except at Beltane. They are wound about with the mysteries of the Goddess and her blossoming sexuality as summer comes. Hawthorn blossom wine is the best ritual drink of all for Beltane.

> 2 LEMONS
>
> 3½ POUNDS SUGAR
>
> 1 CUP BLACK TEA
>
> YEAST AND NUTRIENT
>
> 2 QUARTS HAWTHORN BLOSSOMS

Grate the rinds from the lemons. Boil the sugar and lemon rinds with 4 pints of water for 30 minutes. Put the resulting liquid in a fermenting bin. Add 3 pints lukewarm water and a cup of black tea to the brewing bin and cool to lukewarm. Add the yeast and nutrient. Leave 24 hours, stirring occasionally. Add the flowers and stand for 8 days, stirring daily. Strain into a demijohn and fit an airlock.

HONEYSUCKLE WINE

Honeysuckle is associated with cycles of change. The flowers twist around, following the course of the sun during the day, helping connect with the cycles of change and the energy flow of each new season. Honeysuckle is also an herb of erotic love; the stems twine together like the embrace of two lovers, and thus it makes a perfect drink at handfastings.

2 PINTS HONEYSUCKLE BLOSSOMS

3 POUNDS SUGAR

JUICE OF 2 LEMONS

2 PINTS GRAPE JUICE

YEAST AND NUTRIENT

½ PINT BLACK TEA

Wash the flowers and pour 4 pints of cold water over them. Stir in the sugar, lemon juice, and grape juice, and keep stirring till the sugar has dissolved. Stand 24 hours and add the yeast, nutrient, and tea. Stand in a warm place for 7 days, stirring daily. Strain into a demijohn and top up with enough cold water to make up to a gallon.

Note: Honeysuckle flowers are edible, but the berries are poisonous.

RED CLOVER WINE

Clover is an herb of balance and relates to all the elements. The wine is particularly useful for fairy contacts at Beltane and Midsummer.

2 QUARTS RED CLOVER FLOWERS

3 LEMONS

2 ORANGES

YEAST

2 POUNDS SUGAR

Put the flowers in a brewing bin and pour 1 gallon of boiling water over them. Add the juice of the oranges and lemons. Cool to lukewarm (20°C) and add the yeast. Ferment for 5 days. Pour the sugar into the demijohn, strain the liquid over it, and fit an airlock.

. . . .

ROSE PETAL WINE

The rose is associated with the goddess of love in all her guises. Roses were once thought to be an aphrodisiac, which makes the wine suitable for use in rituals of love (of all kinds), handfastings, and Beltane, when it symbolises the love of the God and Goddess, which renews the world.

4 PINTS ROSE PETALS

2 POUNDS SUGAR

YEAST

Pour 1 gallon of boiling water over the rose petals and allow to infuse until the water becomes scented. Strain. Dissolve the sugar into the liquid. Transfer to a demijohn and add the yeast. The longer this wine is kept, the stronger the rose perfume becomes.

. . . .

ELDERFLOWER WINE

It is said that where the elder grows, the Goddess is not far away. At Midsummer the sweet elder blossom acquires potent magical powers, and it can be gathered to make wine for the Midsummer ritual. Sacred to elves and fairies, it is said to be under the protection of the fairy queen. It is particularly good for rituals involved with fairy contacts.

1 PINT ELDERFLOWERS (WITHOUT STALKS)

2 POUNDS RAISINS

JUICE OF 1 LEMON

YEAST AND NUTRIENT

¾ POUND SUGAR

Place the flowers in a brewing bin with 1 gallon of hot water. Stir, pressing the petals against the sides of the bin. Wash and chop the raisins and add, together with the lemon juice. Stir well and cool to lukewarm (20°C). Add the yeast and nutrient. Cover and keep in a warm place for 10 days. Strain into a demijohn. Stir in the sugar. Fit an airlock and leave to ferment out.

. . . .

JACKANAPES

Marigolds were considered an aphrodisiac and are sacred to the goddess of love in many of her aspects. They are also sacred to sun gods and goddesses and make a suitable drink for Midsummer. This wine can be bottled after nine months. This is a very old recipe that suggests once fermentation has ceased, one pint of French brandy can be added to improve the flavour!

6 POUNDS SUGAR

1 EGG WHITE, BEATEN

15 PINTS MARIGOLD (CALENDULA OFFICINALIS) PETALS ONLY

RIND AND JUICE OF 2 ORANGES

1 POUND CHOPPED RAISINS

YEAST

Heat 2½ gallons of water and dissolve the sugar in it. Add the whisked egg white and skim any scum from the surface. Pour the hot syrup over the petals, oranges, and raisins in a brewing bin. Stand for 2 days, stirring daily. Transfer to demijohns and add the yeast. Fit an airlock.

. . . .

COLTSFOOT WINE

This is one of the traditional ritual drinks of Ostara. Coltsfoot is sometimes called "son-afore-the-father" as the sunshine yellow flowers appear before the leaves, heralding the growing strength of the sun at the vernal equinox.

5 PINTS COLTSFOOT FLOWERS

2 LEMONS

2 POUNDS SUGAR

YEAST

Pour three pints of boiling water over the flowers, squash with a spoon, and cover. Leave 24 hours in a warm place, strain, and add the lemon juice. Boil the sugar in 3 pints of water and add to the flower juice. Cool to lukewarm (20°C) and add the yeast. Cover, leave for 3 days, and transfer to a demijohn. Add water to make up to 1 gallon. Fit an airlock.

. . . . .

GORSE WINE

Gorse is one of the first shrubs to flower and heralds in the spring. It also makes one of the best flower wines. Gorse is strongly associated with the Goddess at the vernal equinox (Ostara).

- 1 GALLON GORSE FLOWERS
- 2 POUNDS SUGAR
- 3 ORANGES
- 1 LEMON
- 1 CUP BLACK TEA
- YEAST AND NUTRIENT

Put the flowers in a jelly bag and drop it into 1 gallon of boiling water. Simmer for 15–20 minutes. Remove the bag, making sure you squeeze all the liquid out of it. Dissolve the sugar in the flower water and add the juice of the oranges and lemon and their grated rinds. Cool to lukewarm (20°C) and pour into a brewing bin; add the tea, yeast, and nutrient. Cover and keep in a warm place for 3 days, stirring daily. Strain into a demijohn and fit an airlock.

DANDELION WINE

The dandelion's golden flowers are very much associated with solar energies and bright life force and vitality. The traditional time to make dandelion wine is St. George's Day, 23 April. St. George may well be a Christian incarnation of a much earlier vegetation deity who overcame the dragon of winter and ushered in the summer around Beltane. Dandelion wine is a suitable drink for the Beltane festivities. The flavour of this wine is much improved with keeping, and it should not be drunk for at least a year (I like to keep mine for three years).

6 PINTS DANDELION FLOWER HEADS

3 POUNDS SUGAR

JUICE AND RINDS OF 2 LEMONS

JUICE AND RINDS OF 1 ORANGE

1 CUP BLACK TEA

YEAST AND NUTRIENT

1 POUND RAISINS

Gather the flowers when you are ready to use them fresh. Boil 1 gallon of water and pour over the flowers; stand for 2 days, stirring daily. Boil with the sugar and citrus fruit rinds for 60 minutes. Put it back in the brewing bin and add the citrus fruit juice. Cool to lukewarm, then add the tea, yeast, and nutrient. Cover the bin and leave in a warm place for 3 days, stirring daily. Strain into a demijohn and add the raisins. Fit an airlock.

BORAGE WINE

Borage was one of the magical herbs of the Celts, and the common name could be derived from the Celtic word borrach, *meaning "person of strong courage or bravery." The wine is used at Lughnasa, when we explore challenges and the path of the warrior. It can also be employed in rituals honouring warrior gods.*

2 PINTS BORAGE FLOWERS AND LEAVES

2 POUNDS SUGAR

1 POUND RAISINS

1 CUP BLACK TEA

JUICE AND GRATED PEEL OF 1 LEMON

YEAST

Wash and chop the flowers and leaves. Put into 5 pints of water and bring to boil. Simmer for 5 minutes, remove from the heat, and leave to infuse for 24 hours. Bring 1½ pints of water to boil and add the sugar, stirring until dissolved. Strain the infused mixture into a fermentation bin and add the sugar mixture. When cool, add the raisins, tea, juice and grated peel of lemon, and the yeast. Cover and leave for a week, stirring daily. Strain into a demijohn and top up with cold boiled water. Fit an airlock and leave to ferment out. When fermentation is completed, siphon into a clean, sterilized demijohn, being careful not to transfer any sediment, and leave to clear.

MEADOWSWEET WINE

Meadowsweet was one of the three most sacred herbs of the Druids. The folk name of mead-wort comes from the fact that it was used to flavour mead. It is sacred to the goddess of summer and her gifts of love, marriage, fertility, and plenty. Meadowsweet wine can be used for the ritual cup at Midsummer, as well as at handfastings.

1 GALLON MEADOWSWEET FLOWERS

1 POUND RAISINS, CHOPPED

3 POUNDS WHITE SUGAR

1 CUP BLACK TEA

JUICE OF 1 LEMON

YEAST AND NUTRIENT

Put the flowers, chopped raisins, and the sugar in a brewing bin. Boil 1 gallon of water and pour over, stirring to dissolve the sugar. Add the tea and lemon juice. Cool to lukewarm (20°C) and add the yeast and nutrient according to manufacturer's instructions. Stand in a warm place for 10 days, stirring twice a day. Strain into a demijohn and fit an airlock. Bottle when clear.

Wine from Vegetables

THE BASIC METHOD

Wash the vegetables and cut off any bad parts. Chop them and simmer them in just enough water to cover them until they are just softening. If you like, you can add some spices to the water. Strain into a brewing bin and add some citric acid or lemon juice, sugar, and either chopped raisins or grape juice. When cool enough, add the yeast and nutrient according to manufacturer's instructions, cover, and stand in a warm place to ferment for three days. Strain into a demijohn and fit an airlock.

. . . .

PUMPKIN WINE

What better wine for Samhain?

7 POUNDS PUMPKIN

JUICE AND RIND OF 2 LEMONS

1 POUND RAISINS

1 PIECE OF GINGER ROOT, BRUISED

10 CLOVES

1 CUP BLACK TEA

1 TEASPOON MALIC ACID

PECTIC ENZYME

YEAST AND NUTRIENT

2 POUNDS SUGAR

Wash and chop the pumpkin and cut into cubes—do not peel or remove the seeds. Put it in a brewing bin with the lemons, raisins, ginger, cloves, tea, malic acid, and pectic enzyme. Add 1 gallon of water, cover, and stand in a warm place for 24 hours. Start the wine yeast by putting it in a cup with a teaspoon of sugar and a tablespoon of lukewarm water; leave to go frothy, then add it to the bin. Stand for 4 days, then strain into a demijohn and add the sugar. Fit an airlock and leave to ferment out.

Beetroot and Ginger Wine

This is a great winter warmer.

4 POUNDS RAW BEETROOT

2 OUNCES GINGER ROOT, PEELED AND CHOPPED

2 POUNDS BROWN SUGAR

JUICE OF 2 LEMONS

YEAST AND NUTRIENT

Wash and chop the beetroot into a brewing bin. Pour 6 pints of boiling water over it and add the ginger. Cover and leave for 4 days, stirring daily. Strain into a demijohn and add the sugar, lemon juice, yeast, and nutrient. Fit an airlock and leave to ferment out in a dark place or wrap in brown paper to prevent the colour fading. It is best to use dark bottles when it comes to bottling this wine.

Parsnip Wine

4 POUNDS PARSNIPS

JUICE OF 1 LEMON

3 POUNDS SUGAR

YEAST AND NUTRIENT

Wash and chop the parsnips, boil them in 1 gallon of water until tender, strain, and keep the liquor. Add to it the lemon juice and sugar. Cool to lukewarm (20°C) and pour into a brewing bin. Add the yeast and nutrient. Cover and keep in a warm place for 10 days. Strain into a demijohn, fit an airlock, and leave to ferment out.

PEA POD WINE

5 POUNDS PEA PODS

3 POUNDS SUGAR

YEAST

Boil the pea pods in 4 pints of water until tender. Strain into a brewing bin. Boil 4 pints of water and dissolve the sugar in it. Add to the pea pod liquor. When cool to lukewarm (20°C), add the yeast, and cover. Leave in a warm place for 24 hours. Pour into a demijohn and fit an airlock. Leave in a warm place to ferment out.

Herb and Leaf Wines

. . . .
NETTLE WINE

The nettle is a plant that is allied to all three realms—the heavens, earth, and underworld. It is a "venomous" plant with a fierce sting and may not be plucked easily. It teaches the lesson of transmutation. Though it appears antagonistic, once assimilated it is totally beneficial, full of vitamins and minerals. Those spiritual and life experiences that are the most difficult and testing are those that make us grow most. The power of the nettle demonstrates that all things have their place in creation, and those things that may be experienced as painful can be integrated and transmuted. Nettle wine may be taken sacramentally at the rites of passage of birth, initiation, and death.

½ GALLON NETTLE TOPS

1 PIECE GINGER ROOT

JUICE AND GRATED RIND OF 1 LEMON

3 POUNDS SUGAR

1 CUP BLACK TEA

YEAST AND NUTRIENT

Wash the nettle tops and remove any stalks. Put the nettles in a pan with the ginger and juice and grated rind of the lemon. Boil and simmer for 30 minutes. Strain into a demijohn. Dissolve the sugar in 2 pints of hot water and add the tea. Pour into the demijohn. Top up to the gallon mark with water, then add the yeast and nutrient according to the manufacturer's instructions. Leave in a warm place for 7 days, strain off into a clean demijohn, and fit an airlock. Leave to ferment out. Store at least 6 months before drinking.

PARSLEY WINE

Parsley is an herb of the underworld, dedicated to the death goddess. It makes a suitable wine for rituals of underworld journeys, funerals, and for Samhain, the death time of the year.

1 POUND PARSLEY

1 POUND RAISINS

RIND AND JUICE OF 2 LEMONS

RIND AND JUICE OF 2 ORANGES

2 POUNDS SUGAR

YEAST AND NUTRIENT

Chop the parsley and place in a brewing bin. Pour 1 gallon of boiling water over, cover, and leave for 24 hours. Strain and add the raisins and the rinds and juice of oranges and lemons. Add half the sugar and stir to dissolve. Add the yeast and nutrient according to manufacturer's instructions, cover, and keep in a warm place for 5 days, stirring daily. Strain and stir in the rest of the sugar, then pour into a demijohn, fit an airlock, and leave to ferment out in a warm place.

CLARY SAGE WINE

In Britain clary sage was used as a substitute for hops and made a very intoxicating drink, famous for its slightly narcotic properties. Magically it is used to enhance the sight during rituals of divination, particularly at the full moon.

3½ POUNDS SUGAR

4 PINTS CLARY SAGE BLOSSOMS

8 OUNCES CHOPPED RAISINS

YEAST

Mix the sugar and water and heat very gently till the sugar has dissolved. Remove from the heat and cool to lukewarm. Pour into a fermentation bin and add the blossoms (no green parts) and raisins. Add the yeast and stand in a warm place for 5 days, stirring daily. Strain into a demijohn and fit an airlock. Bottle the wine when it is clear, and store for 12 months before drinking.

AGRIMONY WINE

Agrimony is regarded as a protective counter-magic herb, which makes this a useful wine for use in rituals of protection and shielding.

4 OUNCES LUMP GINGER

LARGE BUNCH OF AGRIMONY (*AGRIMONIA EUPATORIA*)

7 POUNDS SUGAR

6 ORANGES, SLICED

3 LEMONS, SLICED

YEAST AND NUTRIENT

Crush the ginger and place in a pan with the agrimony and 2 gallons of water. Boil until the water is a good yellow colour. Strain the liquid over the sugar, add the sliced oranges and lemons, yeast, and nutrient, and leave in a brewing bin for 3 days, stirring daily. Strain into a demijohn and fit an airlock.

YARROW WINE

Yarrow is one of the sacred herbs of Midsummer and makes a suitable drink at the solstice ritual. It also promotes clairvoyance.

3 QUARTS YARROW FLOWERS

4 POUNDS WHITE SUGAR

RIND AND JUICE OF 4 ORANGES

YEAST AND NUTRIENT

Pour 1 gallon of boiling water over the flowers and soak for 5 days. Strain the liquid into a pan with the sugar and orange rind. Simmer for 20 minutes. Slice the rest of the oranges into a brewing bin and pour the liquid over. When cooled to lukewarm (20°C), add yeast and nutrient according to manufacturer's instructions. Ferment for 14 days, then strain into a demijohn and fit an airlock.

OAK LEAF WINE

The oak's ogham name of duir *links it not only with the word for door but also with the root of the word "druid"—in other words, a Druid is a person of oak knowledge. The oak symbolises the world tree in some mythologies, with its roots in the underworld and branches in the heavens, connecting all three realms. It is connected to the power of the God and the power of the waxing year.*

3½ POUNDS SUGAR

1 GALLON OAK LEAVES

JUICE OF 2 LEMONS

YEAST AND NUTRIENT

Dissolve the sugar in 4 pints of boiling water. Pour it, still boiling, over the leaves. Stand for 12 hours and strain into a demijohn. Add the lemon juice, yeast, and nutrient. Top up with lukewarm water and fit an airlock. Keep in a warm place until the fermentation is finished. When it is clear, siphon off into another clean demijohn and bottle after another 2 months.

VINE LEAF WINE

1 GALLON FRESH VINE LEAVES (PRUNINGS CAN BE USED)

JUICE AND GRATED PEEL OF 2 ORANGES

2½ POUNDS SUGAR

YEAST

Wash the leaves and place in a fermentation (brewing) bin. Boil 5 pints of water and pour over the leaves. Add the juice and grated peel of 2 oranges. Cover and leave for 3 days, stirring daily. Strain into a demijohn. Boil 1 pint of water and dissolve the sugar in it. Add to the demijohn. When tepid add the yeast and top up with cool boiled water. Fit an airlock and leave to ferment out. Rack into a clean demijohn and leave to clear. Bottle.

GOLDENROD WINE

Use in rituals of prosperity and money-drawing.

1 GALLON GOLDENROD FLOWERS (*SOLIDAGO* SPP.)

3 POUNDS SUGAR

JUICE AND GRATED RINDS OF 2 ORANGES

JUICE AND GRATED RINDS OF 2 LEMONS

1 CUP BLACK TEA

YEAST AND NUTRIENT

Boil 1 gallon of water. Put the flowers in a jelly bag or a cotton pillowcase. Knot the top and drop it into the water. Simmer for 20 minutes. Remove from the heat. When cool enough to touch, take out the bag, squeezing it well to extract all the liquid. Dissolve the sugar in the flower liquor. Add the juice from the lemons and oranges and the grated rinds. Place in a brewing bin. When cool to lukewarm (20°C), add the tea, yeast, and nutrient. Cover and keep in a warm place for 3 days, stirring daily. Strain into a demijohn. Fit an airlock. Keep in a warm place for 2 months. Rack off into a clean demijohn and put in a cooler place for a further 6 months.

AND AN ODD ONE . . .

BIRCH SAP WINE

Birch represents the power of cleansing and purification in preparation for the new beginnings. When the tree is opened to extract the sweet sap, the essence of the tree is released to give its power to the waxing year and the strengthening sun at the vernal equinox, when the light begins to gain on the dark. Opening the tree can form part of the ritual of Ostara. Honour the sun god with birch sap wine the following year.

8 PINTS BIRCH SAP (*BETULA* SPP.)

2 POUNDS SUGAR

½ POUND RAISINS

JUICE OF 3 LEMONS

YEAST

Boil the sap and add the sugar. Simmer for 10 minutes. Pour the liquid over the raisins and lemon juice. Cool the mixture to lukewarm (20°C) and add the yeast. Ferment in a brewing bucket for 3 days, then strain into a demijohn and fit an airlock.

To obtain the sap, bore a small hole into the tree, just inside the bark, and insert a narrow tube, sloping downwards. Sap should start running from the tree (if it doesn't, it is the wrong time of year). Put the free end of the tube into your container (a plastic soda bottle works), which you can tie onto the tree. Don't take too much from one tree. When you have what you need, remove the tube and put a piece of cork into the borehole; the birch tree will seal itself after a short while. In very early spring (late February or early March here in the UK, depending on the weather) you should be able to draw off enough sap for a gallon of wine in a day.

Sparkling Wine

THE BASIC METHOD

To make a sparkling wine, the wine must undergo a second fermentation. The wine is made in the usual way, but after racking the wine is put in a cool place for six months to mature. Now more sugar must be added to begin a new fermentation at the rate of 2½ ounces sugar per gallon. Take a little wine from the jar and dissolve the sugar in it before returning it to the demijohn. Add some activated champagne yeast and wait for the process to start, which will take a few hours. The wine should then be siphoned into sterilised bottles with a gap of 2 inches at the top and fitted with wired corks. The bottles are then laid on their sides. It will take a few days for fermentation to complete, but the wine should be stored on its side for a further 6–12 months before drinking. The stored wine bottles should be rotated (turn the bottom side to the top) at least once a month.

. . . .

NETTLE CHAMPAGNE

JUICE AND PEEL OF 1 LEMON

2 PINTS NETTLE TOPS

3 POUNDS SUGAR

CHAMPAGNE YEAST AND NUTRIENT

Peel the lemon, being careful to leave the bitter white pith behind. Put the peel and juice of the lemon in a pan with the nettle tops and 1 gallon of water. Simmer for 45 minutes, add the sugar, then strain into a demijohn. Cool to lukewarm (20°C), then add the yeast and nutrient. Fit an airlock and leave to ferment out. Put in a cool place for a month, then syphon into strong sparkling wine bottles, add a teaspoon of sugar to each bottle, and cork tightly. Keep in a warm place for 7 days, by which time a secondary fermentation should have started. Store in a cool place and treat the bottles with care—do not shake or knock.

. . . . .

RHUBARB CHAMPAGNE

4 POUNDS YOUNG RHUBARB STALKS

½ POUND SULTANAS

RIND OF 1 ORANGE

1 TEASPOON PECTIC ENZYME

CHAMPAGNE YEAST AND NUTRIENT

2 POUNDS SUGAR

Wash and chop the rhubarb stalks, then put them in a brewing bin with the sultanas and orange rind. Pour over 1 gallon of water, which should be hot but not boiling. Cover. When cool add the pectic enzyme and leave for 24 hours. Add the champagne yeast and nutrient according to manufacturer's instructions and ferment for 5 days, stirring daily. Strain and discard the pulp. Add the sugar, pour into a demijohn, and fit an airlock. Leave to ferment out, then rack off into a clean jar to clear. After 6 months add 2 ounces of sugar and more champagne yeast and nutrient. As soon as the fermentation begins (after a few hours), siphon into strong bottles and cork tightly. Lay the bottles on their sides in a warm place for 6 days, then remove to a cooler place and store on their sides for another 6 months before drinking.

ELDERFLOWER CHAMPAGNE

This is a very hit-or-miss old recipe: sometimes it works and sometimes it doesn't. If there is no sign of the natural yeast working after a day or two, try adding a little yeast.

1½ POUNDS WHITE SUGAR

1 LEMON

4 PINTS ELDERFLOWER HEADS

2 TABLESPOONS WHITE WINE VINEGAR

2 CAMPDEN TABLETS

Dissolve the sugar in the gallon of warm water and allow it to cool. Squeeze the juice from the lemon and chop the rind roughly. Place the flowers in a bowl and add the vinegar, pour on the water, and add the Campden tablets. Steep for 4 days. Strain the infusion well, so that all trace of matter is excluded, and bottle in screw-topped bottles. The elderflower champagne will be ready to drink in 7 days.

GOOSEBERRY CHAMPAGNE

3 POUNDS GOOSEBERRIES

PECTIC ENZYME

1 CUP BLACK TEA

JUICE OF 1 LEMON

½ PINT WHITE GRAPE JUICE CONCENTRATE

CHAMPAGNE YEAST AND NUTRIENT

2 POUNDS 3 OUNCES SUGAR

Put the gooseberries in a brewing bin and pour on 1 gallon of boiling water. When cool, mash them up and add the pectic enzyme, tea, and lemon juice. Cover and stand for 24 hours, then add the grape juice, yeast, and nutrient. Ferment in the bin for 3 more days. Strain off into a demijohn and add 2 pounds of sugar. Fit an airlock and ferment out. Rack off into a clear demijohn and leave to clear. Add 3 ounces of sugar and more champagne yeast and nutrient. Refit the airlock and leave in a warm place. When the fermentation starts, siphon into strong bottles and cork tightly. Lie on their sides for 2 weeks in a warm place, then move to a cool place and store on their sides for another 6 months before drinking.

Mead

THE BASIC METHOD

A mead is really a wine made with honey instead of sugar. Add water to the honey and bring to a boil, skimming off any scum. Add some cold black tea. When cool enough (20°C or lukewarm), add the yeast and nutrient. Pour into a demijohn, fit an airlock, and leave in a warm place until the mead has finished fermenting. When it has cleared, syphon into sterilised bottles and cork.

METHEGLINS AND MELOMELS

A metheglin is a mead made using herbs and spices. Melomels are meads made using fruit. Fruit can be added during the primary fermentation in the brewing bin. I generally make meads and metheglins in the winter, and melomels in the summer and early autumn months as the various fruits become ripe.

• • • •

MEAD

This should be matured for at least a year before drinking—if you can resist it that long!

4 POUNDS HONEY

1 ORANGE

1 LEMON

YEAST AND NUTRIENT

PECTIC ENZYME

Put 1 gallon of water and the honey into a pan and bring to boil. Allow to cool to lukewarm (20°C). Add the juice of the orange and lemon as well as the yeast and nutrient. (A nutrient must be used, as modern honey is deficient in important minerals.) Pour into a demijohn and fit an airlock. Allow to ferment out and bottle.

SWEET MEAD

4½ POUNDS HONEY

JUICE OF 2 LEMONS

YEAST AND NUTRIENT

Boil half a gallon of water with the honey, stirring until the honey has dissolved. Remove from the heat. Allow to cool to 20°C or lukewarm and add the lemon juice and nutrient. Add half a gallon of water and transfer to a demijohn. Add the yeast and fit an airlock. When a layer of sediment settles at the bottom of the jar, rack off into a clean demijohn. Keep for at least a year before drinking.

ROSEHIP MELOMEL

3 POUNDS ROSEHIPS

4 POUNDS HONEY

JUICE OF 2 LEMONS

YEAST

Boil the rosehips in 1 gallon of water for 5 minutes. Cool and mash. Strain carefully through two layers of muslin or a jelly bag to remove the irritant hairs. Add the honey and lemon juice and stir until honey is dissolved. Add the yeast, put into a demijohn, and fit an airlock. Keep for as long as you can resist it before drinking.

Blackcurrant Melomel

4 POUNDS BLACKCURRANTS

2 POUNDS HONEY

YEAST AND NUTRIENT

½ PINT RED GRAPE CONCENTRATE

¼ OUNCE MALIC ACID

Mash the blackcurrants and put them in a brewing bin. Boil 1 gallon of water and add the honey to it, stirring to dissolve. Pour this over the blackcurrants and cool to 20°C or lukewarm. Add the yeast and nutrient and stand for 3 days in a warm place, stirring daily. Add the concentrate and malic acid, strain into a demijohn, and fit an airlock.

Redcurrant Melomel

4 POUNDS REDCURRANTS

2 POUNDS HONEY

YEAST AND NUTRIENT

½ PINT RED GRAPE CONCENTRATE

¼ OUNCE MALIC ACID

Mash the redcurrants and put them in a brewing bin. Boil 1 gallon of water and add the honey to it, stirring to dissolve. Pour this over the redcurrants and cool to 20°C or lukewarm. Add the yeast and nutrient and stand for 3 days in a warm place, stirring daily. Add the concentrate and malic acid, strain into a demijohn, and fit an airlock.

Gooseberry Melomel

6 POUNDS OVERRIPE GOOSEBERRIES

2 POUNDS HONEY

YEAST AND NUTRIENT

1 CUP BLACK TEA

Mash the gooseberries. Boil 6 pints of water and dissolve the honey in it. Cool to lukewarm, then add the nutrient and tea. Put the mixture in a brewing bin with the gooseberries. Cover and stand for 24 hours, then add the yeast. Stand for 3 days, stirring daily. Strain into a demijohn, fit an airlock, and leave to ferment out.

. . . .

GOOSEBERRY AND ROSE MELOMEL

6 POUNDS OVERRIPE GOOSEBERRIES

2 POUNDS HONEY

1 CUP BLACK TEA

½ PINT ROSE PETALS

1 PINT WHITE GRAPE CONCENTRATE

YEAST AND NUTRIENT

Mash the gooseberries. Boil 6 pints of water and dissolve the honey in it. Cool to lukewarm, then add the nutrients and tea. Put the mixture in a brewing bin with the gooseberries and rose petals. Cover and stand for 24 hours, then add the yeast and concentrate. Re-cover and stand in a warm place for a further 2 days, strain into a demijohn, and fit an airlock.

. . . .

RASPBERRY MELOMEL

If a sweeter melomel is required, add another quarter pound of honey when the fermentation slows.

2 POUNDS HONEY

4 POUNDS RASPBERRIES, MASHED

CAMPDEN TABLET

YEAST AND NUTRIENT

½ PINT RED GRAPE CONCENTRATE

Boil ¾ gallon of water and dissolve the honey in it. Remove from the heat and add the mashed raspberries. Put the mixture into a brewing bin and add a campden tablet. Stand for 24 hours. Add the yeast and nutrient. Stand for 3 more days in a warm place and strain into a demijohn. Add the concentrate and fit an airlock.

. . . . .

. . . .
METHEGLIN

4 POUNDS HONEY

3 PINTS WATER

½ OUNCE GINGER

2 CLOVES

YEAST

1 OUNCE HOPS

Boil the honey, ginger, and cloves in 3 pints of water until the liquid is reduced by one quarter. Skim off the scum and cool to 20°C or lukewarm. Add the yeast. Boil the hops in 3 pints of water. Cool to lukewarm and add to the rest. Pour into a brewing bin and stand for 6 weeks. Strain into a demijohn. The metheglin will be ready to drink in 6 months.

. . . .
SACK

This is a traditional English mead drink, mentioned by Shakespeare and others.

3 FENNEL ROOTS

4 POUNDS HONEY

2 SPRAYS RUE

JUICE OF 2 LEMONS

YEAST AND NUTRIENT

1 GALLON WATER

Wash the fennel roots and boil them for 40 minutes in 3 pints of water. Strain and return the liquor to the pan with the honey and boil for 2 hours. Skim off any scum. Cool to 20°C or lukewarm and add 3 pints of water, lemon juice, yeast, and nutrient. Strain into demijohns and fit an airlock. This dry sack will be ready for drinking after a year.

CYSER

An ancient honey and apple drink, cyser is another term for an apple melomel.

4 PINTS APPLE JUICE

JUICE OF 1 LEMON

1 POUND HONEY

1 POUND BROWN SUGAR

YEAST AND NUTRIENT

Put 1 pint of water in a pan, add the apple juice and lemon juice, and simmer for 20 minutes. Meanwhile, dissolve the honey in another pint of hot water. Start off the yeast by putting it in a cup with a teaspoon of sugar and a tablespoon of lukewarm water and letting it get frothy. Put the syrup, dissolved honey, brown sugar, and apple juice into a demijohn and top up with another pint of water. Add the yeast and nutrient, fit an airlock, and leave in a warm place to ferment out. Siphon off into a clean demijohn and top up to the gallon mark with cold water, cork, and leave to mature for 3–4 months before bottling. The taste improves with keeping.

Ciders and Perries

THE BASIC METHOD

Making cider is quite hard work, but it's worth it. You will need about twenty pounds of apples to produce a gallon of apple juice. It is best to use a mixture of different varieties, but if you only have one, don't worry; it will still work. Windfalls produce more juice as they are riper. Discard any brown or rotten ones.

Wash the apples and remove any bad parts. If you want to make a lot of cider, you can invest in a cider press or it may be possible to hire one. I only make small quantities, so I use my juicer—be warned, though: I burned out the motor in one making cider. You could also put the fruit in a plastic bucket, smash the apples with a piece of timber, then put the pulp into a muslin bag and press out the remaining juice. This is a very messy business that is best done outside.

Put the juice in a demijohn and add a Campden tablet. Plug the neck of the demijohn with cotton wool. Fermentation will probably start from the wild yeast on the apples, but add some yeast after 24 hours and fit an airlock. When fermentation has finished, rack into a clean demijohn. When the brew has cleared, siphon off into screw-topped bottles. This will make a very dry cider. If you prefer a sweeter one, add some sugar during the fermentation process. If you want a sparkling cider, add ½ to 1 teaspoon sugar to each bottle after bottling.

PERRY AND PEAR CIDER

A perry is a cider made with pears. The method is the same. A pear cider is made with both apples and pears.

· · · · · · · · · · · · · · ·
OLD-FASHIONED CIDER

10 POUNDS SWEET APPLES

10 POUNDS CRAB APPLES

CHAMPAGNE OR CIDER YEAST

2 CAMPDEN TABLETS

Remove any bad parts from the apples, wash them, and press them either through a cider press or a juicer. Put the juice in a demijohn and add the yeast and a Campden tablet. Fit an airlock and leave in a cool room until the first rapid fermentation ceases. Rack off into a clean jar, add another Campden tablet, and leave for 8 weeks until the cider clears. Bottle in screw-topped bottles. If you want sparkling cider, add a teaspoon of sugar to each bottle.

Sweet Cider

15 POUNDS APPLES

2½ POUNDS SUGAR

YEAST AND NUTRIENT

Chop the apples and place them in a brewing bin, peels, cores and all. Just remove the stems. Cover with water and leave for 2 weeks, stirring daily. Strain off the juice and put into a large saucepan and warm to 20°C (lukewarm—do not boil). Add the sugar to dissolve. Put into a demijohn and add the yeast and nutrient. Fit an airlock and leave to ferment out.

Perry

Pears are sacred to goddesses of the moon, fertility, and the harvest, and the drink may be used in their rites.

FIRM, RIPE PEARS

YEAST AND NUTRIENT

FOR EACH GALLON OF JUICE, ADD 2½ POUNDS RAISINS
   AND 3 POUNDS SUGAR

Chop up the pears and pound into a pulp. Strain through muslin into a brewing bin. Leave for 24 hours, then add the sugar, yeast, and nutrient. After 3 days pour into a demijohn along with the raisins and fit an airlock.

Brewing Beer and Ale

THE BASIC METHOD

Traditionally, beer meant a drink brewed with hops, whereas ale had no hops, though this distinction has largely disappeared. Beers are generally brewed from malt extract, sugar, hops, and yeast, though other beverages (such as ginger beer) are called beers as they are alcoholic and ready to drink faster than wine.

There are various types of yeast to produce ale, bitter, stout, and lager. The malt extract is dissolved in warm water in the brewing bin. The hops are boiled for around three-quarters of an hour, and the liquor is strained into the bin with the malt extract and sugar. When the liquid is cool enough, the started yeast is added and the bin covered and left to ferment in a warm place for 5–7 days. After this, the bin is removed to a cool place for a day or two, then bottled. Unlike wine, beers can be drunk a short time after brewing, but they usually improve with keeping for 3–4 weeks.

. . . .

BEER

Beer and ale may be used for the ritual cup, and their energy is more earthy and basic than that of wine. The hop is associated with the wild wolf, which in Celtic mythology ruled over the winter months of the dead time. February was called the wolf month; thus the wolf is associated with Brighid and Imbolc. The wolf has connections with underworld deities and stands beside Cernunnos on the Gundestrup cauldron.

2 PINTS HOPS

1 POUND SUGAR

YEAST

1 POUND MALT

Activate the yeast: put it in a cup with a teaspoon of sugar and a tablespoon of lukewarm water and leave to go frothy. Put the hops in a large pan and cover with 2 pints of water. Boil for 15 minutes, then strain the liquid into a brewing bin. Add the sugar and malt and stir to dissolve. Add 6 pints of water. When cooled to 20°C, add the yeast, cover, and stand for 5 days. Bottle in screw-topped bottles and leave for 7 days before drinking.

. . . . .

. . . .

STOUT

2 OUNCES DRIED HOPS

4 OUNCES BLACK MALT GRAINS

1 POUND BROWN SUGAR

1 POUND MALT

YEAST

Activate the yeast. Put half a gallon of water in a pan and bring to boil. Add the hops, malt grains, and sugar, and simmer for 30 minutes. Add the malt and stir to dissolve. Add half a gallon of water and, when lukewarm (20°C), the yeast. Cover and leave in a warm place for 5 days. Bottle in screw-topped bottles, adding half a teaspoon of brown sugar to each pint of liquid. Leave for a month before drinking.

. . . .

GINGER BEER

This is alcoholic!

PEEL AND JUICE OF 2 LEMONS

2 OUNCES GINGER ROOT, BRUISED

1 POUND SUGAR

½ OUNCE CREAM OF TARTAR

YEAST AND NUTRIENT

Peel the lemons, removing all the white pith. Place the peel in a brewing bin with the ginger, sugar, and cream of tartar. Pour on 2 pints boiling water and stir to dissolve the sugar. Allow to cool before adding the lemon juice, yeast, and 6 pints of water. Stir well, cover, and keep in a warm place for a week. Siphon off into pint bottles and add ½ teaspoon sugar to each bottle. Seal them tightly and keep in a warm place for 3 days, then remove to a cool place for storage.

. . . . .

HONEY BEER

This can be drunk after seven days.

1 PIECE OF GINGER ROOT

1½ POUNDS HONEY

JUICE OF 3 LEMONS

YEAST AND NUTRIENT

Boil 2 pints of water with the ginger for 30 minutes. Meanwhile, put the honey into a brewing bin with the lemon juice and 4 pints of cold water. Add the boiling water/ginger mixture. Allow to cool to 20°C, then add the yeast and nutrient. Cover and stand for 24 hours. Strain and bottle.

NETTLE BEER

Some sediment may collect at the bottom of the bottle—pour gently so as not to disturb this. Store the bottles in a cool place. Serve chilled.

8 OUNCES SUGAR

1 POUND BREWING MALT EXTRACT

3 POUNDS NETTLE TOPS

BEER YEAST

4 TEASPOONS SUGAR

Mix the sugar and malt extract with 2 pints of warm water and stir until dissolved. Wash the nettles and boil in 4 pints water for 30 minutes. Allow to cool, then strain onto the malt mixture. Add the yeast, cover, and leave in a warm place, stirring daily, skimming off any scum as it appears. Continue until fermentation finishes; this should take about a week. Stand in a cool place for 48 hours to settle, then siphon into a clean brewing bin. Add 4 teaspoons sugar and stir well, then decant into beer bottles. Make sure you leave a 1½-inch air space at the top. Seal tightly and leave in a warm room for a week before drinking.

DANDELION BEER

The beer is ready to drink in seven days.

8 OUNCES DANDELION PLANTS, INCLUDING ROOTS

½ OUNCE BRUISED GINGER ROOT

RIND AND JUICE OF 1 LEMON

1 POUND BROWN SUGAR

1 OUNCE CREAM OF TARTAR

1 OUNCE YEAST

Wash the dandelions and place them in a pan with the ginger, lemon rind, and 3 pints of water. Boil for 15 minutes. Strain into a brewing bin, add the sugar and cream of tartar, and stir to dissolve the sugar. Add the rest of the water and the lemon juice and yeast. Cover and leave in a warm place for 5 days, stirring daily. Strain into screw-topped bottles.

HEATHER ALE

The Picts brewed a legendary ale from heather using a secret recipe. Invading Norsemen tortured the guardians of the secret to obtain the recipe, but it was to no avail. Heather is a sacred plant of Midsummer and represents the spirit of the vegetation god.

2 PINTS HEATHER SHOOTS

1 POUND SUGAR

1 POUND MALT

YEAST

Put the heather in a pan, cover with water, and boil for 15 minutes. Strain into a brewing bin and add the sugar and malt. Stir to dissolve. Add enough water for a total of 2 gallons and cool to 20°C. Activate the yeast by putting it in a cup with a teaspoon of sugar and a tablespoon of lukewarm water and letting it get frothy; add to the brewing bin and cover. Stand for 5 days and bottle into screw-top bottles. Ready to drink after 7 days.

Meadowsweet Ale

2 OUNCES MEADOWSWEET BLOSSOMS

2 OUNCES RASPBERRY LEAVES

2 OUNCES BETONY

2 OUNCES AGRIMONY

3 POUNDS WHITE SUGAR

YEAST

Place the herbs in a large pan and cover with water. Bring to boil and simmer for 10 minutes. Remove from the heat and strain. Dissolve the sugar in the liquid and top up with enough water for 2 gallons. Add the yeast, cover, and stand for 3 days. Bottle in screw-topped bottles.

Dandelion and Burdock Beer

2 LARGE BURDOCK ROOTS

2 LARGE DANDELION ROOTS

1 POUND WHITE SUGAR

1 TABLESPOON BLACK TREACLE (OR MOLASSES)

JUICE OF 1 LEMON

YEAST

Wash and chop the roots into small pieces. Boil for 30 minutes in 1 gallon of water. Remove from the heat and add the sugar, treacle and lemon juice. Stir to dissolve. Strain into a fermentation bin and add the yeast. Leave 5 days and bottle in screw-topped bottles. Store 7 days before drinking.

OATMEAL ALE

2 POUNDS BREWING MALT EXTRACT

4 OUNCES BLACK MALT

1 POUND FLAKED OATS

2 OUNCES HOPS

1 POUND BROWN SUGAR

STOUT YEAST AND NUTRIENT

Put 4 pints of water into a pan and bring to a boil. Stir in the malt extract, black malt, oats, and hops. Cover and boil for 45 minutes. Strain into a brewing bin. Put the solids into a sieve over the bin and keep pouring boiling water over them until all the goodness is washed back into the brew before discarding them. Add the sugar and stir to dissolve. Top up to 2 gallons with cold water and cool to 20°C. Add the yeast and nutrient and stir well. Cover and keep in a warm place for 3 days, stirring and skimming off scum daily. Leave to continue fermenting (this should take about a week), then siphon off into demijohns. Leave in a cool place for 2 days. Siphon off into beer bottles, leaving 1½ inches head room, and add ¼ teaspoon brown sugar to each. Seal tightly and keep in a warm place for a week, then remove to a cooler place for storage. Ready to drink after 6 weeks.

Making Liqueurs

BASIC METHOD

Making a liqueur is very simple: fruit, flowers, or other flavouring ingredients are steeped in spirits such as rum, brandy, whiskey, gin, or vodka, sometimes with the addition of sugar, left for a period so the flavour can develop, then strained off and bottled.

. . . .

SLOE GIN

I always put sloes in the freezer for 24 hours, as this helps the cells break down and release their juice. You can use this recipe for other fruit gins such as strawberry, blackberry, blackcurrant, and so on, but halve the amount of sugar—sloes need a lot as they are very sour. In Ogham lore, blackthorn (from which sloe berries come) is "the increaser of secrets" and "the rune of the great wheel," demonstrating its importance. The berries are ripe around the time of Samhain and are used to make a potent drink for that festival, echoing the plant's paradoxical themes of strife, death, and fertility.

> 8 OUNCES SLOES
>
> 14 FLUID OUNCES GIN
>
> 4 OUNCES SUGAR

Remove the stalks and wash the fruit. Prick the sloes and put them into a screw-top jar (they should take up no more than half the space). Add the sugar and top up with gin. Put on the lid and shake to dissolve the sugar. Stand for 14 days, shaking daily, by which time the gin should have turned a rich red colour. Strain and bottle after 3 months. Leave to mature, preferably for 12 months, though it can be drunk after a few weeks.

. . . . .

BEECH LIQUEUR

YOUNG BEECH LEAVES

GIN OR VODKA

SUGAR

Fill a jar with young beech leaves. Top up with gin or vodka and leave for 10 days. Strain off the spirit and add a pound of sugar and ½ pint water per pint of spirit. Dissolve over a low heat (do not boil the alcohol off) and bottle.

MALLOW GIN

1 PINT GIN

4 OUNCES SUGAR

2 PINTS MALLOW LEAVES, BRUISED

Mix together the gin, sugar, and 1 pint mallow leaves in a glass jar and leave in a dark place for 2 weeks, shaking daily. Strain, wash the jar, and return the liquor to it with a freshly picked batch of leaves. Leave in a dark place for 2 weeks, shaking daily. Strain and bottle.

HOLLY LIQUEUR

Tradition has it that holly should be gathered for magical purposes on the winter solstice eve at midnight. The holly represents eternal life, as it survives the whole year round and fruits in the winter. This liquour would be a suitable drink for Yule, which celebrates the rebirth of the sun.

2 OUNCES FRESH HOLLY LEAVES

¼ PINT BRANDY

2 PINTS RED WINE

Macerate the leaves in the brandy for 24 hours. Add the wine and leave for another 24 hours. Strain and bottle.

Apricot Brandy

This recipe also works well with peaches, blackberries, Morello cherries, and blackcurrants. Use the same recipe for strawberry brandy, but add some lemon zest. You can also make it with pineapple, but add 2 ounces more sugar per pound of fruit.

RIPE APRICOTS

4 OUNCES SUGAR FOR EACH POUND OF APRICOTS

BRANDY

Halve the apricots and take out the stones. Pack them into a large glass jar and add the sugar and enough brandy to cover them completely. Cover tightly and leave for 4 months, shaking the jar occasionally. Strain into sterilised bottles.

Plum Vodka

1 PINT VODKA

1 POUND PLUMS, HALVED AND STONED

8 OUNCES WHITE SUGAR

Place the vodka, plums, and sugar in a large saucepan. Heat gently until the sugar has dissolved, but do not boil or you will evaporate all the alcohol. Allow to cool. Put in a large jar (or two) and store in a dark, cool place for 3 months. Strain into sterilised bottles.

Limoncello

8 UNWAXED LEMONS

1½ PINTS VODKA

1½ POUNDS WHITE SUGAR

Zest the lemons, taking care not to include any bitter white pith, and put all the zest in a large glass jar with the vodka. Leave for 7 days, shaking daily. Put the sugar in a heatproof bowl and pour 1½ pints of boiling water over it, stirring until the sugar has dissolved. Add the vodka and peels and leave for a further week, shaking the jar regularly. Strain into decorative sterilised bottles, adding a few strips of lemon peel to each bottle.

MINT LIQUEUR

1 PINT FRESH MINT LEAVES (WHICHEVER VARIETY YOU PREFER), SEPARATED FROM THE STEMS

1½ PINTS VODKA OR GIN

8 OUNCES WHITE SUGAR

1 TEASPOON GLYCERINE

Chop the mint leaves and pack into a glass jar. Cover them with the vodka and cover tightly. Leave in a cool place for 2 weeks, shaking occasionally. Strain and throw the leaves on the compost heap. Put the sugar and ½ pint of water in a saucepan and heat until the sugar dissolves. Remove from the heat and allow to cool completely. Combine with the minty vodka and add the glycerine. Leave for 2 months before bottling and 1 more month before drinking.

LEMON BALM LIQUEUR

You can also make this with lemon verbena, but use slightly fewer leaves.

½ PINT CHOPPED FRESH LEMON BALM (*MELISSA OFFICINALIS*) LEAVES

1½ PINTS VODKA

2 TEASPOONS FRESH LEMON ZEST

1 TEASPOON CRUSHED CLOVES

8 OUNCES WHITE SUGAR

Put the chopped leaves in a jar and top up with the vodka, lemon zest, and crushed cloves. Leave for 2 months, shaking occasionally. Strain into another jar and add the sugar. Leave for another 4 weeks before bottling.

Blackberry Whiskey

This recipe also works well with cherries.

BLACKBERRIES, LIGHTLY CRUSHED

2 CLOVES PER POUND OF BLACKBERRIES

1½ OUNCES SUGAR PER POUND OF BLACKBERRIES

CINNAMON STICK

WHISKEY

Put the lightly crushed blackberries into a large glass jar until it is half full. Add the cloves, sugar, and cinnamon, then fill up to the top with whiskey. Leave for 2 months. Strain into sterilised bottles.

Herby Honeyed Rum

This is good for coughs and sore throats too!

1 TEASPOON FRESH THYME LEAVES

1 TABLESPOON FRESH SAGE LEAVES

1 TABLESPOON FRESH MINT LEAVES

15 FLUID OUNCES DARK RUM

½ POUND HONEY

Chop the herbs and cover them with the rum in a clean glass jar. Cover tightly and leave 10 days. Strain, add the honey, and leave in a clean jar for another week or two before bottling.

Chilli Vodka

1 PINT VODKA

3 CHILLIES

Prick the chillies, put them in a bottle, and top up with the vodka. Leave to infuse for a week, then strain off the vodka into a sterilised bottle.

MARROW RUM

If you have ever grown courgettes/zucchini and forgotten to pick them, you will know that they become huge—they turn into marrows. Marrows are courges in French and zucchi in Italian, so courgettes and zucchini are both names for diminutive marrows, though in reality separate varieties are grown to produce courgettes and marrows. Once popular, the marrow has rather fallen out of favour, though some gardeners do still grow them. They have been dubbed a useless vegetable and—it has to be admitted—don't have much flavour, so they are generally stuffed or turned into jam, but an interesting alternative is to turn them into alcohol.

This is a very old-fashioned recipe, once made in farm labourer's cottages, and there are many variants on it. Some call for adding actual rum, while the poor man's version doesn't. Be warned, it gets messy and needs patience.

I've also made this by packing the marrow with brown sugar and pouring in a cup of dark rum. Once I made it with a mangel-wurzel, a type of root vegetable grown exclusively for feeding livestock!

Take a large marrow (or a seriously overgrown zucchini) with a firm rind, cut off the top, and carefully scoop out the seeds. Fill the cavity with dark brown sugar (a good-sized marrow will hold about 2 pounds). Replace the top. Using a skewer or knitting needle, make a hole in the bottom. Suspend it upright over a bowl. I do this by putting it into a nylon stocking and hanging it from a nail in an outbuilding. Fermenting brown liquid will drip out of the bottom into the bowl. Leave it dripping for two weeks to a month. As the sugar ferments, it eats up the marrow and drips alcoholic "rum" into the bowl. Put the resulting brown liquid into bottles, and leave to mature for six months before drinking.

This method depends on the natural yeasts in the marrow, and you may get better results by adding some yeast and a handful of raisins in with the brown sugar. Add a piece of ginger root, too, for improved flavour.

Cider Vinegar

Raw cider vinegar is full of enzymes, vitamins, probiotics, and minerals that pasteurised cider vinegars do not have, as they are destroyed by the heating process. All the healing benefits you have read about with cider vinegar are absent from processed products. Raw cider vinegar is best for all the recipes in this book, and if you have ever tried to buy it, you will know that it is very expensive compared to the heavily processed kind. Luckily, it is really easy to make.

1. Sterilise a large wide-necked jar.

2. Wash and chop your apples, including the cores and peel (you can make this recipe just using the cores and peel after making an apple pie), but remove the stalks. A mixture of different varieties makes a better-tasting cider vinegar, but don't worry if you can't manage this.

3. Put them in the jar, making sure it is half to three quarters filled.

4. Cover them with water that has been boiled and cooled to lukewarm.

5. Stir in a little sugar or honey to help the fermentation process start.

6. Cover the jar. When making wine we use an airlock to keep out the bacteria that will cause it to turn to vinegar, but when making vinegar we actually want to encourage them, so just cover the jar with cheesecloth secured by an elastic band.

7. Stir daily for a week. It will begin to bubble and ferment from the natural yeasts in the apples, and you will be able to smell this happening.

8. Strain out the apple pulp.

9. Return the liquid to the jar and cover again with cheesecloth. Leave in a warm, dark place for 4–6 weeks, stirring occasionally. The alcohol will transform into acetic acid, or vinegar. A small amount of sediment will fall to the bottom, and what is called a "mother culture" of dark foam will form on top; don't worry about this, it is normal.

10. Taste it to determine if it is ready starting after 4 weeks, as it will get stronger the longer you leave it, and you can choose how you like it.

11. Strain once more into clean glass jars or bottles. Store out of direct sunlight. Don't worry if another mother culture forms on top; it isn't going bad. Just strain again.

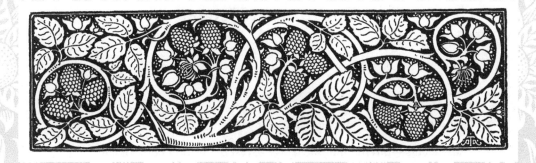

CHAPTER 4

Preserving

I f you are growing your own fruit and vegetables, you will know that you have a glut of produce in the late summer and early autumn but very little in the winter. Our ancestors overcame this by developing techniques for preserving food. Fruit and vegetables were bottled, dried, and salted or made into jams, chutneys, pickles, and jellies. Wonderful treats could then be produced at Yule or Twelfth Night, an otherwise dark and gloomy time with nothing fresh to eat.

Even if you don't have a garden, a hedgerow to forage, or even a window box, making your own preserves is fun and satisfying with cheap seasonal produce from shops and markets. Preserves make wonderful gifts too, especially if you tie a ribbon round the jar or cut out a round of pretty cloth or paper to cover the lid.

Equipment Needed

- Large pan

- Double boiler (for some recipes)

- Kitchen scales

- Sugar thermometer (useful, but not necessary)

- Clean saucers—put them in the fridge to test the setting point of jam if you have no sugar thermometer

- Wooden spoons

- Glass jars with lids (save all your old ones and wash them out)

- Waxed discs (available from supermarkets, kitchen shops, and online), which help prevent bacteria and microorganisms from entering the jar and spoiling the preserves

- Jelly bag (for making clear jellies)

- Nylon sieve

- Plastic funnel (for pouring the preserves into the jars)

TO STERILISE JARS

If you want your preserves to store, you will need to sterilise the jars and bottles you pour them into, even if the jars are new; otherwise you may introduce harmful bacteria into your produce. The traditional way to do this is in the oven, but if you are using the jars that come with rubber seals, these need to be removed first and sterilised separately.

1. Wash the jars using warm, soapy water and rinse thoroughly. Do not towel dry.

2. Put a sheet of baking parchment on the lowest shelf of your oven (never put the jars on the bottom of the oven itself) and load the jars onto the shelf, making sure they're not touching each other.

3. Now turn on the oven and heat to 140°C/210°F/gas mark 1 and dry out the jars for around 15–20 minutes.

4. Carefully remove them using oven gloves. Now they are ready to be filled with hot jam.

There is an alternative method if you have a dishwasher: just put the jars in and run the hottest programme. If your dishwasher has a steam option, this is even better. Lids and rubber seals can be put in boiling water to sterilise them.

SAFETY FIRST

When bottling jam or other preserves, the most important thing to remember is that if you pour hot food into a cold glass jar, it will shatter. If you pour cold food into a hot jar, it will shatter. Make sure your jar is roughly the same temperature as the food you are putting into it.

A NOTE ON MEASUREMENTS

The measurements in this chapter are in UK imperial measures. Check appendix 4 for metric and US measures.

Jams

Jams are the most popular preserves. To make the best jam, you need to pick the fruit when it is only just ripe and in perfect condition. Wash it and remove any stalks and cores. Some fruits have very little pectin, the enzyme responsible for making the jam set. This is easily remedied by adding a chopped apple or the soaked rind of a lemon to your recipe, both being rich in pectin.

THE BASIC METHOD

1. Place the prepared fruit in a pan along with a tiny amount of water if necessary.

2. Bring it to a boil and simmer until the fruit is soft.

3. Stir in the sugar until it dissolves.

4. The jam should then be heated to a rolling boil; this means it is boiling so hard it spits.

5. Continue boiling, stirring only occasionally, until the setting point is reached on a sugar thermometer. To test for set without a sugar thermometer, spoon a little jam onto a cold saucer. Leave a minute and tip the saucer. If the jam is set, it will stay put and not trickle away. Keep testing till you get to the setting point.

6. Remove the pan from the heat and allow it to stand for a few minutes.

7. Remove any scum that has formed on the surface, together with any fruit stones. A knob of butter added at this time will help to eliminate any scum that remains and add a shine to the jam, but this is optional.

8. Stir once and pour the jam into warmed, sterilised jars (warming is necessary, as cold jars are likely to shatter).

9. Cover the surface of the jam with a waxed disc and put the lid on firmly. If lids are not available, cellophane covers can be used and held in place with an elastic band.

NOTE: The only thing that can go wrong is missing the setting point—
if you overcook the jam, it will go dark and the flavour will be spoiled.
If you undercook the jam, it will be too runny and may even start
to ferment with keeping. Keep testing as it is cooking!

Blackberry and Apple Jam

4 POUNDS BLACKBERRIES

1½ POUNDS COOKING APPLES, PEELED AND CORED

½ PINT WATER

6 POUNDS SUGAR

Wash the blackberries and simmer with ½ cup of water. In a separate pan, simmer the apples with ½ cup of water. Mash the apples and combine with the blackberries, add the sugar, and boil until the setting point. Pour into clean, warmed jars and seal.

Rosehip and Apple Jam

2 POUNDS ROSEHIPS

2 POUNDS APPLES

1¾ POUNDS SUGAR

Wash the hips and simmer in 3 pints of water until pulpy. Mash and strain through a jelly bag to remove the irritant fibres; this is important! Peel and core the apples, chop them roughly, and place in a pan. Just cover with water and simmer until mushy. Remove from the heat and add the rosehip juice and sugar. Stir well to dissolve. Boil until the setting point is reached. Pour into clean, warmed jars and seal.

Damson Jam

5 POUNDS DAMSONS

6 POUNDS SUGAR

Wash the damsons and simmer in ½ pint of water for 30 minutes until reduced. Add the sugar and boil rapidly until the setting point, removing the stones as they rise to the surface. This jam will keep better if a few stones are left in. Pour into clean, warmed jars and seal.

. . . .

Pear Jam

3 POUNDS PEARS

RIND AND JUICE OF 1½ LEMONS

1¼ POUNDS SUGAR

Peel, core, and chop the pears; set aside the chopped pears. Boil the pear cores and peels and lemon rinds in ¼ pint of water for 10 minutes. Strain and add to the lemon juice and pear chunks. Simmer until tender. Add the sugar and boil until the setting point is reached. Pour into clean, warmed jars and seal.

. . . .

Grape Jam

1 POUND GRAPES

1 POUND SUGAR

Wash the grapes and put them in a pan with a tiny amount of water. Simmer gently for 5 minutes. Add the sugar, stirring until dissolved, and then boil fast until the setting point is reached. Pour into clean, warmed jars and seal.

. . . .

Marrow and Ginger Jam

4 POUNDS MARROW, PEELED AND SEEDED

4 POUNDS SUGAR

1 OUNCE GINGER ROOT

RIND AND JUICE OF 3 LEMONS

Cut the marrow into ½-inch cubes and weigh them. Place in a basin, sprinkle with about a quarter of the sugar, and stand overnight. Next day, bruise the ginger and tie in muslin with the lemon rind. Place in a pan with the marrow and lemon juice and simmer for 30 minutes. Add the remaining sugar and boil gently until transparent and the setting point is reached. Remove the muslin bag. Pour into clean, warmed jars and seal.

ROSE PETAL JAM

4 OUNCES ROSE PETALS

1½ POUNDS SUGAR

1 TABLESPOON LEMON JUICE

5 FLUID OUNCES ROSE WATER

5 FLUID OUNCES WATER

Put the rose petals in a heatproof bowl and set aside. Meanwhile, put the sugar, lemon juice, rose water, and water in a pan and bring to a boil. Reduce the heat and simmer 5 minutes, then pour over the rose petals. Stand overnight. Put the mixture into a pan and simmer gently for 30 minutes until it thickens.

STRAWBERRY JAM

2 POUNDS STRAWBERRIES

JUICE OF 1 LEMON

1½ POUNDS SUGAR

Remove the stalks from the strawberries and cut off any bruised parts. Put in a pan with the lemon juice and heat slowly until boiling. Add the sugar and stir continuously. Boil until setting point is reached.

PINEAPPLE JAM

Jam sugar has added pectin, used for fruits that contain little pectin of their own.

1 PINEAPPLE

10 OUNCES JAM SUGAR

JUICE OF 2 LIMES

Grate the flesh of the pineapple (you should have about 450 grams). Put into a pan with 8 fluid ounces of water and cook for about 30 minutes till soft. Add sugar and lime juice and cook until thick, about 45–60 minutes. Spoon into sterilised jars and keep in fridge.

Jellies

In jellies only the juice is used and the fruit pulp is discarded; jellies should be clear.

THE BASIC METHOD

1. Wash and roughly chop the fruit—there is no need to peel or core it.

2. Simmer it in a large pan (you may need to add a tiny amount of water if the fruit is not immediately juicy) until the juice is extracted.

3. Strain through a jelly bag suspended from a hook or beneath a chair into a large jug or bowl. This will take quite a while (you can leave it overnight) but do not squeeze the bag as this will force through fibres that will cloud the jelly.

4. Return the juice to the pan. For every pint of juice (20 fluid ounces), add 1 pound of sugar.

5. Bring to a boil and continue boiling until the setting point is reached (see #5 on page 122).

6. Remove the pan from the heat and allow it to stand for a few minutes. Remove any scum that has formed on the surface.

7. Pour the jelly into warmed, sterilised jars.

8. Cover the surface of the jelly with a waxed disc and put on a lid or cellophane cover, held in place with an elastic band.

NOTE: You can use the fruit pulp that you have collected
in the jelly bag to make a fruit butter (see page 134),
but do sieve it first and add a little water.

. . . .

MINT JELLY

2½ POUNDS COOKING APPLES

2 LEMONS

2 OUNCES MINT SPRIGS

2 OUNCES CHOPPED MINT LEAVES

2 POUNDS SUGAR

5 FLUID OUNCES WHITE WINE VINEGAR

Chop the apples—do not peel or core them—and put them in a pan with the lemons and mint sprigs. Cover with 2 pints of water and bring to a boil. Simmer 30–40 minutes until the apple has turned into a liquid pulp. Strain through a jelly bag overnight.

Measure the liquid, return it to the pan, and add 1 pound of sugar per pint of liquid. Add the vinegar and bring to a boil; continue boiling until the setting point is reached. Remove from the heat. Stir in the chopped mint leaves. Pour into warmed, sterilised jars.

. . . .

CRAB APPLE JELLY

Crab apple jelly turns a beautiful shade of pink. You can also make this with cultivated apples.

CRAB APPLES

SUGAR

Gather as many crab apples as you want, remove the stems, and chop the apples roughly. Stew them in their own juice until soft. Strain through muslin and collect the juice. Add one pound of sugar for every pint (20 fluid ounces) of juice, and boil together until the setting point is reached. Pour into warmed, sterilised jars.

. . . . .

ELDERBERRY JELLY

2 POUNDS ELDERBERRIES

2 POUNDS APPLES

SUGAR

Strip the elderberries from their stems with a fork. Wash and chop the apples and put the fruits in separate pans with enough water to cover until cooked. Combine the fruits and strain through a jelly bag. Measure the liquid, add one pound of sugar per pint, and stir to dissolve. Boil until setting point is reached. Pour into warmed, sterilised jars.

BASIL JELLY

Other herbs can be substituted for the basil. You can add a couple of the herb's leaves to each jar when the jelly has cooled.

15 FLUID OUNCES APPLE JUICE

2 TABLESPOONS LEMON JUICE

8 OUNCES SUGAR

12 SPRIGS BASIL

Put the apple and lemon juice in a pan. Add the sugar and stir until dissolved. Add the basil sprigs and boil till the setting point is reached. Strain into warmed, sterilised jars.

HAWTHORN BERRY JELLY

HAWTHORN BERRIES

A FEW CRAB APPLES

1 PIECE OF GINGER ROOT

SUGAR

Simmer the fruit and ginger in enough water to cover until cooked. Strain through a jelly bag and measure the liquid. Add one pound of sugar per pint of liquid and return to the pan. Boil until the setting point is reached, skimming off the scum as you go. Pour into warmed, sterilised jars.

Marmalades

. . . .

ORANGE MARMALADE

3 POUNDS SEVILLE ORANGES

6 POUNDS SUGAR

Peel the oranges and cut the rind into very fine strips. Remove the pips from the fruit pulp, put them into a bowl by themselves, and cover them with 1 pint of boiling water. Cut the pulp into small pieces. Put the rind and pulp into a large bowl and pour 5 pints of boiling water over them. Leave both bowls overnight. The next day there will be a filmy jelly on top of the pip bowl, which is what we want. Using a colander rather than a fine sieve, pour the pip juice and film through it into the pulp and rind. Discard the pips. Boil the rind, pulp, and water mixture until the rind is soft. Add the sugar, stir to dissolve, and boil until the setting point is reached. Bottle and seal.

. . . .

CARROT MARMALADE

JUICE AND PEEL OF 3 LEMONS

2 POUNDS CARROTS, PEELED AND FINELY CHOPPED

2 POUNDS SUGAR

Tie the lemon peel in a muslin bag and put in a bowl with the lemon juice and 1 pint of water and stand overnight. Put the liquid and the muslin bag in a pan with the carrots. Cook until the carrots are tender, then add the sugar, stirring until it dissolves. Remove the muslin bag and boil until the carrot marmalade reaches setting point.

Curds

Curds are sweet preserves with eggs added to create a creamy texture. Because of this, they need to be cooked in a double boiler. Most people only know lemon curd, but curd can be made with a wide variety of fruits. Homemade curds will keep in the fridge for about two weeks.

. . . .
APRICOT CURD

8 OUNCES APRICOTS

8 OUNCES CASTOR SUGAR

2 OUNCES BUTTER

JUICE AND ZEST OF 1 LEMON

2 EGGS, BEATEN

Slit the apricots and put in a pan with a tiny amount of water. Simmer gently until tender. Remove the stones. Liquidise the apricots and put in a double boiler with the sugar, butter, lemon zest and juice, and stir until dissolved. Add the eggs, whisking continually until the mixture thickens. Immediately pour into warm, sterilised jars and seal.

. . . .
BLACKBERRY CURD

12 OUNCES BLACKBERRIES

4 OUNCES APPLES

JUICE OF 1 LEMON

15 OUNCES BUTTER

1 POUND SUGAR

4 EGGS, BEATEN

Wash the fruit. Peel and core the apples and put them in a pan with the blackberries. Simmer gently till tender, then push through a sieve to get the juice or process in a blender before straining out the juice. Put into a double boiler and add the lemon juice, butter, and sugar; stir till dissolved. Add the beaten eggs and cook slowly until the mixture thickens. Pour into warm, sterilised glass jars and seal.

LEMON CURD

2 OUNCES BUTTER

4 OUNCES SUGAR

JUICE AND ZEST OF 1 LEMON

3 EGGS, BEATEN

Put the butter, sugar, and lemon juice and zest in a double boiler and cook slowly, stirring until the sugar dissolves completely. Remove from the heat and add the eggs a little at a time, stirring continuously. Return to the heat and keep stirring until thick. Bottle and seal.

Fruit Cheeses

All types of edible fruit are suitable for making fruit cheeses, which resemble an intensively flavoured cross between a jam and a jelly. They are great served with savoury foods. Fruit cheeses may be spiced with ginger, cinnamon, or nutmeg and should be poured into wide-necked jars or moulds so they can be turned out and sliced.

THE BASIC METHOD

1. Wash and chop the fruit; there is no need to peel or core them.

2. Put the fruit in a saucepan and just cover with water.

3. Simmer gently until soft.

4. Rub the fruit through a sieve to obtain the pulp.

5. Weigh the pulp.

6. Put the pulp in a fresh pan.

7. Add an equal weight of sugar and simmer gently for about an hour.

8. You can test whether it is ready by pulling a wooden spoon across the pan. It should leave a clear line.

9. The cheese can be poured into moulds or small wide-necked pots.

10. Seal well with a wax disc and keep the cheese in the fridge for two months before using to allow the flavour to develop. Once the seal has been removed, keep refrigerated and use within two weeks.

. . . .

DAMSON CHEESE

You can serve this as a dessert, studded with almonds and with port poured over it.

3 POUNDS DAMSONS OR OTHER SMALL, DARK PLUMS

12 OUNCES SUGAR TO 1 POUND PULP

Wash the damsons and remove the stems. Simmer in ¼–½ pint of water until very soft. Push through a sieve using a wooden spoon. Weigh the pulp and add the sugar. Boil gently until thick, stirring regularly. Brush straight-sided jars with glycerine and pour in the damson cheese—this is so that you can turn the cheese out as whole. Seal.

. . . . .

. . . .
BLACKBERRY CHEESE

1 POUND APPLES

2 POUNDS BLACKBERRIES

SUGAR

Chop the apples (no need to peel) and put them in a pan with the washed blackberries and ½ pint of water. Simmer till soft, then sieve off the excess liquid. Measure the pulp and return it to the pan with 1 pound of sugar per 1 pound of pulp, stirring till dissolved. Boil rapidly to set. Pour and seal.

. . . .
BLACKCURRANT CHEESE

BLACKCURRANTS

SUGAR

Weigh the fruit. Put it in a pan with ½ pint of water per 1 pound of fruit. Simmer gently till tender. Sieve or liquidise and weigh the pulp. Return to the pan with 12 ounces sugar per 1 pound of pulp. Stir till the sugar dissolves, stirring occasionally till the mixture thickens. Pour and seal.

. . . .
GOOSEBERRY CHEESE

GOOSEBERRIES

SUGAR

Top and tail the gooseberries. Put them in a pan with just enough water to cover. Simmer until tender and sieve or liquidise. Measure the pulp and return to the pan with 1 pound of sugar per pint of water, stirring until the sugar dissolves. Simmer over a low heat until the mixture becomes thick. Pour and seal.

. . . . .

Fruit Butters

These have a creamier consistency than the fruit cheeses but don't keep as long. They are delicious spread on hot desserts. Keep refrigerated and use within seven days.

APPLE BUTTER

APPLES

CIDER

CLOVES

ALLSPICE

CINNAMON

Peel, core, and chop the apples. Put everything but the stalks in a pan, cover with cider, and add spices to taste. Bring to a boil, mashing the fruit as you go. It will turn brown and buttery, and when it does, pour into warmed, sterilised jars and seal.

APRICOT BUTTER

2 POUNDS APRICOTS

1 LEMON

8 OUNCES SUGAR

CINNAMON

CLOVES

ALLSPICE

Peel the apricots and remove the stones. Put the apricots in a pan with a tiny amount of water and simmer till soft. Put them through a sieve or liquidise them. Measure the resulting pulp; for each pint, add the grated zest and juice of a lemon, 8 ounces sugar, and a pinch of the spices to taste. Cook gently until thick. Pour into warmed, sterilised jars and seal.

DAMSON BUTTER

DAMSONS

SUGAR

WATER

Wash the damsons and slit the sides of the fruits. Put them in a pan with a tiny amount of water and simmer till tender. Remove the stones (they will float to the top). Put through a sieve and measure the resulting puree. Add 1 pound sugar to each pint of puree, stirring until the sugar has dissolved. Cook over a low heat until the butter thickens to a stiff consistency. Pot and seal.

Fruit Syrups

THE BASIC METHOD

1. Use any ripe fruit in good condition. Wash the fruits carefully and remove any bad parts.

2. Mash the fruit in a bowl.

3. Put the bowl over a pan of simmering water until the juice begins to flow out.

4. Mash the fruit again.

5. Strain through a jelly bag overnight.

6. Measure the juice and add 12 ounces sugar to each pint of juice.

7. Stir until the sugar dissolves in the cold juice.

8. Strain again through a jelly bag and pour it into screw-topped bottles.

9. The bottles must then be sterilised. Screw on the lids of bottles to be sterilised, without tightening.

10. Place them on a trivet in the bottom of a large pan. Add warm water to cover the bottles up to the neck (the water must be higher than the top of the syrup inside the bottles) and gently heat the water so that it begins to simmer after about half an hour.

11. Continue simmering for 30 minutes.

12. Remove from the saucepan and tighten the lids.[29]

---

29 Plant foods with a low acidity (most vegetables) need sterilisation under high temperature (116–130°C), which requires a pressure canner, but this method is suitable for most fruits.

ELDERBERRY SYRUP

ELDERBERRIES

WHITE SUGAR

Strip the fruit from the stems; the easier way to do this is with a fork. Wash the fruit and remove any unripe berries. Mash the fruit in a bowl. Put the bowl over a pan of simmering water until the juice begins to flow out. Mash the fruit again and strain through a jelly bag overnight. Measure the juice and add 12 ounces sugar to each pint of juice. Stir until the sugar dissolves in the cold juice. Strain again through a jelly bag and pour it into screw-top bottles. Sterilise the bottles as per above instructions.

ROSEHIP SYRUP

2 POUNDS HIPS

1 POUND SUGAR

Pick red hips, mince them, and put them straight into boiling water, allowing 3 pints of water per 2 pounds hips. Boil, then remove from heat and stand 15 minutes. Strain through muslin (reserve the liquid) and return the hips to the pan. Add another 1½ pints of water, boil, stand 10 minutes, and strain. Reserve the liquid and combine it with the first batch and boil until reduced to 1½ pints. Add 1 pound sugar and stir until dissolved. Boil 5 minutes. Strain into bottles and seal immediately. Sterilise as described previously but boil for 5 minutes rather than 30 minutes (a longer boiling would destroy the vitamin C content in this instance).

Pickling

Although the most popular pickling vegetable in the UK is the onion, virtually any edible fruit or vegetable can be pickled. Utensils can be of any material with the exception of copper and brass, as vinegar reacts with these metals. The easiest method of pickling is to put your produce in vinegar with a blend of pickling spices, which may vary according to the fruit or vegetable being pickled.

THE BASIC METHOD

1. The vegetables should be soaked in brine (2 ounces salt per pint of water) overnight.

2. Rinse and pack into jars.

3. Put the spices and vinegar into a pan and heat it up a little (do not boil).

4. Remove from the heat and pour over the vegetables, making sure to cover them completely.

5. Screw the lid on tightly and leave to cool.

6. Store in a cool, dry place.

. . . .
BASIC SPICED VINEGAR

For a mild flavour, use ½ ounce each of cinnamon, cloves, mace, allspice, and white peppercorns to every 4 pints of malt or spirit vinegar.

. . . .
PICKLED CAULIFLOWER

SMALL CAULIFLOWER FLORETS

BRINE

SPICED VINEGAR

To make the brine, combine 8 ounces salt and 1 pint boiling water and stir until the salt is dissolved, then add 1 pint cold water. Allow to cool. Cover the florets with brine and stand for 24 hours. Drain and pack into jars. Cover with the spiced vinegar and put on the lids.

. . . .
PICKLED CUCUMBER

4 ONIONS, SLICED

3 LARGE CUCUMBERS CUT IN FINGERS 3-4 INCHES LONG

3 TABLESPOONS SALT

1 PINT WHITE OR MALT VINEGAR

6 OUNCES SUGAR

1 TEASPOON CELERY SEED

1 TEASPOON MUSTARD SEED

Put the onions and cucumbers in a bowl and sprinkle the salt over them. Stand for an hour. Rinse thoroughly. Heat the other ingredients and cook for 3 minutes until the sugar has dissolved. Pack the vegetables into jars, cover with hot vinegar, and screw the lids on tightly. Leave for 2 weeks before eating.

. . . .
PICKLED CARROTS

These are excellent with cheese.

2 POUNDS BABY CARROTS

1¼ PINTS DISTILLED VINEGAR

8 OUNCES SUGAR

3 LEVEL TEASPOONS PICKLING SPICE IN MUSLIN

Scrub the carrots, cover with cold water, and simmer for 10 minutes until parboiled. In another pan place the vinegar, 6 tablespoons water, sugar, and spices. Boil for 10 minutes and remove the spices. Add the carrots and boil for 4 minutes. Pack into hot jars and pour the vinegar over.

. . . .
PICKLED MUSHROOMS

1 POUND SMALL MUSHROOMS

2 BLADES OF MACE

½ TEASPOON WHITE PEPPER

1 TEASPOON SALT

1 TEASPOON GROUND GINGER

1 VERY SMALL ONION, CHOPPED

WHITE VINEGAR

Wash the mushrooms in salt water and drain well. Place them in a pan with the other ingredients and cover with vinegar. Cook until the mushrooms are tender and shrunken. Lift them out and pack into jars. Cover with the hot vinegar.

. . . .
PICKLED NASTURTIUM SEEDS

Pickled nasturtium seeds are peppery and yummy sprinkled over a green salad.

WHITE VINEGAR

A PINCH OF SALT

1 BAY LEAF

BLACK PEPPERCORNS

NASTURTIUM SEEDS (FRESH ONES FROM THE PLANT)

Put the vinegar in the pan with a pinch of salt, a bay leaf, and a scant few peppercorns. Boil, strain, and allow to cool. Wash the nasturtium seeds and spread on kitchen paper (paper towels) to dry thoroughly. Pack them into jars, cover with the cold spiced vinegar, and put the lids on. Leave for 3 months before using.

PICKLED ONIONS

I generally pickle all the tiny onions I've grown that are too small to be of any other use, but there are varieties of small onions especially for the purpose. I haven't given quantities, as you can do as many as you have or want, but you need to have enough to fill a jar at least.

SMALL ONIONS

BRINE

SPICED VINEGAR

Peel the onions and put them whole into a bowl. To make the brine, combine 8 ounces salt and 1 pint boiling water and stir until the salt is dissolved, then add 1 pint cold water. Allow to cool. Cover the onions in brine and leave 24 hours. Drain and rinse really well. Pack them into jars and cover with spiced vinegar (see page 138). Put the lids on. Leave for 2 months before using.

Chutneys

Chutneys are like savoury jams. They are made from fruit and vegetables chopped and cooked with spices, sugar, and vinegar, then served with savoury foods such as cheese and salads. The flavour improves with keeping; they can be shelf stored, unopened, for up to three years. Refrigerate once opened and eat within three months.

THE BASIC METHOD

1. The fruit and vegetables should be washed, peeled, cored, and finely chopped.

2. They are put into a pan with vinegar and gently cooked until soft.

3. More vinegar, sugar, and spices are added, and the whole is simmered for 1–2 hours uncovered to reduce until the chutney has thickened to the required consistency.

4. It is then bottled in the same way as the jam.

5. The flavour improves with keeping, and they can be shelf stored for up to three years.

SPICY APPLE AND TOMATO CHUTNEY

2 POUNDS APPLES, PEELED AND SLICED

2 POUNDS RIPE TOMATOES, SKINNED AND SLICED

¾ POUND ONIONS, CHOPPED

1 CLOVE GARLIC, CRUSHED

½ POUND RAISINS

¾ POUND DEMERARA SUGAR

½ OUNCE MUSTARD SEEDS IN MUSLIN

½ OUNCE CURRY POWDER

1 LEVEL TEASPOON CAYENNE PEPPER

1 OUNCE SALT

1½ PINTS MALT VINEGAR

Stew the apples in a little water. Add the other ingredients and bring to a boil. Reduce the heat and simmer until thick, with no free liquid. Cool, spoon into clean glass jars, and seal.

. . . .

Apricot Chutney

2 POUNDS COOKING APPLES

4 OUNCES DRIED APRICOTS OR 8 OUNCES FRESH

½ POUND ONIONS

8 OUNCES SULTANAS

8 OUNCES SOFT BROWN SUGAR

½ PINT VINEGAR

1 TEASPOON SALT

½ TEASPOON CAYENNE PEPPER

If using dried apricots, soak overnight in water before draining and chopping. Peel and slice the apples (and apricots if using fresh) and put all the fruit in a pan with the other ingredients. Bring to a boil and simmer for 30 minutes or until thickened. Pour into warm, sterilised glass jars and seal.

. . . .

Walnut and Apple Chutney

2 POUNDS APPLES

1 ORANGE

1 LEMON

2 OUNCES WALNUTS, CHOPPED

8 OUNCES SULTANAS

1 POUND SOFT BROWN SUGAR

15 FLUID OUNCES VINEGAR

2 CLOVES

Peel, core, and chop the apples. Grate the zest from the orange and lemon and reserve. Juice the orange and lemon. Put the apples and the citrus fruit zest and juice into a pan with all the other ingredients, bring to a boil, then simmer gently for an hour or until thickened. Pour into warm, sterilised glass jars and seal.

. . . . .

. . . .

CUCUMBER CHUTNEY

The spices are not removed from this chutney, so the longer it is kept, the stronger the flavour will become.

1 MEDIUM CUCUMBER

1 COOKING APPLE

4 SMALL ONIONS

½ PINT WHITE WINE VINEGAR

½ POUND RAISINS

½ TEASPOON WHITE MUSTARD SEEDS

1 TEASPOON MIXED PICKLING SPICES

1 POUND SUGAR

Chop the cucumber, apple, and onions, and place in a large saucepan with the vinegar, raisins, mustard seeds, and spices, reserving about an eighth of the cucumber. Boil until the cucumber is soft. Remove from the heat and liquidise. Return to the pan and stir in the sugar until it dissolves. Boil for 40 minutes. Add the remaining chopped cucumber and simmer for a further 20 minutes. Turn into warmed jars.

. . . .

PEPPER CHUTNEY

1 TEASPOON PEPPERCORNS

½ TEASPOON MUSTARD SEEDS

3 RED PEPPERS

3 GREEN PEPPERS

1 POUND TOMATOES, QUARTERED

12 OUNCES ONIONS, CHOPPED

1 POUND APPLES, PEELED, CHOPPED, AND CORED

8 OUNCES DEMERARA SUGAR

1 TEASPOON ALLSPICE

¾ PINT MALT VINEGAR

. . . . .

Tie the peppercorns and mustard seeds in a muslin bag. Chop the peppers finely. Combine all the ingredients in a pan, bring to a boil, and simmer for around 1½ hours until soft and pulpy. The mixture should reduce considerably by the end of cooking. Remove the spice bag and turn into clean, warm jars.

· · · · · · · · · · · · · · ·

GREEN TOMATO CHUTNEY

2 OUNCES GINGER ROOT

4 RED CHILLIES (HOT), SEEDS REMOVED, CHOPPED

1 TEASPOON PICKLING SPICE

4 POUNDS GREEN TOMATOES, CHOPPED

2 POUNDS COOKING APPLES, SLICED

1 POUND ONIONS, DICED

½ PINT VINEGAR

1 POUND BROWN OR DARK BROWN SUGAR

Bruise the ginger root, place it in a square of muslin with the red chillies and pickling spice, and tie round with string. Place in a large pan with the other ingredients except the sugar. Bring to a boil and simmer. Add the sugar, stirring until dissolved. Simmer until the mixture thickens (1–2 hours), tasting occasionally. When the required strength of flavour is obtained, remove the spice bag. Turn into clean, warmed jars and seal.

Ketchups and Sauces

Ketchups are made of the juice of one or two vegetables or fruits, the best known being tomato, but other vegetables can be used; mushrooms work well. Sauces are made in the same way but have more than two kinds of vegetable or fruit in them.

THE BASIC METHOD

1. Simmer the fruits or vegetables until soft.

2. Rub through a sieve to obtain a puree. Retain the puree.

3. For every pint of puree, add ½ pint vinegar, 2 ounces sugar, and whatever spices are called for in the recipe. (If you wish to retain the colour of the fruit or vegetable, then white vinegar should be used. Malt vinegar will give a brown colour.)

4. Return to the pan and simmer until it thickens.

5. Pour into warmed bottles, which must then be sterilised (see the previous instruction for fruit syrups on page 136) and sealed.

. . . .
MUSHROOM KETCHUP

4 POUNDS MUSHROOMS

4 OUNCES SALT

4 CLOVES GARLIC

2 PINTS WINE VINEGAR

½ TEASPOON GINGER

½ TEASPOON CLOVES

A PINCH OF PEPPER

4 TABLESPOONS BRANDY

Slice the mushrooms and layer in a bowl with the salt overnight. Wash thoroughly and put in a pan with the chopped garlic, vinegar, and spices. Simmer for 60 minutes. Strain through a jelly bag and add the brandy. Pour into bottles and sterilise.

· · · · · · · · · · · · ·
Red Tomato Ketchup

6 POUNDS RIPE TOMATOES, SLICED

8 OUNCES SUGAR

½ PINT DISTILLED VINEGAR

1 TABLESPOON TARRAGON VINEGAR

A PINCH OF CHILLI POWDER

1 TEASPOON PAPRIKA

2 TEASPOONS SALT

1 TEASPOON PICKLING SPICES IN MUSLIN BAG

Cook the tomatoes very gently until liquid. Reduce by boiling until the sauce thickens. Liquidise and return to the pan with the remaining ingredients. Boil until the desired consistency is reached (really thick!) and remove the spice bag. Pour into hot bottles and sterilise.

· · · · · · · · · · · · ·
Wellington Sauce

1 POUND GREEN TOMATOES

1 ONION

1 LEMON

2 POUNDS APPLES, PEELED AND CORED

½ OUNCE MIXED SPICE (SEE PAGE 26)

2 TEASPOONS SALT

6 OUNCES BROWN SUGAR

4 PINTS VINEGAR

1 TEASPOON SOY SAUCE

Chop the tomatoes, onion, and fruit. Place in a pan with the spice, salt, and sugar. Cover with vinegar and bring to the boil. Simmer for 3 hours. Sieve and add the soy sauce. Return to the heat and boil. Bottle and sterilise.

Spiced Apple Ketchup

1 TEASPOON MUSTARD SEEDS

2 CLOVES

2 POUNDS OF PEELED, CORED APPLES

1 ONION

1 CLOVE GARLIC

1 TEASPOON SALT

½ TEASPOON CURRY POWDER

½ TEASPOON CAYENNE PEPPER

½ TEASPOON TURMERIC

2 FLUID OUNCES MALT VINEGAR

4 OUNCES SUGAR

Put the mustard seeds and cloves into a muslin bag. Put the apples, onion, garlic, spices, and vinegar into a pan, add the muslin bag with the cloves and mustard seeds, and cook until the apples turn into a thick pulp. Remove the muslin bag and sieve or liquidise the pulp. Return the pulp to the pan, add the sugar, and boil for 10 minutes. Pour into warm, sterilised bottles and seal.

Drying

Drying is the oldest method of preserving food and has been used throughout the world for thousands of years. In hot countries foods such as the wonderful sun-dried tomatoes are still dried by leaving them in an airy place.

OVEN DRYING

To preserve food in this way, spread your fruit in a single layer over a cooling rack which has been covered with muslin. Place it in the oven with the door open (this applies to all oven drying) at 110°C/225°F/gas mark ¼. Leave it until the juices have evaporated. Remove the tray from the oven and cover it with a cloth. Leave the fruit to cool for 12 hours and pack it in a box lined with greaseproof paper. This method is suitable for apricots, peaches, plums, apples, grapes, and pears. Preserved in this way, fruit will keep for several months. You can eat the dried fruits as they are or rehydrate them for pies and such by soaking them in water for a few hours.

AIR DRYING

Several fruits and vegetables air dry successfully. To dry apple rings, core good, unblemished apples and cut the apple into rings ⅛-inch thick. Put them into a bowl containing a solution of salt (1½ ounces salt to 6 pints water) and steep for 10 minutes. Thread them onto a bamboo cane over a heat source such as a wood burning stove, AGA cooker, or in an airing cupboard (watch out for drips). They will dry in 2–3 days and feel slightly leathery. Take down and store in an airtight container. To dry chillies, thread them on a cord using a needle, hang in a warm place to dry, then take down and store in an airtight container.

DEHYDRATORS

I was recently given an electric dehydrator that has stackable shelves and a fan that moves warm air though it to dry out food. Some people rave about them for making fruit leathers and drying out other produce. To be honest, I've had mixed results with it. It takes more work than usual preparing food to put in it, the shelves have to be rotated regularly, and it takes a long time to dry things out, much longer than in a low oven and nearly as long as air drying in some cases. I have used it for some herbs and apples with good results.

ONION OR APPLE RINGS

Onions and cored apples can also be dried as rings. Cut them into slices (dip the apple slices in salted water to prevent browning), thread them onto short canes, and hang the canes in the open oven at 130°C/250°F/gas mark ½. Leave them to dry out thoroughly (about 4 hours).

DRIED MUSHROOMS

Mushrooms should be washed, de-stalked (the stalks can be used in soups and stews), threaded onto a string with a knot between each, and hung up somewhere warm and dry, such as in an airing cupboard, for a couple of days to dry out. They can then be packed into jars.

DRYING HERBS

Any fresh herbs can be dried. They should be picked and tied in small bunches. Hang them in the kitchen or a well-ventilated shed to dry. Once dried out they should be crumbled into jars and stored in a dark place.

Fruit Leathers

Fruit leathers are delicious and healthy snacks made from pureed fruit that is then spread out and dried. You can use a single fruit or a mixture of any fruits you have (they are a good way of using up very ripe fruit) and add spices to taste. You can even use the pulp from your juicer.

THE BASIC METHOD

1. Wash the fruit and remove any damaged parts.

2. Chop large fruit such as apples and bananas; smaller fruit such as raspberries, blackcurrants, etc., can be left whole.

3. Put in a pan and add a little water (generally 1 tablespoon water to 2 cups fruit).

4. You can add spices such as cinnamon, ginger. etc.

5. Simmer until the fruit is soft.

6. Put through a sieve to remove any pips or seeds.

7. Return to the pan; here you can add some sugar or honey to taste, which will help the keeping properties. Stir over a low heat until dissolved.

8. Turn out onto a baking tray lined with greaseproof paper. Your fruit leather should not be more than a third of an inch (1 cm) thick.

9. Dry thoroughly in a dehydrator or a very, very low oven (as low as it will go) for 6–8 hours or until they no longer feel sticky.

10. Store in the fridge for up to 6 months.

. . . .

STRAWBERRY AND BANANA FRUIT LEATHER

Wash, dry, and cut up your strawberries and bananas. Liquidise until completely smooth. Spread out onto the prepared baking tray (see above). Bake for 6–8 hours or until the fruit is set but still slightly tacky. Cool and cut into pieces.

Bottling

Bottling preserves the colour and flavour of fruits. The best jars for the purpose are the ones with screw lids and rubber seals. Most fruits are suitable for bottling, with the exception of figs. Tomatoes (which are a fruit, not a vegetable) can be bottled.

Thoroughly clean and sterilise your bottles in boiling water for 10 minutes before use. They must be hot when you add the fruit. During heating, air is forced from the jars to create a germ-proof vacuum. Any flaws in the rubber or faults in a metal lid will destroy this vacuum and spoil the contents of the jar.

Fruit can be bottled in syrup, water, or brine solution, but it is most commonly bottled in syrup to preserve the colour and flavour.

THE BASIC METHOD

1. Make a syrup from 1 pound sugar to each pint of water.

2. Bring the syrup to boil and add another pint of water.

3. Pack the fruit into scalded jars and pour the syrup over. Do not fill the jars to the top, as you must allow space for expansion.

4. Screw on the lids firmly, then loosen by half a turn to allow any expanding air to escape when the jars are being sterilised.

5. Place them on a towel in the bottom of a large saucepan, which should have sides taller than the bottles. Place cotton kitchen towels between the bottles to prevent them touching.

6. Add warm water to cover the jars and gently heat it so that it begins to simmer after about half an hour.

7. Continue simmering for a time according to the following table.

8. Remove the bottles from the pan and tighten the lids.

9. As the jars cool, carefully tighten the lids two or three times more to be sure of a good seal.

SIMMERING TIMES	
SLICED APPLES	2 MINUTES
BLACKBERRIES	2 MINUTES
CURRANTS	2 MINUTES
GOOSEBERRIES	2 MINUTES
RASPBERRIES	2 MINUTES
STRAWBERRIES	2 MINUTES
DAMSONS	10 MINUTES
PLUMS	10 MINUTES
PEACHES	10 MINUTES
APRICOTS	10 MINUTES
WHOLE PEARS	40 MINUTES

· · · · · · · · · · · · ·

BOTTLED GOOSEBERRIES

2 POUNDS GOOSEBERRIES

1 POUND SUGAR

1 VANILLA POD, SPLIT

Wash, top, and tail the gooseberries. Put the sugar, split vanilla pod, and pint of water into a pan. Stir over low heat until the sugar has dissolved. Boil for a minute, remove the vanilla pod, and add a pint of water. Put the fruit into hot jars, pour on the syrup, and proceed as in the basic method.

Bottled Fruits in Alcohol

Fruits can also be bottled in spirits such as rum, brandy, or whiskey. It's an easy process. Just fill a jar with fruit, cover it in the alcohol of your choice and some spices if you wish, add a couple spoonfuls of sugar (sour fruits need more), and pop on the lid. Shake it every now and then over the course of the next month or two. You can use the now-boozy fruit in muffins, trifles, and cakes, and, naturally, you can drink the fruity alcohol!

PLUMS IN BRANDY

PLUMS, STONED AND SLICED

BRANDY

SUGAR

CINNAMON STICKS

Put everything in a jar and leave for a month.

BRANDIED APRICOTS

16 OUNCES DRIED APRICOTS

8 OUNCES SUGAR

¼ PINT BRANDY

Soak the fruit in cold water overnight. Place the fruit and water in a pan and bring to a boil. Cover and simmer for 15 minutes. Strain the liquid into a measuring jug and return the fruit with ¼ pint of liquid to the pan. Stir in half the sugar and bring to a boil. Simmer without stirring for a couple of minutes. Using a slotted spoon, remove the fruit and pack it into jars. Add the remaining sugar to the pan and stir until dissolved. Boil for 4 minutes and remove it from the heat. Cool the syrup, measure it, and add an equal amount of brandy. Pour the mixture into the jars, covering the fruit. Seal.

Salting

Salting is another very old method of keeping food. To cook salted vegetables, place them in a colander, rinse them in cold water, then put them in a bowl of cold water for two hours to draw out the salt. Do not leave them any longer as they will then begin to reabsorb the salt. Give them a final rinse before cooking.

THE BASIC METHOD

1. Vegetables are dry salted in cooking or coarse salt, rather than refined table salt.

2. The vegetables should be washed, sliced, and packed into sterilised earthenware, enamel, or glass jars in alternate layers with the salt, which then dissolves with the juices of the vegetables to form a brine.

3. The top of the jar should be securely tied with greaseproof paper.

Nuts can also be salted in the same way. Never use a metal container or metal spoons for salting, as metal reacts with the salt.

. . . .
SALTED GREEN BEANS

GREEN BEANS

COARSE SALT

Top and tail the beans and slice them. Pack them into a container, layering them with the salt up to the rim and finishing with a layer of salt. Cover with a weighted lid. After 7 days, check the container; you will probably be able to add another layer of beans and salt as the contents pack down. Rinse well before using.

Dry Sugar Preserving

THE BASIC METHOD

Sugar can be used to preserve fruit in the same way that salt is used to preserve vegetables, though rinsing the fruit before eating is obviously not so necessary. Fruit preserved this way will keep for at least six months.

1. Just wash, slice, and pack fruit into earthenware, enamel, or glass jars in alternate layers with the sugar, which then dissolves with the juices of the fruit to form a syrup.

2. The top of the jar should be securely tied with greaseproof paper.

SUGARED APPLES

Peel, core, and slice your apples. Layer them alternately with sugar, finishing with a layer of sugar.

SUGARED BLACKBERRIES

Wash and pick over the berries, removing any stems or bad fruit. Allow them to drain before packing them into a jar, layering alternately with sugar. Finish with a layer of sugar.

Conserves

The making of conserves, another method of sugar preserving, is used for flowers.

THE BASIC METHOD

1. Grind 1 pound flowers or flower petals into 2½ pounds sugar.

2. The conserve should be pressed into clean, dry jars and sealed well.

. . . .
COSTMARY CONSERVE

1 POUND COSTMARY PETALS

2½ POUNDS SUGAR

On a dry day pick the costmary flowers. Remove and weigh the petals. Place them in a large mortar and pound in 2½ pounds sugar for every 1 pound of petals. Press them into pots and seal.

. . . .
NETTLE FLOWER CONSERVE

1 POUND DEAD NETTLE (*LAMIUM* SPP.) FLOWERS

2½ POUNDS SUGAR

Put the flowers into a mortar and beat in the sugar. Pot in jars and seal well.

. . . .
LAVENDER SUGAR

10 LAVENDER FLOWER HEADS

5 OUNCES (¾ CUP/150 GRAMS) CASTER (SUPERFINE) SUGAR

Put the flower heads and sugar in a jar, put on the lid, and leave for 3 days. Remove the flowers. The sugar will be infused with a subtle lavender flavour (and when using lavender in cooking, the key is subtlety!), which can then be used to make cakes and cookies.

Freezing

DRY FREEZING FRUIT

Strawberries, raspberries, loganberries, blackberries and other soft berries can be dry frozen by spreading them on trays, which are then put in the freezer until the fruit is firm. To dry freeze apples, blanch them first to prevent browning by cooking them briefly in boiling water. The fruit can then be packed into plastic tubs or bags and stored in the freezer, where it will keep for six to nine months.

SUGAR FREEZING FRUIT

Soft berry fruits can also be frozen in containers layered with sugar, and this is called sugar freezing. Sugar freezing is also suitable for apples, and in this case the apples do not need blanching.

Fruits without much natural juice—such as figs, melons, peaches, and plums—should be frozen in syrup. To make a syrup, dissolve 1 pound sugar in 2 pints water for every 3 pounds fruit and allow it to cool. Put the fruit into containers and cover with the syrup. Seal and freeze.

FREEZING VEGETABLES

Vegetables for freezing should be of good quality and frozen as soon as possible after picking. To prevent loss of colour and flavour they must be blanched, or cooked briefly in boiling water. They should then be rinsed in running water to cool them, drained, and packed in containers or polythene bags.

FREEZING HERBS

Herbs can be frozen by simply putting the sprigs in polythene bags and placing them in the freezer. They can also be put into ice cube trays, topped up with water, and frozen, and then when you want to make a soup or stew, just drop one in.

Fruit and Herb Vinegars

FRUIT VINEGARS

Cover a pound of soft fruit (blackberries, raspberries, blackcurrants, gooseberries, etc.) with 1 pint white wine vinegar and stand 4–5 days. Strain and put the liquid into a pan with ½ pound sugar per pint of liquid. Boil 10 minutes, bottle, and seal. There is no need to keep this in the fridge, and it will last about a year.

HERB VINEGARS

Crush the herbs (you can use basil, marjoram, mint, sage, tarragon, thyme, lavender flowers, etc.) in a pestle and mortar or with a rolling pin, pack them into a jar to half full, and then fill the jar with cold white wine or malt vinegar. Store for 6 weeks, shaking now and then. Strain and rebottle the resulting liquid.

. . . .

BLACKBERRY VINEGAR

The same method can be used to make elderberry vinegar. Many people find this very good for coughs—drink a tablespoon of blackberry or elderberry vinegar in hot water with a little honey.

2 POUNDS BLACKBERRIES

2 PINTS MALT VINEGAR

Place the washed blackberries in a bowl and break them up slightly with a wooden spoon. Pour on the malt vinegar. Cover with a cloth and stand for 3–4 days, stirring occasionally. Boil for 10 minutes, cool, strain, and bottle the resulting liquid. Quantities can easily be increased, allowing 1 pound blackberries to 1 pint vinegar.

. . . .

RASPBERRY VINEGAR

1 PINT RED WINE VINEGAR

1 PINT WATER

1 TEASPOON SUGAR

1 POUND RASPBERRIES

Place all the ingredients in a pan and bring slowly up to a simmering point. Cook for 10 minutes, strain, and bottle the liquid.

. . . . .

Nonalcoholic Cordials

Cordials are a good way to use up surplus ripe fruit and make a refreshing drink that is redolent of summer. You can use all kinds of soft fruits and apples, as well as some flowers. Some fruits, such as raspberries, are good on their own, while fruits that are lower in acid, such as blackberries, can be blended with tarter fruits like elderberries.

Cordials don't store for very long and once opened must be kept in the fridge and used within a week. To use your cordial, dilute to taste with iced water, sparkling water, or white wine. You can also add a dash of lemon juice, a sprig of mint, or a few fresh fruits.

THE BASIC METHOD

1. Wash the fruit and remove any bad parts.

2. Put it in a large pan. Add ¼ pint of water per 1 pound of fruit.

3. Bring to a boil and simmer gently until the fruit is reduced to a liquid pulp. This can take 30 minutes or more.

4. Strain through a jelly bag overnight. Never squeeze the bag.

5. Measure the liquid and return to the pan.

6. Add 6–10 ounces sugar (or 7 ounces honey) per pint of liquid.

7. Heat gently to dissolve the sugar and then simmer for a few minutes to thicken the cordial, but do not boil for more than 5 minutes or it will turn into jelly.

8. Adding a couple of teaspoons of citric acid (available online) at this stage will increase the shelf life.

9. Remove from the heat and let it stand for a few minutes.

10. Pour the cordial into warm, sterilised glass bottles. See the "To Sterilise Jars" section on page 120.

· · · · · · · · · · · · · · · · · ·

BLACKCURRANT CORDIAL

Pick the blackcurrants when they are very ripe and strip off the stalks. Simmer the blackcurrants in a tiny amount of water gently for 30–45 minutes until they are reduced to a pulp. Strain through a jelly bag overnight and measure the liquid. For each pint (20 fluid ounces), add 8 ounces sugar. Heat gently to dissolve the sugar but do not boil. Cool a little and pour into warm, sterilised bottles.

· · · · · · · · · · · · · · · · · ·

RHUBARB AND GINGER CORDIAL

2 POUNDS RHUBARB

JUICE OF 2 LEMONS

ZEST AND JUICE OF 1 ORANGE

2 INCHES OF GINGER ROOT, PEELED AND CHOPPED

2½ POUNDS GRANULATED SUGAR

2 TEASPOONS CITRIC ACID (OPTIONAL)

Peel and chop the rhubarb. Put it in a pan with 2 pints of water. Add the lemon juice and zest and the orange juice and the ginger. Bring to a boil, then turn down the heat and simmer until the rhubarb is mushy. Remove from the heat and strain through a jelly bag overnight. Return the juice to the pan and add the sugar. Stir over a low heat until it has dissolved. Add the citric acid if desired. Cool a little and pour into sterilised bottles. Keep in the fridge and use within a week.

· · · · ·

ELDERFLOWER CORDIAL

4 POUNDS SUGAR

ZEST AND JUICE OF 2 LEMONS

50 ELDERFLOWER HEADS

2 OUNCES CITRIC ACID

Put the sugar into a plastic brewing bin or large bowl and pour on 2½ pints of boiling water. Stir to dissolve and add the lemon zest and juice, elderflower heads, and citric acid. Leave overnight. Strain through muslin into warm, sterilised bottles. This does not store well and is best kept in the fridge.

APPLE AND BLACKBERRY CORDIAL

2 POUNDS APPLES

1 POUND BLACKBERRIES

JUICE OF 1 LEMON

SUGAR

Wash the apples, cut out any bad bits, and chop them roughly; there is no need to peel or core them. Wash the blackberries and add them to the apples in a large pan. Add enough water to cover the fruit halfway up. Bring to a boil, then turn down the heat and simmer until the fruit is a liquid pulp. Remove from the heat and add the lemon juice. Strain overnight through a jelly bag. Measure the liquid and return it to the pan. Add 12 ounces sugar for each pint of juice. Stir over a low heat until the sugar has dissolved, then boil for 5 minutes. Pour into warm, sterilised bottles.

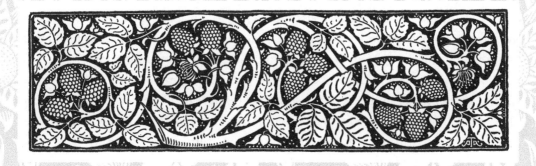

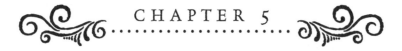

CHAPTER 5

The Witch's Home

Any self-respecting (and earth-respecting) Pagan avoids actions that harm the environment. When you shop, consider the following in relationship to any purchase:

- Does it endanger your health or the health of others?

- Does it damage the environment during its manufacture, use, or disposal?

- Does it have wasteful or nonrecyclable packaging?

- Does it use materials from threatened environments or species?

- Does it involve animal testing?

Look in the cupboard under your sink. I bet it is full of the many and varied cleaning products you use to fight dirt, kill germs, and mask odours to keep your home sparkling clean and protect your family. The big trouble is, those products are full of hazardous chemicals. Look at the labels—do they say *hazardous to humans and domestic animals, danger, warning, poison, vapours harmful,* or *may cause burns on contact*? They might take away dirt and kill bacteria, but they leave behind health-damaging substances.

The average household contains about sixty-two toxic chemicals that are likely to be inhaled as they linger in the air, ingested via the residues on dishes and absorbed by the skin (which, unlike the digestive system, has no safeguards against toxins). Various ingredients can cause asthma, headaches, chronic fatigue, stuffy noses, coughing, itchy eyes, and other mysterious health conditions that your GP might be at a loss to explain. We can tolerate these chemicals in low doses with occasional exposure, but when we are in contact with them in our soaps, detergents, air fresheners, "antibacterials," and cleaning products day after day, week after week, over the course of a lifetime, they can gradually build up in the tissues of our bodies, and many now believe some are linked to heart and lung problems, hormone disruption, liver and kidney damage, low sperm count, and various cancers. There is often no legal requirement for damaging chemicals to be listed on a product label. One-third of the substances used in the fragrance industry are toxic, but they are just listed on the label as "fragrance."

You might think that you are doing the right thing and protecting your family by using products labelled "antibacterial," but there is growing concern that such aggressive antibacterial agents actually promote the growth of drug-resistant bacteria, and that's how microbes develop resistance, not just to these household antibacterials but also to the medicinal antibiotics that we need.

When we wash our cleaning products down the drain, they are treated along with sewage and waste water, and then discharged into nearby waterways. Some break down into harmless substances but others do not, threatening water quality or fish and other wildlife.

The plastic bottles used to package cleaning products pose another environmental problem by contributing to the mounds of solid waste that must be landfilled, incinerated or, in not enough cases, recycled.

Be wary of ecological claims on commercial products. "Natural" or "biodegradable" doesn't actually mean anything; most substances will eventually break down if given enough time and the right ecological conditions.

Natural Alternatives

The good news is that proprietary chemicals are not necessary to keep your home spotlessly clean. Below are some natural recipes that you might like to try. If not, remember that you can obtain more ecologically friendly household products from health food stores and most supermarkets.

CASTILE SOAP is pure vegetable soap made from olive oil. It can be purchased in liquid form and in flakes, powders, or bars. It is biodegradable and may be used to wash dishes, in the laundry, or even to make your own shampoo and shower gels.

BAKING SODA AKA BICARBONATE OF SODA cleans, deodorizes, softens water, and scours. It is a nontoxic cleaner that is safe on most surfaces and fabrics. It has numerous household uses, but it should be used fresh—replace old boxes frequently. Baking soda will clean many surfaces without scratching: mix to a paste with water and use to scrub grills, hobs, fridges, deep fat fryers, irons, plastic buckets, bowls and sinks, barbecues, stained tea and coffee cups, etc.

BORAX (SODIUM BORATE) is a naturally occurring mineral that is antibacterial, deodorising, inhibits the growth of mould and mildew, removes grease, is a disinfectant, and can be used as a laundry booster. It is not harmful to the environment but it should not be ingested, and it is best to wear rubber gloves when using it and avoid inhaling the fumes.

WASHING SODA (SODIUM CARBONATE OR SODA ASH) is made from common salt and limestone or found as natural mineral deposits. It contains no phosphates, enzymes, or bleaches. Washing soda cuts grease, removes stains, softens water (use as a pre-soak for laundry), and cleans walls, tiles, sinks, and bathtubs. A strong solution will clear a blocked drain. Unlike baking soda, the slightly stronger washing soda can't be ingested; wear rubber gloves when handling it. Do not use on aluminium.

LEMON is one of the strongest food acids and is effective against most household bacteria. The acid in lemon juice removes dirt and rust stains. It can be used to sanitise cooking surfaces and chopping boards. Lemon breaks down limescale and can be used as a mild bleach in the laundry.

WHITE VINEGAR cuts through grease and removes mildew, odours, and some stains and wax buildup. It inhibits the growth of mould, mildew, and some bacteria, such as E. coli and salmonella. In a 5 percent solution it can kill 99 percent of bacteria,

82 percent of mould, and 80 percent of viruses. It is also completely safe, unlike commercial antibacterial sprays, which are toxic in large doses. Make a stronger solution to clean limescale from taps and appliances or to clean windows effectively without smearing. Use in the kitchen and bathroom to eliminate mould and as a natural fabric softener that removes soap residue in the rinse cycle and helps to prevent static cling in the dryer. (Don't be tempted to use the brown malt vinegar, which will stain and also smells much stronger.)

CORN STARCH AKA CORNFLOUR can be used to clean windows, polish furniture, or shampoo carpets and rugs.

OLIVE OIL dislodges dirt, diminishes scratches and imperfections, and nourishes wood, as well as shines stainless steel.

SALT makes a good scouring agent, especially when combined with borax. Combine with baking soda and white vinegar to unblock drains. Table salt, sea salt, and coarse salt can all be used, but cooking salt is the cheapest option.

ESSENTIAL OILS such as tea tree, lavender, eucalyptus, or lemongrass are antibacterial, antifungal, and antiseptic. Natural oils made from fruit, flowers, and barks are a much better scenting option than the nasty chemicals that comprise synthetic petroleum-based fragrances in most commercial products.

NOTE: Do not ingest essential oils, and do not
apply them undiluted to the skin.

Polishes

Many commercial brands contain nerve-damaging petroleum distillates, and some formulations may contain formaldehyde, a suspected carcinogen. Aerosol spray furniture polishes are easily inhaled into lung tissue.

DRY DUST

Do you really need to use a polish every time, when all you want to do is remove the dust? Microfiber cloths are brilliant little helpers that lift off dirt and dust without the need for chemicals of any kind. They can be washed and reused over and over again.

LEMON FURNITURE POLISH

12 DROPS LEMON ESSENTIAL OIL

3 TABLESPOONS LEMON JUICE

A FEW DROPS OF OLIVE OIL

Dip a soft duster in the mixture and wipe over wooden furniture.

BEESWAX WOOD POLISH

½ PINT REAL TURPENTINE

3 OUNCES BEESWAX

1 OUNCE PURE SOAP FLAKES

10 DROPS LEMON OIL

In a double boiler heat the turpentine and flaked wax until dissolved. Boil ¼ pint of water, add the soap, and allow to dissolve and cool a little. Pour into the wax and stir continuously as it cools and emulsifies. Add the lemon oil and pour into jars. Substitute lavender or another essential oil if you wish.

NUT POLISH

A fresh nut is oily enough to polish furniture beautifully. Cut it in half and rub over the surface. Walnuts work particularly well—a single walnut is enough to polish a coffee table—but you can use hazels, almonds, chestnuts, and beech nuts.

HERB POLISH

As well as nuts, some herbs are oily enough to impart a polish to wooden furniture. Try the leaves of the mock orange (*Philadelphus coronarius*) and just follow up with a clean duster afterwards. The Elizabethans used handfuls of lemon balm (*Melissa officinalis*).

SHOE POLISH

Olive oil with a few drops of lemon juice can be applied to leather shoes with a thick cotton or terry rag. Leave for a few minutes, then wipe and buff with a clean, dry rag.

Bathroom Products

Corrosive ingredients in toilet bowl cleaners are severe eye, skin, and respiratory irritants. Some toilet bowl cleaners contain sulphates, which may trigger asthma attacks. Bathroom cleaners containing sodium hydroxide, sodium hypochlorite (bleach), or phosphoric acid can irritate lungs and burn eyes, skin, and, if ingested, internal organs. Mixing acid-containing toilet bowl cleaners with cleaners that contain chlorine will form lung-damaging chlorine gas. Your safest best is to avoid both ingredients.

TOILET CLEANER

Make a paste of borax and white vinegar and spread it on the toilet bowl. Leave it for a couple of hours, then scrub with a brush.

ANTIBACTERIAL SPRAY

1 PINT WATER

10 DROPS LAVENDER ESSENTIAL OIL

10 DROPS TEA TREE ESSENTIAL OIL

Pour the water into a spray bottle. Add the essential oils and shake. Use on surfaces to kill bacteria—just spray on and wipe over. It will also break down mould and mildew.

SCOURING POWDER

1 OUNCE BAKING SODA

1 OUNCE BORAX

1 OUNCE SALT

Mix together and keep in an airtight container. Use as you would any commercial scouring powder.

BATH CLEANER (ENAMEL AND PORCELAIN)

1 LEMON

COARSE SALT

Halve the lemon. Wet your bathtub and sprinkle the salt around it. Scrub the lemon halves around the bath, making sure that you pick up plenty of the salt with them. Rinse well. You could also use limes or grapefruits, but lemon does seem to work better. If the bath is heavily stained, substitute borax for the salt, but make sure that you wear rubber gloves.

TO REMOVE LIMESCALE ON TAPS

Rub lemon juice onto the taps and leave overnight, then wipe off on a damp cloth. Alternatively, wrap the taps in a cloth soaked in white vinegar and leave overnight.

GROUT CLEANER

Make a paste of fresh lemon juice and cream of tartar. Apply with a toothbrush, scrub, and rinse.

Kitchen Products

. . . .
GENERAL CLEANER

½ PINT WATER

2 TEASPOONS CASTILE SOAP

20 DROPS LEMON ESSENTIAL OIL

Pour ingredients into a spray bottle preferably made of glass. Shake well before use. Store in a cool, dark place.

. . . .
SAINT CLEMENT'S VINEGAR

ORANGE PEEL

LEMON PEEL

WHITE VINEGAR

Take a glass jar and add your fresh orange and lemon peel (just save the peel whenever you use one). Cover with white vinegar and leave to infuse on a sunny windowsill for 2 weeks. Strain into a spray bottle and use to clean and disinfect your kitchen counters, handles, cutting boards, etc.

. . . .
DISHWASHER "DETERGENT"

12 TABLESPOONS BAKING SODA

12 TABLESPOONS BORAX

4 TABLESPOONS COARSE SALT

½ TEASPOON CITRIC ACID (FOOD GRADE)

Combine and store in an airtight container. Use as normal in your dishwasher.

. . . .
SINK CLEANER

Using a paste of baking soda and water, scrub with a sponge to remove stains. If the stains are really tough, sprinkle the baking soda over the sink and spritz white vinegar on it. As it fizzes, scrub with a sponge and then rinse well with hot water.

. . . . .

Easy Microwave Cleaner

Add a tablespoon of white vinegar to a half pint of water in a heatproof jug and microwave on full for 10 minutes. Wait a few minutes before you open the door and remove the jug. Use a cloth dipped in baking soda to scrub any baked-on stains, then wipe down with a clean cloth. You can use the same trick on your conventional oven.

To Clean a Burned Pan

If you have burned the bottom of a saucepan, add an inch or two of water and bring to a boil. Turn off the heat, sprinkle in plenty of baking soda, and leave overnight; it will clean up easily in the morning. To clean tarnished copper pans, sprinkle baking soda on half a lemon and use this to clean the pans.

Dishwasher Stain Remover

½ OUNCE CITRIC ACID (FOOD GRADE)

In an empty dishwasher, put the citric acid powder into the detergent dispenser. Run a wash cycle. If you don't have citric acid, pour white vinegar into the dispenser and run a cycle.

Kettle Limescale Remover

Put 6 tablespoons white vinegar and 1 pint water into the kettle and bring to a boil. Leave a few minutes, then rinse really, really well with warm water.

Broom Spray

To clean a dirty broom, swish broom bristles in warm, soapy water and spray with a mixture of white wine vinegar into which a few drops of tea tree and lavender essential oils have been added.

Windows

Some window cleaners contain nerve-damaging butyl cellosolve. Many contain ammonia, which may irritate airways and will release toxic chloramine gases if accidentally mixed with chlorine-containing cleaners. Even then, many of them are barely more effective than plain water.

WINDOW SPARKLER

Combine bicarbonate of soda (baking soda) and white vinegar with plenty of hot water to get dirty windows sparkling. Rinse with clean water and wipe dry with crumpled newspaper.

Laundry Products

. . . .

SOAP NUTS

Soap nuts are the dried fruits of the Chinese soapberry tree. I was given some as a Yule present last year and discovered that they are wonderful for laundry, leaving it clean and soft. They are naturally rich in saponins—or soapy stuff—and so are nasty-chemical free. You can buy them online or from health food stores, and you just put half a dozen of them into a muslin bag or knotted sock, then put them in the washing machine with your laundry and run your usual programme. The nuts can be used up to six times before they run out of juice. To use them for a hand wash, put them in a muslin bag in a bowl of hot water and allow the soap to come through. You can even use them in the dishwasher—just put a couple in the cutlery holder.

. . . .

LAUNDRY DETERGENT

2 OUNCES WASHING SODA

2 OUNCES BORAX

1 OUNCE GRATED CASTILE SOAP

A FEW DROPS OF LAVENDER ESSENTIAL OIL

A FEW DROPS OF ROSEMARY ESSENTIAL OIL

Combine and store in an airtight container. Use as you would your usual washing powder.

. . . .

ROSE LAUNDRY RINSE

2 PINTS ROSE WATER

1 OUNCE FRESH LAVENDER FLOWERS

2 OUNCES ORRIS ROOT

4 DROPS CLOVE OIL

Place in a large glass jar and leave on a sunny windowsill for 14 days. Strain and add a teaspoonful to the final rinse water of your clothes.

. . . . .

ANTI-STATIC RINSE

Add white vinegar or baking soda to the rinse cycle to prevent static cling. You can add essential oils of your choice to scent your clothes.

SCENTED TUMBLE DRYER SHEETS

Dab a few drops of your favourite oil onto a washcloth and add to the dryer load.

Carpets and Floors

. . . .
CARPET SHAMPOO

2 PINTS WATER

½ PINT LIQUID CASTILE SOAP

8 DROPS PEPPERMINT ESSENTIAL OIL

Rub the foam into soiled areas with a damp sponge. Let dry thoroughly and then vacuum.

. . . .
CARPET DEODORIZER

2 OUNCES BAKING SODA

10 DROPS LEMON ESSENTIAL OIL

10 DROPS ORANGE ESSENTIAL OIL

In a dark glass jar, combine the baking soda and essential oils. Sprinkle the mix over your carpet, wait an hour, and then vacuum.

. . . .
FLOOR WASH

½ PINT WHITE VINEGAR

1 PINT VERY HOT WATER

2 TABLESPOONS LIQUID CASTILE SOAP

40 DROPS PEPPERMINT OIL

Combine and use to wash your floors. Rinse after using or omit the castile soap for a no-rinse cleaner.

. . . .
FLOOR WASH #2

2 FLUID OUNCES LEMON JUICE

1 FLUID OUNCE LIQUID SOAP

Add the solution to a bucket of hot water and mop the floor as usual.

Air Fresheners and Deoderisers

Synthetically fragranced air fresheners, particularly aerosols, contain toxic chemicals that are inhaled and absorbed into the body. They can cause asthmatic or allergic reactions and have been linked to increased incidences of headaches and depression in adults, as well as ear infections and diarrhoea in infants.[30] Some deodoriser blocks contain paradichloroben-zene, a known carcinogen. I can never understand why people use them; they smell artifi-cial and just make your visitors suspect that the deodoriser blocks probably are masking a dirty home.

If there is a persistent smell in your house, you might need to clear a blocked pipe or drain, wash the dog or shampoo the carpet, or maybe you just need to open the windows now and again. If you do need to eliminate cooking or pet odours, you can place small dishes of baking soda or white vinegar (add a splash of lemon juice or lemon/orange essen-tial oil) around the house. However, if you do want to introduce some nice scents into your home, there are natural alternatives:

FRIDGE FRESHENER

Place a saucer of bicarbonate of soda in the bottom of your fridge to prevent odours. Alternatively, cut a lemon—the old wrinkly one you forgot about will do—in half, prick it with a fork several times, and place the two halves in the fridge. The lemon will absorb all the nasty odours.

KITCHEN BIN FRESHENER

If your kitchen bin (garbage can) is a bit smelly, sprinkle baking soda in it. This also works on running shoes and trainers.

CAT LITTER TRAY DEODORISER

Place some baking soda in the bottom of the cat litter tray to absorb the odours.

---

30 *New Scientist Magazine*, issue 2202 (4 September 1999), quoted in *Home Cleaning* by Rachelle Strauss (London: New Holland, 2009).

UPHOLSTERY FRESHENER

To remove odours, simply sprinkle baking soda on the fabric, leave for a few minutes, then vacuum off.

SCENTED SACHETS

2 TABLESPOONS ORRIS ROOT POWDER

1 TABLESPOON DRIED LAVENDER FLOWERS

A FEW DROPS OF LAVENDER OIL

1 TEASPOON GROUND CINNAMON

SEVERAL SQUARES OF 4" X 4" COTTON CLOTH

THREAD

Mix together the orris, lavender flowers and oil, and cinnamon. Place a couple of teaspoonfuls on each piece of cloth, gather it together, and tie it up with the thread. If you are handy with a needle, you can sew up oblongs of cloth into little pouches instead. These will scent your clothes drawers or you can hang one in the wardrobe. You could use aromatic roses, scented geranium leaves, or lemon verbena instead.

ANTI-INSECT POTPOURRI

2 TABLESPOONS DRIED MINT LEAVES

2 TABLESPOONS DRIED SAGE LEAVES

2 TABLESPOONS DRIED WORMWOOD LEAVES

2 TABLESPOONS DRIED ROSEMARY LEAVES

1 TABLESPOON DRIED LEMON PEEL

Mix the herbs together and put into a shallow bowl in a warm place to discourage insects. Discard when the scent has gone.

ROSE AND LAVENDER POTPOURRI

Always make your own potpourri and avoid any storebought ones that list "fragrance" as an ingredient.

DRIED ROSE PETALS

DRIED, SCENTED GERANIUM LEAVES

DRIED LAVENDER FLOWERS

ORRIS ROOT POWDER

A FEW DROPS OF GERANIUM ESSENTIAL OIL

GROUND CINNAMON

WHOLE CLOVES

Dry your flowers on paper for a few days. Mix the ingredients and seal together in a large jar for at least a month before using.

POMANDER

These scent cupboards and wardrobes and make excellent gifts at Yule.

APPLE OR ORANGE

CLOVES

RIBBON

2 TEASPOONS ORRIS ROOT POWDER

2 TEASPOONS NUTMEG

Pomanders are usually made with oranges, though apples work equally well. The fruit must be fresh and unbruised. Press cloves all over the fruit, very close together so that the flesh is not visible between them; it is best to start at the base and work upwards and round in rows. Roll the pomander in the nutmeg and powdered orris root, wrap it up in tissue paper, and put it in the airing cupboard (or a warm place) for a few weeks until it hardens. Shake off the powder and tie a ribbon round it for hanging.

ROSE INCENSE CONES

½ OUNCE GUM TRAGACANTH

ROSE WATER

3 OUNCES GUM ARABIC

2 OUNCES STORAX

1 OUNCE DAMASK ROSEBUDS, DRIED AND GROUND

1 OUNCE SALTPETER

1 OUNCE SANDALWOOD POWDER

Dissolve the tragacanth in a little rose water. Meanwhile, blend the other ingredients. Add the tragacanth. If the mixture is too slack, add more sandalwood so that you can shape it into pyramids or cones. Allow the mixture to air dry completely, then store in an airtight container. To use, just light the pointed end and it should smoulder away nicely. If it doesn't burn well, you can always put it on an ignited charcoal block.

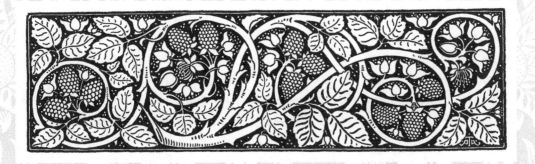

CHAPTER 6

Personal Care

It is said that the average woman is exposed to over 500 chemicals before she even leaves home in the morning. Have you ever really read the label of your favourite personal care products? Ingredients are listed in order of the highest concentrations, and you might be shocked by what you discover, as the safety of many ingredients is being questioned. Numerous studies have shown that long-term exposure to some is deleterious to health and linked to serious medical problems. They may be classified as safe "in small amounts," but if you use half a dozen different products several times a day over a period of time and add in contact with your household chemicals, that toxic effect is compounded.

Almost all commercial skincare products contain synthetic, petroleum-based chemicals. Studies on rodents have found that the topical application of petrochemicals resulted in anaemia, kidney degeneration, and nerve damage to the brain and spinal cord. Artificial fragrances are cheaper for the manufacturer than essential oils, but they are made from petroleum or coal. Is that a rose you smell in your shampoo or is it something that comes from a coal mine? Petroleum products are known disrupters of the nervous system, and some are cancer causing. Some synthetic colours, preservatives, absorbing agents, and degreasers (in cleansers and shampoos) have also been linked to cancer. Other chemicals in shampoos, face creams, and antiperspirants have been linked to allergies, chronic fatigue, depression, dizziness, headaches, joint pain, and insomnia.

The body absorbs as much as 60 percent of what is applied to the skin; indeed, some prescription medications are applied to the skin in the form of a patch. I believe that you shouldn't put anything onto your skin that you wouldn't put into your mouth, so I like to make my own personal care products.

Equipment Needed

- Kitchen scales

- Wooden spoons

- Bottles, jars, and tins

- Large ceramic or plastic bowls

- Double boiler (or a heatproof bowl over a pan of simmering water)

Safety First
DO A PATCH TEST

Even with the most pure and natural ingredients, it is still possible that some people will have an allergic or sensitive reaction. When using any new product or ingredient, it is advisable to carry out a patch test by placing a tiny amount of the product on the inside of your arm and monitoring for any adverse reaction such as itching, reddening, soreness, or a rash. If this occurs, discontinue using the product. If you are on medication or have a health condition, please consult a health professional before using any of the ingredients in this book.

Bath Salts

Bath salts are very easy to make, as you simply stir the ingredients together. Start with the salts; if you really want to colour them (they don't really need it), use natural food colouring as the safest option (go easy—a little goes a long way) and blend it into the salt with the back of a metal spoon. Mix in any essential oils, then you can stir in any dried herbs or flowers. Store in an airtight jar or tin. To use, just add a handful to your bath, lie back, and soak up the loveliness. Bath salts make great gifts, too; put them in a nice bottle or jar and decorate with a ribbon.

NOTE: Diabetics should avoid Epsom salts. Just use cooking
salt instead or double the quantity of sea salt.

RITUAL PURIFICATION BATH

2 OUNCES SALT

A FEW DROPS OF ROSEMARY OIL

A FEW DROPS OF FRANKINCENSE OIL

BLUE FOOD COLOURING (OPTIONAL)

Blend together and store in an airtight container. Use a handful in your bath as a ritual cleansing.

HANGOVER/REVIVING BATH SALTS

1 OUNCE EPSOM SALT

1 OUNCE SEA SALT (OR COOKING SALT)

2 OUNCES BICARBONATE OF SODA (BAKING SODA)

30 DROPS FENNEL ESSENTIAL OIL

10 DROPS GINGER ESSENTIAL OIL

Combine the salts and bicarbonate. Add the oils and stir well. Store in an airtight container.

LAYERED BATH SALTS

1 OUNCE BICARBONATE OF SODA (BAKING SODA)

2 OUNCES EPSOM SALTS

5 DROPS YELLOW FOOD COLOURING

10 DROPS ORANGE ESSENTIAL OIL

5 DROPS RED FOOD COLOURING

10 DROPS JUNIPER ESSENTIAL OIL

Combine bicarbonate of soda and Epsom salts. Divide into two bowls. Add the yellow food colouring and orange oil to one, and the red colouring and juniper to the other. Blend well. Layer in a jar and stopper tightly.

DETOX BATH SALTS

1 OUNCE EPSOM SALTS

½ OUNCE DEAD SEA SALT

10 DROPS ROSEMARY ESSENTIAL OIL

10 DROPS GRAPEFRUIT ESSENTIAL OIL

Blend together and keep in a screw-top jar.

EARTH BATH SALTS

1 OUNCE EPSOM SALTS

1 OUNCE SALT

3 DROPS GREEN FOOD COLOURING

10 DROPS PATCHOULI ESSENTIAL OIL

5 DROPS CYPRESS ESSENTIAL OIL

5 DROPS ROSE ESSENTIAL OIL

Mix the salts and food colouring. Add the oils and blend well. Keep in a screw-topped jar.

LEMON AND LIME FIZZ

1 OUNCE SALT

1 OUNCE BICARBONATE OF SODA (BAKING SODA)

¼ OUNCE CITRIC ACID

5 DROPS LIME ESSENTIAL OIL

5 DROPS LEMON ESSENTIAL OIL

Combine the salt, soda, and citric acid. Add the oils and mix well. Keep in a screw-topped jar.

MERMAID'S DELIGHT

Full of vitamins and minerals, kelp helps your skin to regenerate and retain its elasticity.

1 OUNCE SEA SALT

3 OUNCES BICARBONATE OF SODA (BAKING SODA)

½ OUNCE POWDERED KELP

Combine and keep in a screw-topped jar.

Bath Bombs

Fizzy bath bombs are simple and inexpensive to make. They can be perfumed with which-ever essential oils you like (or feel you need) and tinted with natural food colouring (I have found the powdered kind easier to use for bath bombs). The bombs may incorporate or be decorated with dried rosebuds, sprigs of lavender, dried herbs and flower petals, dried orange and lemon slices, or whatever your imagination can come up with.

You can buy specialist bath bomb moulds, but I use silicone muffin and individual cake moulds, large ice cube trays, or individual waxed-paper cake cases. When you have run your bath, drop in a bomb and watch it sizzle! Homemade bath bombs make wonderful presents for your special friends, too.

THE BASIC METHOD

In a dry ceramic or glass bowl mix the bicarbonate of soda (baking soda) and citric acid pow-der. Add a few drops of food colouring or a sprinkling of food colouring powder (optional) and a few drops of essential oil. Mix thoroughly with the back of a metal spoon. It will only need a little water to bring the mixture together so that the mixture will clump together in your hand, which is why I use a spray bottle. Spoon the mixture into the moulds, press down with the back of the spoon, and leave to set overnight. Turn out of the mould and store in an airtight jar or container.

You can scale up the recipe for a larger quantity by using 1 cup citric acid and 3 cups of bicarbonate of soda—the ratio is always 1:3.

. . . .

BASIC BATH BOMB RECIPE

1 TABLESPOON CITRIC ACID POWDER

3 TABLESPOONS BICARBONATE OF SODA (BAKING SODA)

FOOD COLOURING (OPTIONAL)

A FEW DROPS OF YOUR FAVOURITE ESSENTIAL OIL

WATER IN A SPRAY BOTTLE

Make up as described in the basic method.

MANDARIN BATH BOMBS

Revives and stimulates.

1 TABLESPOON CITRIC ACID POWDER

3 TABLESPOONS BICARBONATE OF SODA (BAKING SODA)

YELLOW FOOD COLOURING

A FEW DROPS OF MANDARIN ESSENTIAL OIL

A PINCH OF DRIED CALENDULA PETALS

Make up as described in the basic method, adding the flower petals last and using a little water to bring the mixture together.

LAVENDER BATH BOMBS

Soothes tired muscles and relaxes the body and mind.

1 TABLESPOON CITRIC ACID POWDER

3 TABLESPOONS BICARBONATE OF SODA (BAKING SODA)

BLUE FOOD COLOURING

A FEW DROPS OF LAVENDER ESSENTIAL OIL

A PINCH OF DRIED LAVENDER PETALS

Make up as described in the basic method.

TROPICAL BATH BOMBS

Soothes tired muscles and stimulates the senses.

1 TABLESPOON CITRIC ACID POWDER

3 TABLESPOONS BICARBONATE OF SODA (BAKING SODA)

A FEW DROPS YLANG-YLANG OIL

A FEW DROPS VETIVER OIL

A FEW DROPS SWEET ORANGE OIL

PINCH OF DRIED HIBISCUS PETALS

Make up as described in the basic method.

Bath Tea Bags

Bath bags allow you to use the therapeutic properties of fresh or dried herbs in your bath. Simply take a piece of fabric, gather up the herbs inside it, secure the top with string or ribbon, and tie it beneath the tap as the bath runs so that the hot water runs through it and activates the herbs. Alternatively, pop the bag into a large jug, add some boiling water, and infuse for 20–25 minutes, strain, and add the infusion to the bathwater.

To make the bags, you can use muslin, cheesecloth, or any loosely woven fabric. I have a little laundry bag that I can zip herbs into, and I drop this into the bath—a handful of rosemary is great for soothing tired muscles after I have been doing some heavy gardening. You could also use the little drawstring organza bags that are sold for wedding and party favours and make up some pretty herbal bath bags for gifts. The bags can be washed out and refilled.

If you are using dried herbs, you can make up a quantity of the mixtures and store in an airtight container. If you are using fresh herbs, they will need to be used straightaway. You can add a few drops of essential oil to the blend if you wish.

RELAXING BATH BAG

1 PART LAVENDER FLOWERS

1 PART CHAMOMILE FLOWERS

1 PART HOPS

SOOTHING BATH BAG

1 PART OATMEAL

½ PART LAVENDER FLOWERS

ELDERFLOWER REFRESHING BATH BAG

Tie a handful of fresh elderflower heads in muslin and hang beneath the hot tap as the bath fills.

· · · · · · · · · · · · · · ·
SLEEPY-TIME BATH BAG

1 PART HOPS

1 PART PASSIONFLOWER

1 PART ROSEBUDS OR PETALS

1 PART CHAMOMILE FLOWERS

· · · · · · · · · · · · · · ·
ENERGIZING BATH BAG

1 PART PEPPERMINT LEAVES

1 PART LEMON PEEL

1 PART GREEN TEA

·
SEVENTEENTH-CENTURY BATH BAG

1 PART ROSES

1 PART ORANGE PEEL

1 PART ORANGE FLOWERS

1 PART JASMINE FLOWERS

1 PART BAY LEAVES

1 PART ROSEMARY LEAVES

1 PART LAVENDER FLOWERS

1 PART MINT LEAVES

Milk Baths

Remember the story of Cleopatra bathing in ass's milk to maintain her legendary beauty? Well, she was no fool. Milk softens and rejuvenates the skin, moisturises, and combats dryness. You can simply add whole milk to your bath, maybe mixed with some honey and olive oil, or you can use dried milk powder for the following recipes. You can also put these blends into bath bags.

CLEOPATRA'S BATH

2 OUNCES DRIED MILK POWDER

1 TEASPOON POWDERED MYRRH

5 DROPS CINNAMON ESSENTIAL OIL

4 DROPS FRANKINCENSE ESSENTIAL OIL

Blend together and store in an airtight container. Add 2 tablespoons to your bath.

RELAXING CHAMOMILE MILK BATH

2 OUNCES POWDERED MILK

2 OUNCES DRIED CHAMOMILE, POWDERED

Blend together and store in an airtight container. Add 2 tablespoons to your bath.

HERBY MILK BATH

2 OUNCES POWDERED MILK

1 OUNCE CORNFLOUR (CORNSTARCH)

½ TEASPOON DRIED ROSEMARY

½ TEASPOON DRIED LAVENDER

½ TEASPOON DRIED SAGE

Combine the ingredients in a blender. Store in an airtight container. Add 2 tablespoons to your bath.

LAVENDER MILK BATH

2 OUNCES POWDERED MILK

1 TABLESPOON DRIED LAVENDER

A FEW DROPS LAVENDER ESSENTIAL OIL

Blend the powdered milk and dried lavender in a blender. Put into a bowl and add the lavender essential oil. Store in an airtight container. Add 2 tablespoons to your bath.

Bubble Baths

I love soaking in a luxurious bubble bath. The base for these recipes is castile soap, which can be purchased in liquid form; alternatively, you can grate up a bar of solid castile soap. I always use essential oils to perfume my bubble baths as they are natural products with therapeutic properties.

Here are a couple of recipes to start you off, but you can use any blend of essential oils you like. If you want to, you can colour the bubble bath with natural food colouring.

ORANGE AND LEMON REVIVING BUBBLE BATH

¼ PINT LIQUID CASTILE SOAP

½ PINT WATER

½ TEASPOON SALT

8 DROPS ORANGE ESSENTIAL OIL

8 DROPS LEMON ESSENTIAL OIL

Pour the liquid soap into a bowl and add the water. Mix and add the salt. Stir well, then add the essential oils. Store in a clean bottle or jar.

LAVENDER BUBBLE BATH

¼ PINT LIQUID CASTILE SOAP

½ PINT WATER

½ TEASPOON SALT

1 OUNCE GLYCERINE

10 DROPS LAVENDER ESSENTIAL OIL

Pour the liquid soap into a bowl and add the water. Mix and add the salt and glycerine. Stir well, then add the essential oil. Store in a clean bottle or jar.

Bath Oils

Make your own pampering bath oils by adding 20 drops of essential oils to 4 tablespoons of carrier oil (see chapter 11 on essential oils). Store in a dark glass jar or bottle and add a teaspoon or two to the bath after it has run. Light oils such as almond, sunflower, grapeseed, or jojoba work best as a carrier oil. Adding a teaspoon of wheat germ oil or vitamin E oil not only helps the storing properties of the bath oil but is great for your skin too. Experiment with your own blends, as one person will love a particular scent while another will hate it.

REVIVING BATH OIL

4 TABLESPOONS CARRIER OIL

7 DROPS ORANGE ESSENTIAL OIL

7 DROPS MELISSA (LEMON BALM) ESSENTIAL OIL

6 DROPS ROSEMARY ESSENTIAL OIL

Blend in a dark bottle.

LUXURY BATH OIL

4 TABLESPOONS APRICOT OIL

10 DROPS JASMINE ESSENTIAL OIL

10 DROPS ROSE ESSENTIAL OIL

Blend in a dark bottle.

RELAXING BATH OIL

4 TABLESPOONS CARRIER OIL

5 DROPS LAVENDER ESSENTIAL OIL

7 DROPS YLANG-YLANG ESSENTIAL OIL

7 DROPS SANDALWOOD ESSENTIAL OIL

Blend in a dark bottle.

ACHING MUSCLE BATH OIL

4 TABLESPOONS CARRIER OIL

5 DROPS BLACK PEPPER ESSENTIAL OIL

7 DROPS ROSEMARY ESSENTIAL OIL

7 DROPS LAVENDER ESSENTIAL OIL

Blend in a dark bottle.

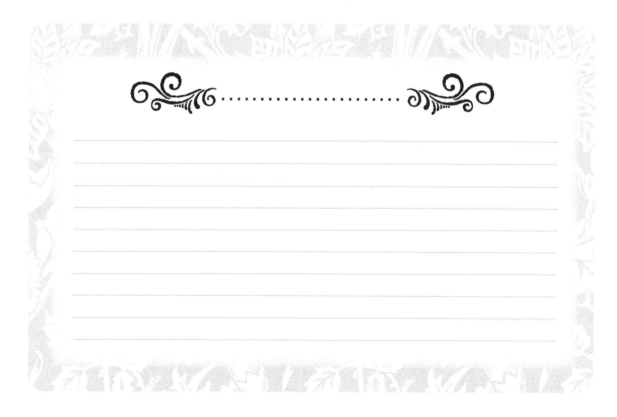

Shower Bags

This is a variation on the bath bags for use in the shower—just scrub yourself with the bag. Make sure the size of the bag is comfortable in your hand, and fill it with:

2 PARTS OATMEAL

2 PARTS DRIED HERBS

1 PART GRATED CASTILE SOAP

Oatmeal contains saponins, or natural soap, as well as being moisturising, exfoliating, and soothing for the skin. You can use whichever herbs you like, such as those listed in the following table:

HERBS FOR THE SHOWER	
CALENDULA	SKIN SOOTHING
CHAMOMILE	CALMING, SOOTHING
HEARTSEASE (PANSY)	SKIN SOOTHING
HOPS	CALMING
HORSETAIL	SPRAINS, IRRITATED SKIN
JASMINE	CALMING, DE-STRESSING
LAVENDER	SOOTHING, CALMING
LEMON BALM	REFRESHING, STIMULATING
LEMON GRASS	ACHING MUSCLES
LINDEN FLOWERS	CALMING, DE-STRESSING
PEPPERMINT	REFRESHING, STIMULATING
ROSE	CALMING, SOOTHING
ROSEMARY	STIMULATING
SAGE	SKIN HEALING, SOOTHING
THYME	STIMULATING, ANTISEPTIC

• • • • •

Shower Wash

LEMON AND LIME SHOWER WASH

½ PINT LIQUID CASTILE SOAP

½ TEASPOON SALT

¼ PINT WATER

10 DROPS LEMON ESSENTIAL OIL

10 DROPS LIME ESSENTIAL OIL

YELLOW FOOD COLOURING (OPTIONAL)

Pour the liquid castile soap into a bowl and add the salt and water. Mix well, add the oils and colouring, bottle, and label. You can substitute any essential oils of your choice.

Soaps

Making soap from scratch is a lengthy process and involves some dangerous chemicals, so I don't propose to go into it here. Instead, here are some easy recipes for homemade soaps using simple herbs or melt-and-pour soap bases.

USING MELT-AND-POUR SOAP BASE

Melt-and-pour soap base is available online and comes in several varieties, from clear glycerine to opaque white and even goat's milk. You simply melt it in the microwave or in a double boiler, add your scent and colouring (optional, but for best results buy special soap colouring) and any dried herbs or flowers, and pour into moulds. I use silicon muffin moulds or you could use cupcake paper cases; for a soap "loaf" that I slice up, I use a silicon loaf mould. Dedicated soap moulds are available online, but they are quite expensive.

Once the soap has set, which will take a few hours, remove it from the mould and package by wrapping in greaseproof paper or cellophane. Homemade soaps make great gifts. If you can't get melt-and-pour soap base, you can use a grated bar of castile soap.

. . . .
SOAPWORT SOAP

A HANDFUL OF SOAPWORT LEAVES, CHOPPED AND BRUISED

½ PINT WATER

Boil together for 30 minutes. Strain off the liquid and retain this. It will be soapy and can be used for washing hands and woollen fabrics. Don't be alarmed by a slightly green stain on fabrics, as it rinses out.

. . . .
LAVENDER SOAP

7 OUNCES GLYCERINE MELT-AND-POUR SOAP BASE

1 TABLESPOON DRIED LAVENDER FLOWERS

10 DROPS LAVENDER ESSENTIAL OIL

A FEW DROPS OF PURPLE SOAP COLOUR (OPTIONAL)

Chop up the soap base and put into a heatproof jug. Microwave on medium high until melted; this will only take a couple of minutes, so keep an eye on it and do not let it boil. Remove from the heat and stir in the lavender flowers, colour, and oil. Pour into moulds.

. . . . .

CITRUS SOAP LOAF

1 POUND GLYCERINE MELT-AND-POUR SOAP BASE

10 DROPS LEMON ESSENTIAL OIL

10 DROPS ORANGE ESSENTIAL OIL

10 DROPS LIME ESSENTIAL OIL

10 DROPS GRAPEFRUIT ESSENTIAL OIL

YELLOW SOAP COLOUR (OPTIONAL)

ORANGE SOAP COLOUR (OPTIONAL)

GREEN SOAP COLOUR (OPTIONAL)

Divide the soap base into four parts. Melt the first part, add lemon oil and yellow colouring, and pour into a silicon loaf mould. When it has almost set, melt the next batch and add orange oil and orange colouring, and pour into the mould. When that has set, melt the third batch, add lime oil and green colouring, and pour into the mould. When that has set, melt the last batch and add grapefruit oil and yellow colouring. Allow the loaf to set fully and turn out. You will have a stripy citrus soap loaf that you can slice and package.

OATMEAL GARDENER'S SOAP

7 OUNCES MELT-AND-POUR SOAP BASE

2 TABLESPOONS COARSE OATMEAL

10 DROPS ROSEMARY ESSENTIAL OIL

Chop up the soap base and put into a heatproof jug. Microwave on medium high until melted; this will only take a couple of minutes, so keep an eye on it and do not let it boil. Remove from the heat and stir in the oatmeal and oil. Pour into moulds.

CALENDULA SOAP

7 OUNCES GLYCERINE MELT-AND-POUR SOAP BASE

1 TABLESPOON DRIED CALENDULA PETALS

10 DROPS CALENDULA ESSENTIAL OIL

A FEW DROPS OF ORANGE OR YELLOW SOAP COLOUR (OPTIONAL)

Chop up the soap base and put into a heatproof jug. Microwave on medium high until melted; this will only take a couple of minutes, so keep an eye on it and do not let it boil. Remove from the heat and stir in the petals, oil, and colour. Pour into moulds.

MORE SOAP COMBINATIONS

Using melt-and-pour soap bases is very straightforward, and you are only limited by your imagination. Here are a few ideas for some herbal combinations to get you started:

SOAP COMBINATIONS
ROSE PETALS & FRANKINCENSE ESSENTIAL OIL
MINT LEAVES & PEPPERMINT ESSENTIAL OIL
STINGING NETTLE LEAVES & ROSEMARY ESSENTIAL OIL
CHAMOMILE FLOWERS & CHAMOMILE ESSENTIAL OIL
LEMON ZEST & ORANGE ESSENTIAL OIL

Lotion Bars

These are solid moisturising bars made from oils and solid vegetable butters. Rub over your damp skin when you get out of the bath or shower, or even add a little piece to your bath-water and let it dissolve for a moisturising bath.

MANGO AND ALMOND LOTION BAR

2 OUNCES MANGO BUTTER

2 OUNCES GRATED BEESWAX

2 OUNCES SWEET ALMOND OIL

30 DROPS ESSENTIAL OIL OF YOUR CHOICE

ORANGE SOAP COLOURING

In a double boiler melt the mango butter and add the beeswax. When this has melted, add the almond oil. Remove from heat and allow to cool slightly before adding the essential oil and colourant. Pour into moulds.

MINTY LOTION BAR

1 OUNCE COCONUT OIL

1 OUNCE COCOA BUTTER

2 OUNCES BEESWAX

20 DROPS PEPPERMINT ESSENTIAL OIL

GREEN SOAP COLOURING

Melt the oil and butter together in a double boiler and add the wax. Allow it to melt, then add the fragrance oil and colour.

Bath Powders

Talcum powder has been linked to some forms of cancer, so here are a couple of natural alternatives.

Arabian Nights

2 OUNCES RICE FLOUR

1 TABLESPOON GROUND DRIED ROSE PETALS

2 TEASPOONS CRUSHED DRIED LAVENDER BLOSSOMS

½ TEASPOON POWDERED MYRRH

A PINCH OF POWDERED CLOVES

½ TEASPOON DRIED POWDERED ROSEMARY

½ TEASPOON POWDERED BENZOIN

Rub everything through a fine sieve and keep in a dark, airtight container.

Herbal Deodorant Powder

2 PARTS CORNFLOUR (CORNSTARCH)

1 PART POWDERED DRIED SAGE LEAVES

1 PART POWDERED DRIED THYME LEAVES

A FEW DROPS SAGE ESSENTIAL OIL

A FEW DROPS LEMON ESSENTIAL OIL

Pulverize herbs in a blender or food processor until they become a very fine powder. Store in an airtight container.

Natural Shampoos

Read the ingredient list on any bottle of commercially available shampoo that has a lovely plant picture on the front of the bottle and claims it contains some herb or fruit, and you might be in for a shock—there will be a scary list of chemicals, petroleum products, and synthetic ingredients, some of them now thought to be toxic or even carcinogenic. The lovely herbs or fruits featured so prominently on the artwork that suggest that the product is "natural" may scrape in at the bottom of a very long list and in a tiny proportion. Here's a mad idea: why not use the real plant?

You can make your own pure shampoos from ingredients including liquid castile soap, herb tinctures, carrier oils, essential oils, cider vinegar, fruits, and vegetables. Homemade shampoos are fiddlier and take some getting used to, but you can do your hair (and health) a favour by caring for it naturally and using what Mother Nature provides. Natural shampoos usually do not lather much or even at all, which can feel very odd at first, but they do clean.

. . . .

ROSEMARY SHAMPOO FOR OILY HAIR

½ PINT DISTILLED WATER

6 TABLESPOONS LIQUID CASTILE SOAP

1 TABLESPOON WITCH HAZEL EXTRACT

1 TABLESPOON ROSEMARY TINCTURE

40 DROPS ROSEMARY ESSENTIAL OIL

1 TABLESPOON FINELY MILLED SEA SALT

Add all the ingredients to a bottle or jar and shake well. This shampoo will keep in the fridge for up to two weeks. To use, shake the bottle well and massage a small amount of the shampoo into wet hair. Rinse with warm water several times.

. . . . .

SOAPWORT SHAMPOO

You can make this without the brandy but it will not keep for more than a few days. It is good for greasy hair.

    1 OUNCE SOAPWORT ROOT, CHOPPED

    ½ PINT DISTILLED WATER

    4 TEASPOONS SALT

    4 TEASPOONS CASTOR OIL

    A FEW DROPS OF TEA TREE OIL

    2 OUNCES BRANDY

Simmer the chopped root in the water for 15 minutes. Leave to cool a little, then strain onto the salt and oils in a jam jar. Shake to dissolve the salt. Use as per a normal shampoo, though it won't lather much.

CHICKPEA SHAMPOO

Chickpea flour (also called gram flour) removes oiliness and helps to maintain healthy and shiny hair.

    2 OUNCES CHICKPEA FLOUR

    ¾ PINT DISTILLED WATER

Gradually add the water to the flour in a pan and simmer very gently for 15 minutes. Use immediately: cool the mixture, work it through the hair, and massage the scalp with it. Rinse very thoroughly.

EGG SHAMPOO

Packed with proteins, amino acids, fatty acids, and vitamins, eggs (particularly the yolks) feed and strengthen your hair and improve its texture and shine, as well as reduce frizz and breakages.

1 EGG

¼ PINT DISTILLED WATER OR RAINWATER

Whisk the ingredients together and immediately massage into the hair and scalp for at least 5–10 minutes. Rinse with lukewarm water—too hot and you will get scrambled eggs!—and add some lemon juice to the final rinse.

HERBAL SHAMPOO (FOR DRY HAIR)

½ OUNCE COMFREY LEAVES

½ OUNCE ELDERFLOWERS

1 PINT BOILING WATER

1 OUNCE LIQUID CASTILE SOAP

Infuse the herbs in the boiling water overnight. Strain and combine with the soap. This should keep for up to a month.

HERBAL SHAMPOO (FOR OILY HAIR)

½ OUNCE MINT LEAVES

½ OUNCE LEMON BALM LEAVES

1 PINT BOILING WATER

1 OUNCE LIQUID CASTILE SOAP

Infuse the herbs in the boiling water overnight. Strain and combine with the soap. This should keep for up to a month.

Dry Shampoos

Dry shampoos are a quick fix when you don't have time to wash your hair. They soak up excess oil and remove dirt when sprinkled on the hair and combed through. Ingredients can include cornflour (cornstarch), arrowroot powder, powdered clays, orris root powder, bicarbonate of soda (baking soda), oat flour, and rice flour. If you have dark hair, you can even use cocoa powder. Scent your dry shampoos with essential oils.

LEMONY DRY SHAMPOO

A FEW DROPS OF LEMON ESSENTIAL OIL

1 OUNCE DRY COARSE-MILLED SEMOLINA

In a mortar and pestle add the lemon oil to the semolina; do not put in a blender. Keep in an airtight container.

REFRESHING PEPPERMINT DRY SHAMPOO

1 OUNCE ARROWROOT POWDER

1 TABLESPOON BICARBONATE OF SODA (BAKING SODA)

20 DROPS PEPPERMINT ESSENTIAL OIL

Mix in a blender and keep in an airtight container.

Hair Rinses

A hair rinse after washing your hair can help to add extra shine and manageability, as well as remove all traces of chemical buildup on your hair.

. . . .

NETTLE ANTI-GREASE HAIR RINSE

Massage this into the scalp before shampooing or use it between shampoos to remove grease by wiping the scalp and hair roots with a little on a cotton wool pad. Regular use will help treat greasy hair.

4 OUNCES FRESH NETTLES

½ PINT VODKA

2 BAY LEAVES

30 DROPS TEA TREE OIL

1 PINT CIDER VINEGAR

Put the nettles in a blender with the vodka until pulped. Place in a jar and leave for 2 weeks, shaking daily. Strain into a clean jar and add the oil and cider vinegar.

. . . .

ANTI-DANDRUFF HAIR RINSE

Shampoo your hair as normal, and add a tablespoon of this to the final hair rinse.

1 OUNCE FRESH NETTLES

1 OUNCE IVY LEAVES, CHOPPED

½ OUNCE SAGE LEAVES, CHOPPED

½ OUNCE ROSEMARY LEAVES, CHOPPED

½ OUNCE THYME, CHOPPED

2 FLUID OUNCES VODKA

1 PINT CIDER VINEGAR

Wash and pat dry the nettles. Place the nettles, along with the chopped herbs, vodka, and cider vinegar, in a jam jar and leave for 2 weeks, shaking daily. Strain into a clean jar.

. . . . .

HAIR TONIC

Use as a final rinse after shampooing.

BUNCH OF ROSEMARY

BUNCH OF NETTLES

1 PINT WATER

1 PINT CIDER VINEGAR

Simmer the herbs in the water and vinegar for 1½ hours. Strain into jars and keep in the fridge for up to 4 weeks.

Colouring Rinses

Herbal hair rinses can add subtle highlights and colour to your hair when used over a period of time, but they won't dye it a different shade. Make a strong infusion or decoction of your one chosen herb, cool, and strain, retaining the liquid. To use it, first wash and rinse your hair clean of shampoo with plenty of running water. Have your colouring rinse ready and, standing at the basin, use a jug to pour the rinse over your hair. Scoop the runoff up from the basin and keep pouring at least a dozen times. Rinse once with clean water. Repeat weekly and the colour will gradually intensify, though it will always be much more subtle than a chemical hair dye.

Colour Rinses for Redheads

ALKANET ROOT

BLACK COFFEE

CALENDULA

CLOVES

RADISH ROOT

RED HIBISCUS TEA

ROSEHIP TEA

SAFFRON

Colour Rinses for Blonds

BROOM FLOWERS

CALENDULA

CHAMOMILE

LEMON JUICE

MULLEIN FLOWERS

RHUBARB ROOT

SAFFRON

TURMERIC

Colour Rinses for Brunettes

BAY LEAVES

BLACK COFFEE

BLACK TEA

CATNIP

ELDERBERRIES

GREEN WALNUT SHELLS

IVY BERRIES

PARSLEY

RASPBERRY LEAVES

ROSEMARY

SAGE

VINE LEAVES

Colour Rinses to Darken Grey Hair

MARJORAM

SAGE

Chamomile Lightener for Fair Hair

1 OUNCE CHAMOMILE FLOWERS

1 OUNCE MARIGOLD FLOWERS

JUICE AND ZEST OF 2 LEMONS

½ PINT WATER

Add the flowers and lemon zest to the water and simmer 10 minutes. Cool and strain through a muslin bag. Add the lemon juice. Apply the mixture to fair hair to lighten it. Cover with a warm towel and leave for 45 minutes, then rinse.

Conditioners

. . . .

MAYONNAISE CONDITIONER

This might sound crazy, but mayonnaise is an excellent hair conditioner. Make your own mayo or buy an organic one, and work a tablespoon of it through your hair. Leave for 5 minutes, then shampoo as usual.

. . . .

FOR DRY, LIFELESS HAIR

A FEW DROPS OF CHAMOMILE ESSENTIAL OIL

1 TABLESPOON SWEET ALMOND OIL

1 TABLESPOON AVOCADO OIL

1 TABLESPOON OLIVE OIL

1 EGG YOLK

4 TABLESPOONS RUNNY HONEY

Mix the oils, egg yolk, and honey. Spread over the head, massaging into the scalp. Cover with a towel and leave for 30 minutes. Rinse with warm water, then shampoo as usual. Your hair will be super soft and shiny.

. . . .

FOR DAMAGED HAIR

3 TABLESPOONS RUNNY HONEY

1 TABLESPOON OLIVE OIL

Shampoo your hair and leave it damp. Mix the honey and olive oil and apply to your hair. Leave for 20 minutes and rinse several times with warm water.

. . . . .

Anti-Dandruff Scalp Treatment

½ OUNCE FRESH MARIGOLD FLOWERS

½ OUNCE FRESH NETTLE

½ OUNCE FRESH SAGE LEAVES

CIDER VINEGAR

2 TEASPOONS WHEAT GERM OIL

Place the herbs in a jar and cover with the cider vinegar. Leave on a sunny windowsill for 14 days, shaking daily. Strain into a clean jar and add the oil. Massage the mixture into the scalp regularly before washing your hair.

Dental Care

. . . .

TOOTHPASTE

5 OUNCES BICARBONATE OF SODA (BAKING SODA)

2 TEASPOONS FINE SALT

3 TEASPOONS GLYCERINE

10 DROPS PEPPERMINT ESSENTIAL OIL

LUKEWARM WATER

Mix the bicarbonate of soda and salt in a bowl. Mix in the glycerine and essential oil. Add the lukewarm water a drop at a time until you reach the required consistency. Put into a wide-topped jar and use for your normal toothpaste. This keeps indefinitely.

. . . .

TOOTH POWDER

3 TABLESPOONS BICARBONATE OF SODA (BAKING SODA)

1 TABLESPOON FINE SALT

A PINCH OF FINELY GROUND DRIED SAGE

3 DROPS PEPPERMINT ESSENTIAL OIL (OPTIONAL)

Combine the ingredients well. Store them in a wide-necked jar. To use the tooth powder, slightly wet your toothbrush and dip it into the powder, then clean your teeth as usual.

. . . .

SAGE TOOTH CLEANER

Using fresh sage leaves, rub over the teeth to clean and whiten.

. . . . .

MOUTHWASH

1 PINT (20 FLUID OUNCES) DISTILLED WATER

1 TABLESPOON FRESH MINT LEAVES

½ TEASPOON WHOLE CLOVES

1 TEASPOON TINCTURE OF MYRRH

Boil the water, remove from the heat, add the mint and cloves, and leave to infuse for 20 minutes. Strain and add the tincture of myrrh (a natural preservative that is also antiseptic). Use as a gargle or mouthwash.

BREATH FRESHENERS

Simply chew fresh parsley leaves or munch on a few fennel seeds to freshen your breath.

Foot Care

SOFTENING FOOT BATH

2 PINTS BOILING WATER

½ OUNCE ROSEMARY (FRESH OR DRIED)

OLIVE OIL

Pour the boiling water over the rosemary and infuse for 15 minutes. Strain into a bowl large enough to soak your feet in and cool a little before soaking your feet for 15 minutes. Dry and moisturise with olive oil.

DEODORIZING FOOT BATH

4 PINTS BOILING WATER

A HANDFUL OF FRESH SAGE LEAVES

6 TABLESPOONS EPSOM SALTS

½ PINT WHITE VINEGAR

Pour the boiling water over the sage leaves and infuse for 15–20 minutes. Strain and add the infusion to a foot bath with the Epsom salts and vinegar. Soak your feet for 15 minutes. Used often, this will help combat the problem of smelly feet.

SAGE DEODORIZING FOOT POWDER

2 OUNCES BICARBONATE OF SODA (BAKING SODA)

½ OUNCE POWDERED DRIED SAGE

10 DROPS SAGE ESSENTIAL OIL

Combine and store in an airtight container. Dust the feet with the powder after bathing, and sprinkle a little in your shoes to prevent odour.

Hand Care

. . . .

LETTUCE HAND CREAM

2 LARGE LETTUCE LEAVES

½ PINT BOILING WATER

2 TABLESPOONS BEESWAX

1 TABLESPOON LANOLIN

4 TABLESPOONS JOJOBA OIL

Place the lettuce leaves in a pan and add the boiling water. Stand for 2 hours and strain. Melt the wax and lanolin in the oil in a double boiler over very low heat. Whisk in the lettuce infusion and continue beating until the mixture is cool and creamy. Try adding the infusion a bit at a time, as there may be too much liquid. Spoon into a clean jar and keep refrigerated.

Note: Some people are allergic to lanolin.

. . . .

ELDERFLOWER HAND CREAM

4 TABLESPOONS ALMOND OIL

2 HANDFULS OF FRESH ELDERFLOWERS

3 TABLESPOONS GRATED BEESWAX

Warm the almond oil (do not boil) in a double boiler and add the elderflowers. Remove from the heat and steep for 45 minutes. Strain through a fine sieve, return to the double boiler, and warm gently, adding the wax until it has melted. Pour into wide-necked jars or pots.

. . . .

WHEAT GERM HOT OIL NAIL TREATMENT

To strengthen weak, brittle nails, soak fingernails in warmed wheat germ oil for about 5 minutes.

Elizabethan Hand Oil

¼ PINT SWEET ALMOND OIL

20 WHOLE CLOVES

Put almond oil into a jar and add the cloves. Put the jar in the airing cupboard for 3 weeks. Strain off into a clean jar.

Age Spot Remover

1 TEASPOON LEMON JUICE

2 TEASPOONS GLYCERINE

Combine and apply to your hands twice a day.

Lavender Hand Cream

4 TABLESPOONS COCOA BUTTER

4 TABLESPOONS OLIVE OIL

4 TABLESPOONS GRATED BEESWAX

20 DROPS LAVENDER OIL

Warm the cocoa butter and olive oil in a double boiler. Remove from the heat and stir in the beeswax until it has dissolved. Allow to cool a little and add the lavender oil. Pour into small, wide-necked jars or pots.

Nail Strengthener

Using a cotton wool pad, rub a little almond oil on your nails each night.

Hand Cleanser

If you have dirty hands from working in the garage or garden, rub them over with half a lemon, then wash with soap in warm water.

Body Scrub

Scrubs help to remove dead skin cells and stimulate the circulatory system, making you glow inside and out.

. . . .

HERBAL BODY SCRUB

Use as a body scrub in the shower, rubbing onto wet skin and then rinsing well.
Follow with a moisturiser.

2 OUNCES FRESH MINT LEAVES

2 OUNCES FRESH ROSEMARY LEAVES

½ OUNCE JUNIPER BERRIES, CRUSHED

1 TEASPOON FRESH GINGER, GRATED

GRATED ZEST OF 1 GRAPEFRUIT

½ PINT SUNFLOWER OIL

1 POUND SEA SALT

5 TEASPOONS VITAMIN C POWDER

Put the mint, rosemary, juniper berries, ginger and zest into a pan with the sunflower oil. Simmer on low heat for 5 minutes. Strain, discarding the pulp and retaining the oil. In another bowl combine the sea salt and vitamin C powder. Add the herb oil, mix well, and store in an airtight jar. This will keep for about 6 months.

Aftershave

· · · · · · · · · · ·
HERBAL AFTERSHAVE

2 FLUID OUNCES CIDER VINEGAR

2 FLUID OUNCES WITCH HAZEL

2 FLUID OUNCES VODKA

6 CLOVES, POWDERED

1 OUNCE SAGE

Put everything in a jar and leave on a sunny windowsill for 14 days. Strain into a clean bottle. You can experiment by using different herbs in the mix.

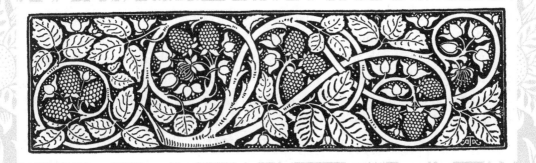

CHAPTER 7

A Witch's Guide to Natural Beauty

We've all been taken in by the claims of expensive skincare formulas that promise so much—they will erase our wrinkles, plump up our skin, and reduce our pores—and then been disappointed when they deliver so little and we end up out of pocket. In truth, the high prices they command pays for the marketing, packaging, and the dividends of the shareholders, but it doesn't reflect the true cost of the ingredients.

I've been making my own beauty products and toiletries in my kitchen for decades (ahem) using natural ingredients. It is reasonably easy and very satisfying to make your own organic, chemical-free and eco-friendly products. They are just as effective at reducing wrinkles and keeping your skin smooth and supple, and they are very much cheaper. Most of these recipes can be made using plants found in the garden or hedgerow. For the purposes of natural cosmetics and toiletries, fresh plants have more concentrated properties than dried ones, but both are fine. We will be using various flower petals, leaves, herbs, and fruits, as well as kitchen ingredients such as vinegar, oil, beeswax, honey, milk, cider vinegar, and so on.

If you want to use such preparations all year round, you will have to get into a rhythm of collecting and drying herbs, and sometimes use different ingredients in the winter to the summer. It takes time and effort to make and use natural products, but you will find it rewarding and well worth the effort. You can work in harmony with what Mother Nature provides. As always, she is the teacher. Be patient; not everything you make will work out and you won't like everything you produce, but every failure will increase your store of knowledge.

Just remember that real beauty is not about conforming to the airbrushed standards of the mass media. It is not about being sliced and diced by cosmetic surgeons to fit some arbitrary archetype or about the price you pay. It is about being happy and glowing in your own skin whatever your age, shape, or size, which is the most attractive thing of all. After all, witches are said to know all the means of enchantment and glamour, and that includes natural methods as well as magic!

Safety First
DO A PATCH TEST

Even with the most pure and natural ingredients, it is still possible that some people will have an allergic or sensitive reaction; anyone can be allergic to anything. When using any new product or ingredient, it is advisable to carry out a patch test by placing a tiny amount of the product on the inside of your arm and monitoring it for any adverse reactions such as itching, reddening, soreness, or a rash. If this occurs, discontinue using the product.

Basic Hygiene

Clean and sterilize all your measuring cups, bowls, containers, sieves, jars, and other tools properly, and your product is much more likely to keep longer.

Equipment Needed

- Double boiler (or a bowl over a pan of boiling water)

- Kettle

- Heatproof jug

- Heatproof bowl

- Sieves

- Coffee filters

- Wooden spoons

- Scales

- Measuring jug

Herbs for Beauty

ALOE VERA (*ALOE BARBADENSIS*) treats burns, soothes irritated skin, moisturises, and reduces wrinkles. Using fresh aloe is better, as commercial products lose some of the vital properties during processing and may be adulterated with alcohol.

BASIL (*OCIMUM BASILICUM*) detoxifies the skin and promotes circulation. In hair products it helps hair grow and reduces tangles. **Note:** Avoid basil essential oil during pregnancy.

BAY (*LAURUS NOBILIS*) fights wrinkles, treats many skin conditions, and makes a stimulating scalp treatment. **Note:** Avoid bay essential oil during pregnancy.

BIRCH (*BETULA* SP.) tones the skin and increases elasticity. **Note:** Avoid birch essential oil during pregnancy.

BLACKBERRY LEAVES (*RUBUS FRUTICOSUS*) can be used as an astringent and toner.

BURDOCK (*ARCTIUM LAPPA*) is an effective skin detoxifier and helps dry, flaky skin.

CALENDULA (*CALENDULA OFFICINALIS*) is good for any skin type but can help dry, acne-prone, and aging skin, soothing, cooling, and plumping it up.

CARROT (*DAUCUS CAROTA*) is revitalizing for mature skin and wrinkles, stimulating the formation of new cells.

CHAMOMILE (*ANTHEMIS NOBILIS*) has soothing properties and is especially useful for sensitive, mature, irritated, or chapped skin. It is an excellent skin softener that improves the texture and elasticity of the skin.

CINNAMON (*CINNAMONUM VERUM*) is filled with antioxidants and nutrients that stimulate hair growth, plump the skin, stimulate collagen growth, and tighten loose skin. **Note**: Avoid cinnamon essential oil during pregnancy.

COLTSFOOT (*TUSSILAGO FARFARA*) promotes blood flow in the scalp, which has a positive effect on greasy hair and reduces dandruff.

COWSLIP (*PRIMULA VERIS*) reduces blemishes and wrinkles.

CUCUMBER (*CUCUMIS SATIVA*) is a gentle astringent that can be used on sensitive skins and for cooling, healing, and soothing.

DANDELION FLOWERS (*TARAXACUM OFFICINALE*) can be used for large pores, age spots, blemishes, sunburn, and chapped skin.

ELDERFLOWERS (*SAMBUCUS NIGRA*) are calming, healing, and soothing, and can be used in astringents, toners, moisturisers, and aftershaves.

EVENING PRIMROSE (*OENOTHERA BIENNIS*) is very moisturising, high in gamma-linolenic acid (GLA), and helps prevent the premature aging of the skin.

EYEBRIGHT (*EUPHRASIA OFFICINALIS*) is a natural astringent effective in tightening porous, oily skin and healing acne. It also brightens the eyes.

GALANGA (*ALPINA OFFICINARUM*) has reddish brown roots that can be dried and used with orris and sandalwood as a "talcum" powder. A decoction helps heal chapped and sunburned skin.

GOTU KOLA (*CENTELLA ASIATICA*) fights wrinkles, keeps skin smooth and supple, stimulates new cell growth, and can help repair connective tissues and smooth out cellulite.

HORSE CHESTNUT FRUITS (*AESCULUS HIPPOCASTANUM*), called conkers, are used in bath oils and bath foams to make the skin soft and supple as well as reduce cellulite.

HORSETAIL (*EQUISETUM ARVENSE*) is high in silica, a constituent of collagen, and has a firming and tightening action on the skin. It can help with sagging skin, wrinkles, and aging skin. It promotes hair growth and repair.

LADY'S MANTLE (*ALCHEMILLA VULGARIS*) helps heal sore skin and prevent wrinkles. A decoction dabbed on the breasts helps to firm them.

LAVENDER (*LAVENDULA* SPP.) helps skin to heal and renew itself, fights wrinkles, and helps prevent acne. It is a natural deodorant.

LECITHIN (*SOYA*) is an emulsifying agent that acts as a deep-action skin restorative.

LEMON (*CITRUS LIMOMUM*) promotes new cell generation and regulates sebum production. It softens the skin, diminishes wrinkles, and fades freckles and age spots.

LEMONGRASS (*CYMBOPOGON CITRATUS*) is an astringent that minimises the pores and tightens the skin. It is useful for oily skin and acne.

LIME (*CITRUS AURANTIFOLIA*) can help remove dead cells from the surface of the skin.

MYRRH (*COMMIPHORA MYRRHA*) is useful for mature skin, balancing and hydrating, promoting tissue repair, and making skin look healthier and more vital.

NETTLE, STINGING (*URTICA DIOICA*) contains many minerals useful for cell regeneration and promoting youthful-looking skin. It is an astringent beneficial for oily skin and blocked pores. It is also good for dry scalps and dandruff.

OATMEAL (*AVENA SATIVA*) soothes irritated skin and is a gentle exfoliant. It can also be used to help fade age spots.

PATCHOULI (*POGOSTEMON CABLIN*) is useful for aging and chapped skin and dandruff.

PEPPERMINT (*MENTHA PIPERITA*) has a cooling effect on the skin. It nourishes dull skin and helps balance out oily skin. **Note:** Do not use peppermint essential oil during pregnancy.

PINE (*PINUS SYLVESTRIS*) helps balance, smooth, and renew skin.

PLANTAIN (*PLANTAGO MAJOR*) has emollient and moistening properties in anti-aging and dry skin formulas.

RICE FLOUR (*ORYZA SATIVA*) is good for blemishes, wrinkles, and uneven skin pigmentations. It has soothing and softening properties.

ROSE (*ROSA* SPP.) is astringent, toning, anti-inflammatory, and regenerative, promoting new cell growth. This makes it excellent for aging, dry, and sensitive skin, rehydrating and smoothing.

ROSEMARY (*ROSMARINUS OFFICINALIS*) prevents hair loss and strengthens the hair, adds lustre to dark hair, and smooths damaged hair shafts. It is also useful for treating acne. **Note:** Avoid rosemary essential oil during pregnancy.

SAGE (*SALVIA OFFICINALIS*) is astringent and also useful for wrinkles. **Note:** Avoid sage essential oil during pregnancy.

SPEARMINT (*MENTHA SPICATA*) is good for acne, dermatitis, and congested skin.

SPRUCE (*PICEA* SPP.) is antimicrobial, high in vitamin C, and useful for acne formulas, enlarged pores, and oily skin.

TURMERIC (*CURCUMA LONGA*) is antioxidant, anti-inflammatory, and antibacterial. It's useful for acne, rosacea, and eczema, as well as being a great cleanser. **Note:** It will temporarily tinge your skin yellow.

VIOLET (*VIOLA ODORATA*) is emollient, mucilaginous, and anti-inflammatory, and the leaves are used in dry skin care and to assist in healing wounds.

Facial Scrubs

Exfoliating—getting rid of the old, dead cells that clog and dull skin—is one of the most important things you can do to improve the condition of your skin. It rejuvenates your skin and leaves it glowing. Afterwards, your moisturiser and skin treatments will be better absorbed. Ground almonds, fine oatmeal and bran, and even fresh ground coffee (the tannin reduces puffiness) can be effectively used as a gentle alternative to commercial chemical products, but please do not use salt on your face, though it is fine for a body scrub. You can experiment by adding carrier oils, eggs, honey, and tiny amounts of essential oils for extra benefits. Always avoid the delicate eye area when using a facial scrub.

ALMOND FACIAL SCRUB

This scrub simply uses the ground almonds you might already have in your kitchen cupboard. Wet your face, then rub on the ground almonds. Rinse off with warm water. Finish by splashing your face with cold water to close the pores.

BRAN FACIAL SCRUB

1 LARGE EGG

½ OUNCE BRAN MEAL

2 TEASPOONS WHEAT GERM OIL

2 DROPS CALENDULA ESSENTIAL OIL

2 DROPS CHAMOMILE ESSENTIAL OIL

Beat the egg and add the bran and oils. Massage into the face with circular movements, avoiding the eye area. Rinse with warm water. The mixture will keep for 2 days in a sealed jar in the fridge.

Facial Steams

Facial steams help to deep cleanse your skin by opening the pores so that impurities are removed. It is especially useful if you have dull skin, blemishes, or clogged pores, and even more effective if you follow the steam immediately with a face mask, then tone and moisturise. You can use hot water alone, but for added benefits you can add herbs (try an herbal tea bag) or a few drops of essential oils.

Start with a clean face. Put a heatproof bowl on a mat and fill it with boiling water, add your chosen herbs, leave them to infuse for a few minutes, and then put a towel over your head and lean over the bowl to let the steam work on your face for about ten minutes, taking a break when you need to. You can then follow with a mask or just wash your face with cool water to close the pores.

HERBAL STEAM TREATMENT

2 PINTS BOILING WATER

1 TABLESPOON ROSEMARY LEAVES

1 TABLESPOON LAVENDER FLOWERS

1 TABLESPOON CHAMOMILE FLOWERS

Pour the boiling water over the herbs, leave to infuse a few minutes, and lean over the bowl, putting a towel over your head to keep in the steam.

ROSE PETAL STEAM FOR MATURE SKIN

2 PINTS BOILING WATER

1 HANDFUL OF ROSE PETALS

Pour the boiling water over the rose petals, infuse for 5 minutes, and then proceed as above.

Face Masks

Face masks have a deep cleansing effect that removes toxins, impurities, and dead skin cells, as well as unclogs your pores. They help to improve skin tone and leave it looking healthy, and they are an important part of any anti-aging or blemish-busting regime. Afterwards, your moisturiser will be better absorbed too. Face masks, especially natural ones, can be very, very messy, so it's a good idea to apply them while you are in the bath. Cleanse your face first, and if possible use one of the herbal steams in this chapter to open your pores. Apply the mask to the damp skin of your neck and face, avoiding the delicate eye area. Relax while the mask sets, leave it for the recommended time, and then wash the mask away with plenty of warm water and a washcloth. Follow with your favourite moisturiser.

SIMPLE HONEY MASK FOR DRY SKIN

Spread runny honey all over your face and neck. Relax for half an hour, and then rinse off with warm water. The honey, as well as having antibacterial properties, will nourish and feed your skin.

SIMPLE MAYONNAISE MASK

Mayonnaise is great for nourishing skin (and hair). Spread natural organic mayonnaise over your face and neck. Relax for 20 minutes and rinse off with warm water. Follow with a moisturiser.

EGG WHITE MASK FOR OILY SKIN

Take one egg and separate the white from the yolk. Whisk up the white and spread over your face. Relax for 20–30 minutes, during which time you will feel the mask tightening. Rinse off well with warm water.

. . . .
YOGURT MASK FOR OILY SKIN

Spread natural plain yoghurt over your face and neck. Leave for 20–30 minutes. Rinse off with warm water. For a mild astringent effect, you can add pureed cucumber to the yoghurt.

. . . .
NOURISHING APPLE AND MARSHMALLOW MASK

4 TEASPOONS RUNNY HONEY

2 TEASPOONS ALMOND OIL

½ OUNCE FRESH MARSHMALLOW LEAVES

4 OUNCES APPLE, PEELED AND CORED

1 EGG WHITE

Put all the ingredients in a blender to make a thick paste. Add some rice flour if it is too thin. Spread the mixture over your cleansed face and leave on for 30 minutes. Rinse off with warm water and pat the skin dry before putting on a moisturiser.

GET FRUITY

Fruits are full of vitamins and minerals. Fresh fruit's natural enzymes exfoliate, protect, and nourish the skin. You've probably heard of the benefits of alpha hydroxy acids and beta hydroxy acids in skin care, both of which are derived from fruit. The mild preparations you make from fresh fruit are safer than some of the more concentrated commercial products available.

Just put the fresh fruit in a blender or mash it by hand. Strain the resulting pulp to get rid of the excess juice. Add a little olive oil or honey to the pulp if you wish; if the fruit seems too slippery to stick to your face, add a little fine oatmeal. Apply the fruit pulp to your face, avoiding the delicate area around your eyes. Relax for twenty minutes and rinse off with warm water.

FRUITS FOR YOUR FACE

APPLE	RICH IN ANTIOXIDANTS AND VITAMINS A AND C, APPLES HELP TO MAKE THE SKIN SOFT AND GLOWING
APRICOT	NOURISHING AND REVITALISING FOR DRY AND MATURE SKIN AND RICH IN VITAMIN A
AVOCADO	RICH IN NATURAL OILS, MINERALS LIKE POTASSIUM, AND VITAMINS A, B, AND C, AVOCADO IS GREAT FOR DRY SKIN
BANANA	RICH IN NATURAL OILS, POTASSIUM AND OTHER MINERALS, AND VITAMINS A, B, C, AND E, BANANA IS SOOTHING, REFINING, CLEANSING, AND MOISTURIZING FOR ALL SKIN TYPES
BLUEBERRY	CONTAINING A VARIETY OF ANTIOXIDANTS, BLUEBERRIES HELP REPAIR DAMAGE FROM THE SUN OR ACNE, AND THEY MAY ALSO HELP THREAD VEINS
CARROT	A RICH SOURCE OF VITAMIN A, WHICH SMOOTHES WRINKLES AND REMOVES SPOTS AND BLEMISHES
CHERRY	RICH IN VITAMIN C, A, AND BETA CAROTENE, ANTIOXIDANTS AND MINERALS LIKE IRON, MAGNESIUM, AND POTASSIUM, CHERRIES HAVE SKIN-LIGHTENING AND ANTI-AGING PROPERTIES
CRANBERRY	GOOD FOR OILY SKIN AND ENLARGED PORES
CUCUMBER	A GENTLE ASTRINGENT WITH COOLING PROPERTIES, CUCUMBER IS GREAT FOR DRY AND SENSITIVE SKIN, AS WELL AS SHAVING RASH
GRAPE	CONTAINS ANTIOXIDANTS AS WELL AS ALPHA HYDROXY ACIDS, WHICH HAVE ANTI-AGING EFFECTS, USE GRAPE TO GET RID OF MINOR ACNE AND OTHER BLEMISHES

KIWI	RICH IN VITAMINS C, E, AND K, BRIGHTENS DULL SKIN AND HAS ANTI-AGING BENEFITS
MANGO	RICH IN VITAMIN C
MELON	RICH IN VITAMINS A AND C, LIGHTLY MOISTURISES AND SOOTHES
PAPAYA	REMOVES DEAD, FLAKY SKIN FOR A GLOWING, HEALTHY COMPLEXION
PINEAPPLE	THE ENZYMES IN THE PINEAPPLE GENTLY STRIP AWAY DEAD SKIN CELLS TO LEAVE THE SKIN FRESH AND GLOWING
PEACH	GOOD FOR TIRED, DULL, AND MATURE SKIN, LEAVING IT SMOOTH AND SOFT
POMEGRANATE	VERY RICH IN ANTIOXIDANTS, POMEGRANATE REJUVENATES AGING SKIN
STRAWBERRY	FULL OF VITAMIN C, REDUCES FINE LINES, WRINKLES, BLEMISHES, AND ACNE
TOMATO	GOOD FOR BOTH OILY AND DRY SKIN, REDUCES ENLARGED PORES AND ACNE
WATERMELON	RICH IN VITAMINS A, B, AND C, AND LEAVES THE SKIN SOFT AND FRESH

. . . .
Fruit Gelatine Mask

Instead of just applying the fresh fruit to your face, you can use it to make a gelatine mask. Take your chosen fruit or combination of fruits, mash them, and then push through a sieve into a double boiler. Mix in one or two sachets of vegetable gelatine. Heat, stirring, until it forms a thick paste. Allow the mixture to cool and then apply the mask to your face, avoiding the eye area. Leave on for 15–30 minutes and rinse well with warm water. The mixture will keep in the fridge for 2 days.

. . . . .

Clay Masks

Natural mineral clays have been used for millennia in face masks that refine pores, cleanse, and revitalise. Clays are rich in minerals, but different clays are suitable for particular skin types:

- red Moroccan clay (sometimes called rose clay) is good for dry or sensitive skin and is rich in magnesium and calcium

- white kaolin clay (also called white China clay) is a cheaper but effective alternative to red clay

- fuller's earth is useful for oily skin, as it has a slightly drying effect

- green clay (also called sea clay) is used to absorb oils and impurities from the skin, is rich in calcium, iron, magnesium, and potassium, and is suitable for normal or oily skin.

Powdered clays are easily sourced on the Internet, but always look for the ones that say "cosmetic grade." You can use them as they are by simply mixing in a very small amount of water, or you can add herbs, fruits, honey, and essential oils for extra benefits.

GREEN CLAY MASK FOR NORMAL SKIN

2 TABLESPOONS GREEN CLAY POWDER

1 TEASPOON HONEY

2 DROPS LAVENDER ESSENTIAL OIL

Combine all ingredients and add a very small amount of water to make a paste. Apply to the skin and allow to dry for 15–25 minutes. Rinse off with warm water, then splash your face with cold water and apply a moisturiser.

RED CLAY MASK FOR DRY SKIN

1 TABLESPOON RED CLAY POWDER

1 TABLESPOON OATMEAL

1 TEASPOON HONEY

1 TEASPOON AVOCADO OIL

1 DROP ROSE ESSENTIAL OIL

1 DROP SANDALWOOD ESSENTIAL OIL

Combine all ingredients and add a very small amount of water to make a paste. Apply to the skin and allow to dry for 15–25 minutes. Rinse off with warm water, then splash your face with cold water and apply a moisturiser.

MASK FOR OILY SKIN

2 TABLESPOONS FULLER'S EARTH POWDER

½ TEASPOON SUNFLOWER OIL

1 DROP LEMON ESSENTIAL OIL

1 DROP TEA TREE ESSENTIAL OIL

Combine all ingredients and add a very small amount of water to make a paste. Apply to the skin and allow to dry for 15–25 minutes. Rinse off with warm water, then splash your face with cold water and apply a moisturiser.

Facial Cleansers

We all know that soap is pretty harsh on the skin of the face, and most of us use proprietary cleansers. It's possible to use a facial scrub rather than a lotion or cream cleanser, but you might also like to try some of these recipes.

USING MILK

Ever wondered why some cleansers are called cleansing milks? It's because our great-grand-mothers actually used milk. To remove makeup, you can apply milk or plain yogurt to your face with a cotton ball, then rinse. It will leave your skin increasingly soft and smooth if you use it daily.

. . . .

DEEP CLEANSER

Use when your skin is tired and dull. This cleanser also helps reduce wrinkles.

SMALL POT (4 OUNCES/120 GRAMS) NATURAL LIVE YOGHURT

2 TEASPOONS RUNNY HONEY

1 TEASPOON OLIVE OIL

1 SMALL APPLE, PEELED AND CORED

1 EGG WHITE

5 DROPS ROSEMARY OIL

5 DROPS LEMON OIL

Place all the ingredients in a blender and blend on a low setting. Massage the mixture over the face. Rinse thoroughly with warm water. Place any remaining mixture in a screw-top jam jar and keep in the fridge for up to 3 days.

CUCUMBER AND HONEY CLEANSER

This potion moisturises, cleanses, and clarifies the skin.

1 OUNCE RUNNY HONEY

2 PINTS DISTILLED WATER OR RAINWATER

4 OUNCES CUCUMBER

Place the ingredients in a blender and blend on a low setting. Massage over the face and rinse with warm water.

ELDERFLOWER CLEANSER

6 ELDERFLOWER HEADS

¼ PINT NATURAL LIVE YOGHURT

1 TABLESPOON RUNNY HONEY

Wash the elderflower heads and cut off as much of the green stem as possible. Place them with the yoghurt in a pan and simmer over a very low heat for 30 minutes. Remove from the heat and leave for 4 hours. Reheat the mixture, then strain and add the honey, whipping as the mixture cools. Apply to the face with cotton wool and rinse off with warm water. Keep in airtight jars in the fridge for up to 7 days.

CLEANSING MILK

¼ OUNCE FRESH LETTUCE LEAVES

¼ OUNCE FRESH CHAMOMILE FLOWERS

¼ PINT DISTILLED WATER OR RAINWATER

2 FLUID OUNCES FULL FAT COW'S MILK

2 FLUID OUNCES RUNNY HONEY

1 TEASPOON WHEAT GERM OIL

½ OUNCE FINE CORNFLOUR (CORNSTARCH)

Place the herbs in the water and simmer for 10 minutes and allow to cool. Place in a blender with the other ingredients. Massage into the skin with your fingers and rinse off with warm water. This will keep for 2 days in a screw-top jar in the fridge.

. . . .

HEAVENLY FLUID

This sixteenth-century recipe cleanses the skin and smoothes wrinkles.

3 OUNCES RYE BREADCRUMBS

2 EGG WHITES

1 PINT CIDER VINEGAR

5 DROPS BENZOIN OIL

Put all the ingredients in a blender and blend on high speed for 1 minute. Strain through a muslin bag into a clean screw-top jar. Smooth over the skin and rinse with warm water. It will keep for 6–7 days in the fridge.

. . . .

EGGY CLEANSER

This will feed the skin as it cleanses and reduces wrinkles.

1 EGG YOLK

½ TEASPOON SUGAR

1 TABLESPOON CIDER VINEGAR

4 FLUID OUNCES EXTRA VIRGIN OLIVE OIL

Whip the egg yolk. Add the sugar and vinegar and then the oil a drop at a time, whisking vigorously until a paste is obtained. Use with a cotton wool pad and rinse off with warm water. Will keep for 3 days in the fridge.

. . . . .

Olive Oil Cleansing Cream

1 TABLESPOON BEESWAX

2 TABLESPOONS LANOLIN

3 TABLESPOONS OLIVE OIL

1 TABLESPOON SWEET ALMOND OIL

Melt the wax in a double boiler, then stir in the lanolin and oils. Remove from the heat and the double boiler and beat until cool and creamy. Spoon into clean jars. It will keep for several months.

To use, dab some onto a cotton ball and use to wipe over your face to remove dirt and impurities.

Note: Some people are allergic to lanolin.

Eye Makeup Remover

1 TABLESPOON SESAME OR OLIVE OIL

2 TEASPOONS GLYCERINE

3 TABLESPOONS ROSE WATER

Blend all ingredients together. Apply with tissue or cotton ball to remove makeup on and around the eyes.

Skin Toners

Using a toner after cleansing helps to remove any oily residue left by your cleanser as well as tone and refine the skin. You can use rose water on its own for dry, mature, and normal skin. If your skin is very oily, you can use witch hazel, though this is very astringent and you may want to dilute it with rose water or cider vinegar.

VIOLET MILK

¼ PINT MILK

A HANDFUL OF FRESH VIOLET FLOWERS

Warm the milk but do not boil. Pour it over the flowers, infuse for several hours, strain into a sealed bottle, and keep refrigerated; it will keep for 3 days. Soak cotton wool in the milk and pat over the face twice a day to improve the complexion.

GLYCERINE AND ROSE WATER FOR MATURE SKIN

1 PART GLYCERINE

1 PART ROSE WATER

Combine in a bottle and use a cotton ball to wipe over the skin after cleansing. This will keep indefinitely. If you wish, you can add a couple of drops of essential oils of your choice. Sandalwood or rose works well.

ROSE WATER AND WITCH HAZEL TONER FOR OILY SKIN

100 MILLILITRES ROSE WATER

25 MILLILITRES WITCH HAZEL

Combine in a bottle and use a cotton ball to wipe over the skin after cleansing. This will keep indefinitely. If you wish, you can add a couple of drops of essential oils of your choice. Juniper and cypress work well.

QUEEN OF HUNGARY WATER

Queen of Hungary Water first appeared in the early 1300s in Europe. There are many legends of its origin, but some say it was created by an alchemist for an aging queen of Hungary. It worked so well that a young duke asked for her hand in marriage! It was sometimes distilled as a perfume and sometimes applied to heal and tone the skin. This recipe is for a skin toner. It will tone, tighten pores, and normalise the pH of the skin. It especially benefits oily complexions.

1 PART ROSES

1 PART LAVENDER

1 PART ROSEMARY

1 PART SAGE

1 PART ORANGE PEEL

1 PART LEMON PEEL

2 PARTS MINT

CIDER VINEGAR

ROSE WATER

Pack the fresh herbs into a jar and cover with cider vinegar. Leave on a sunny windowsill for 2 weeks, shaking daily. Strain through a coffee filter and dilute half and half with rose water.

After cleansing your skin, dab a little Queen of Hungary toner on a cotton bud and wipe gently over your face, avoiding the delicate under-eye area. Follow with a moisturiser.

Moisturisers

Most people include a moisturiser in their daily skincare regimes. By making your own moisturisers, it is possible to tailor the ingredients for specific skin types and problems. However, don't expect your creams to have the same texture or shelf life that commercial creams have, though they will be made from pure and natural ingredients.

A cream or lotion is basically a mixture of water and oil. As we all know from school, oil and water don't mix, so they will need another agent to bind them together, and this is called an emulsifier. I generally use beeswax, but there are other options. You can make a basic cream just from vegetable oil, water, and emulsifying wax. Of course, you'll want to add other ingredients for their properties and natural perfumes. You can substitute herb and flower infusions or purchased floral waters (hydrosols) for the plain water, vary the oils and emulsifiers used, and add essential oils, aloe vera gel, honey, glycerine, and so on.

You can add a preservative to make your product store longer, though most of the natural creams in this book have a very short shelf life or will need to be kept in the fridge. I suggest you make small quantities and use them up quickly. Because the cost is so much less than a shop-bought cream, you can afford to use them on your body as well as your face.

THE BASIC METHOD

1. Prepare the oil part and the liquid part separately before bringing them together.

2. Combine the emulsifying wax and oil(s) in a double boiler. Most creams use a combination of pouring oils (such as grapeseed or almond) and more solid oils (such as coconut or shea butter).

3. Your water needs to be warmed in a separate pan but must reach the same temperature as the oils, as this will help the two elements combine when they come together.

4. Then the water part is dripped into the oil part very slowly as you whisk constantly with a wooden spoon, hand whisk, or electric whisk until they are fully combined and emulsified.

5. The cream is then allowed to cool down a little.

6. Now you can add other ingredients such as essential oils, glycerine, preservatives, etc.

7. Stir and quickly transfer to your storage jars before it thickens too much.

TROUBLESHOOTING

MY CREAM WON'T EMULSIFY. The two parts of your cream, the oil mix and the water mix, need to be at the same temperature. If it doesn't work the first time, allow the mixture to separate out, pour them off, and try again.

MY CREAM HAS GONE MOULDY. Using fresh or dried plant-based material in your creams is great for your skin and has many benefits, but it usually means that the cream will not last more than a few days, or a couple of weeks in the fridge. In addition, it is vital that all your equipment, including the final jars and their lids, are sterilised to prevent mould. If the recipe calls for water, distilled water is best, as tap water can contain bacteria. If using tap water, boil and cool it first.

. . . .

Basic Cream

3 FLUID OUNCES ALMOND OR GRAPESEED OIL

2 TABLESPOONS COCONUT OIL OR SHEA BUTTER

½ OUNCE BEESWAX OR EMULSIFYING WAX, GRATED

5 FLUID OUNCES ROSE WATER (ROSE HYDROSOL)

A FEW DROPS OF ESSENTIAL OIL (OPTIONAL)

In a double boiler combine the oils and wax and heat gently until they melt. Allow to cool a little without setting. Warm the rose water slightly—do not boil—until the two liquids are the same temperature. Add the rose water to the oil and wax mixture, whisking constantly as the mixture cools and thickens. Spoon into sterilised jars. Because this cream has no fresh plant material, providing that you have sterilised all your equipment, it should keep well for months.

VIOLET MOISTURISER FOR DRY SKIN

2 TABLESPOONS BOILING WATER

A HANDFUL OF FRESH VIOLET (*VIOLA ODORATA*) FLOWERS AND LEAVES

5 EVENING PRIMROSE CAPSULES

1 TEASPOON APRICOT OIL

1 TEASPOON LANOLIN

¼ OUNCE EMULSIFYING WAX

2 DROPS ROSE ESSENTIAL OIL (OR ESSENTIAL OIL OF YOUR CHOICE)

Pour the boiling water over the violet flowers and leaves and leave to infuse for 20 minutes. Meanwhile, prick the evening primrose capsules with a pin and add the resulting oil to the apricot oil, lanolin, and emulsifying wax in a double boiler. Strain the violet infusion, discarding the pulp and retaining the liquid. Gradually, drop by drop, add the warm violet infusion to the oil mixture, whisking constantly. Pour into glass jars and stopper tightly. Will keep in the fridge for up to 2 months.

MINT MOISTURISER FOR COMBINATION SKIN

A HANDFUL OF FRESH MINT

½ PINT BOILING WATER

3 TABLESPOONS COCONUT OIL

2 TABLESPOONS JOJOBA OIL

1 TABLESPOON GRAPESEED OIL

1 TEASPOON BEESWAX

½ TEASPOON POWDERED MYRRH RESIN

Infuse the mint in boiling water for 2 hours. Strain and retain the liquid. Place the oils and wax in a double boiler and melt over a low heat. Separately warm the mint infusion again and dissolve the myrrh into it. Gradually add this to the oils, remove from heat, and whisk until cool and creamy. Keeps in the fridge for up to 2 weeks.

. . . .

LINDEN MOISTURISER FOR MATURE SKIN

½ OUNCE LINDEN (*TILIA CORDATA*) LEAF BUDS,
    PICKED BEFORE THEY UNFURL

½ PINT GLYCERINE

3 FLUID OUNCES VODKA

¼ OUNCE BEESWAX

½ OUNCE COCOA BUTTER

1 OUNCE SWEET ALMOND OIL

5 TEASPOONS JOJOBA OIL

2 TEASPOONS RUNNY HONEY

10 DROPS ROSE OIL

10 DROPS JASMINE OIL

Put the crushed linden buds in a clean screw-top jam jar and cover with the glycerine and vodka. Leave for 2 weeks, shaking daily, and then strain into a clean jar. Keep this in the dark and it will store indefinitely.

Use 1 fluid ounce of the resulting linden maceration for this recipe. In a double boiler (or heatproof bowl over a pan of boiling water) melt the wax into the cocoa butter and almond and jojoba oils. Gradually add the warmed linden maceration and honey. Remove from the heat and continue to beat the mixture until it is completely cool; it will thicken as it cools. Lastly, stir in the essential oils and spoon into clean screw-top jars. Keeps in the fridge for up to 2 months.

. . . .

ROSE NIGHT CREAM FOR MATURE SKIN

2 TABLESPOONS LANOLIN

½ TABLESPOON RUNNY HONEY

½ TEASPOON GLYCERINE

1 TABLESPOON WHEAT GERM OIL

½ TABLESPOONS BEESWAX

3 TABLESPOONS ROSE WATER

10 DROPS ROSE ESSENTIAL OIL

Place everything in a pan except the rose water and rose essential oil. Put it over a very low heat, beating with a wooden spatula until the wax has melted and the ingredients are blended together. Add the rose water and continue to beat until smooth. Remove from the heat and continue beating until the mixture is cool and creamy. Add the rose oil. Bottle in an airtight jar.

Note: Some people are allergic to lanolin.

Anti-Wrinkle Serum

1 TABLESPOON LANOLIN

2 TABLESPOONS JOJOBA OIL

2 TABLESPOONS SESAME OIL

1 TABLESPOON WHEAT GERM OIL

1 TABLESPOON APRICOT OIL

1 TABLESPOON AVOCADO OIL

2 TABLESPOONS CIDER VINEGAR

4 DROPS LEMON OIL

In a double boiler melt the lanolin in the oils over a very low heat. Remove from the heat and add the cider vinegar. Keep whisking until the mixture is cool and add the lemon oil. Apply to the skin and leave for 30 minutes to 1 hour before wiping off any excess. Use regularly to achieve the best effects. The mixture will keep for a few weeks in an airtight jar.

JUST ADD ESSENTIAL OILS

If you don't want to go to the bother of making your own face creams from scratch, another option is to simply add essential oils to a bought moisturiser. For a 50 millilitre pot, don't add more than 3 drops in total. Carrot seed, chamomile, frankincense, rose, myrrh, and neroli are all great for the skin; see chapter 11 on essential oils for oils to treat your particular problem.

Eye Treatments

· · · · · · · · ·
For Puffy Eyes

½ OUNCE EYEBRIGHT (*EUPHRASIA OFFICINALIS*)

½ PINT BOILING WATER

Infuse the eyebright in the boiling water for 15 minutes, strain, and dab the cooled liquid around closed eyes with a cotton ball. An alternative to the eyebright is to use rose petals.

· · · · · · · · · ·
For Dark Circles

½ GRATED RAW POTATO

Put the grated raw potato on the affected area for 15 minutes, then rinse with cold water.

· · · · · · · · ·
For Tired Eyes

2 SLICES FRESH CUCUMBER

Place a slice of fresh cucumber over each closed eye for 10 minutes.

Neck Treatments

TOMATO NECK MASK

For an aging neck, cut a tomato into fine slices, spread over the neck, and relax for 30 minutes.

RICH NECK OIL

2 TABLESPOONS SESAME OIL

1 TABLESPOON AVOCADO OIL

1 TABLESPOON MACADAMIA OIL

40 DROPS VITAMIN E OIL

5 DROPS GERANIUM ESSENTIAL OIL

10 DROPS MYRRH ESSENTIAL OIL

10 DROPS CARROT SEED ESSENTIAL OIL

Combine the ingredients in a dark glass bottle or jar. Shake well before using. Spread over the neck, leave for 30 minutes, and wipe off any excess.

Lip Salves

Honey Lip Salve

7 TABLESPOONS OLIVE OIL

2 TEASPOONS RUNNY HONEY

6 TABLESPOONS BEESWAX, GRATED

Warm the oil and honey together (do not boil) in a double boiler. Remove from the heat and stir in the wax until it has melted. Pour into small pots and seal.

Grapefruit Lip Salve

6 TABLESPOONS BEESWAX, GRATED

7 TABLESPOONS OLIVE OIL

15 DROPS GRAPEFRUIT ESSENTIAL OIL

Warm the oil (do not boil) in a double boiler. Remove from the heat and stir in the wax until it has melted. Allow it to cool slightly and add the grapefruit essential oil. Pour into small pots and seal. You can substitute any essential oil of your choice, but stick to the ones that are derived from foodstuffs.

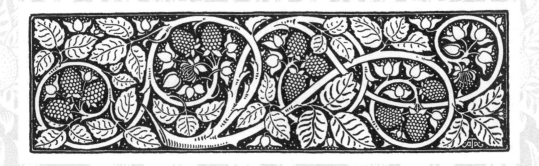

CHAPTER 8

The Witch's Garden

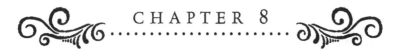

Traditionally, the wise woman's garden contained plants for healing, plants to attract and feed familiars, plants to contact the spirits, plants for divination and spells, and trees such as rowan and holly for protection.

Gardening helps us to attune to the ebb and flow of the earth's energy in its seasonal turning. I love to grow as much of what I eat as possible, plus all of my herbs for healing and magic. I know that my produce has been grown organically and that it has not been covered in toxic insecticides and weed killers.

I'm lucky enough have a fairly big garden plus a plot of land for growing vegetables, but even if you only have a patio, a couple of pots outside the front door, or simply a window box or kitchen windowsill, it is still worthwhile to grow some herbs of your own. Gardening teaches you about the magic of hope, growth, and renewal. It requires patience and observation to be in tune with your plants, and there is nothing better to teach you about herb craft.

Gardening can become a magical act in itself as you plant your seeds with intent, care for them with love, and open yourself to communicating with their spirits. The plants you grow will be much more powerful for your magical and healing practice than any you buy. This is magic in its rawest form, the meeting of human and plant spirit, and it should benefit both.

I like to have a god and goddess statue in the garden and plenty of green man representations to look after my charges.

What to Grow

What you decide to grow will depend on two things: what you want your plants for and how much space you have. You might want to grow good things to eat or focus on herbs for healing, plants for vegetable dyes, or plants to help you with your magic. You could grow elemental plants for your incenses and invocations, plants for divination and scrying, or plants for smudging.

Even if you only have a windowsill, you can grow some herbs for magical and culinary uses. In a small paved back yard you can install some pots and growbags for herbs and flowers and even raise tomatoes, beans, and salad leaves. The flavour of food picked and eaten within minutes is completely different to that of food purchased from the supermarket, which may be days or even weeks old. You are getting the full life force of the plant when it is fresh, as well as the satisfaction in knowing you have grown it yourself.

Some say you can be self-sufficient in fruit and vegetables on a 40 by 40-foot plot with good planning and a big freezer. I have a small orchard with apple, pear, plum, and cherry trees, soft fruit bushes including gooseberries, raspberries, redcurrants, blackcurrants, and loganberries, rhubarb, and two strawberry beds. In my deep beds I grow potatoes, celery, carrots, Jerusalem and globe artichokes, cauliflowers, sprouting broccoli, brussels sprouts, onions, leeks, asparagus, squashes, peas, broad beans, French beans, runner beans, and garlic, as well as a variety of herbs. In my polytunnel (sometimes called a hoophouse or a cold frame) I grow tomatoes, peppers, chillies, aubergines (eggplants), melons, cucumbers, and other less hardy plants and herbs, as well as several large herb plots where I grow healing and magical herbs, and I've just started a plot for dye plants. What you can grow will depend on the climate where you live; while I have struggled to grow oranges, lemons, and tropical herbs in my greenhouse here in England, and I have to keep my aloe vera indoors, you might be lucky enough to have them in your warmer garden, but then you might have difficulty growing the plants that do well on my plot.

Here are a few suggestions for different kinds of herb gardens:

MAGICAL GARDEN	
ANGELICA	ANISE
BASIL	BETONY
BLUEBELL	BORAGE
CINQUEFOIL	ELDER
FOXGLOVE	HAWTHORN
HAZEL	HOLLY
IVY	LAVENDER
LEMON BALM	MUGWORT
MULLEIN	PERIWINKLE
ROSE	ROSEMARY
ROWAN	SAGE
ST. JOHN'S WORT	THYME
VERVAIN	WORMWOOD
YARROW	

WINE MAKER'S GARDEN

ALECOST	ANGELICA
APPLES	BLACKBERRY
BORAGE	CALENDULA
CLOVE PINKS	COWSLIPS
GRAPE	HAWTHORN
HYSSOP	JUNIPER
LEMON BALM	MEADOWSWEET
NETTLE	PEPPERMINT
PRIMROSE	RASPBERRY
ROSEMARY	SWEET CICELY
SWEET WOODRUFF	THYME
VIOLETS	

DYER'S GARDEN

COREOPSIS	DYER'S CHAMOMILE
DYER'S WOODRUFF	DYER'S GREENWEED
HOLLYHOCK	LADY'S BEDSTRAW
MADDER	PURPLE LOOSESTRIFE
RHUBARB	ST. JOHN'S WORT
SNEEZEWORT	SUNFLOWERS
TANSY	WELD
WOAD	YARROW

HEALING GARDEN

ALOE VERA	ARNICA
CALENDULA	CHAMOMILE
CHICKWEED	DANDELION
FENNEL	FEVERFEW
GARLIC	GINGER
HEARTSEASE (PANSY)	LAVENDER
LEMON BALM	MARSHMALLOW
NETTLE	PEPPERMINT
ROSEMARY	ST. JOHN'S WORT
SKULLCAP	YARROW

COSMETICS GARDEN

ALOE VERA	CALENDULA
CHAMOMILE	CUCUMBER
DAISY, ENGLISH	ELDERFLOWER
FENNEL	LAVENDER
LEMON	MARSHMALLOW
MINT	NETTLES
PINE	ROSE
ROSEMARY	SAGE
STRAWBERRY	VIOLET

An Elemental Garden

A magical way to grow your herbs is to create an elemental garden, with herbs arranged according to whether they fall under the rulership of earth, air, fire, or water. You could have four separate beds or one round bed divided into the quarters of the compass, with the herbs planted in the relevant quadrant. You'll need a compass to work this out accurately or you can get a handy app on your phone. You can't really do this using the sun, since the sun only rises due east at the vernal equinox and only sets due west at the autumn equinox.

PLANTS FOR EAST AND AIR

AGRIMONY	ALECOST
BERGAMOT	CHERVIL
CHICORY	CLARY SAGE
COMFREY	DANDELION
DILL	DOCK
ELECAMPANE	FENUGREEK
FERN	HOREHOUND
HOUSELEEK	LAVENDER
LEMON VERBENA	LILY OF THE VALLEY
MARJORAM	MINT
PARSLEY	SAGE
SWEET CICELY	SWEET PEA
WORMWOOD	

PLANTS FOR SOUTH AND FIRE

ANGELICA	AVENS
BASIL	BAY
BETONY	CENTAURY
CINQUEFOIL	CUCKOO PINT
CORIANDER	DILL
FENNEL	GARLIC
HYSSOP	LILY OF THE VALLEY
MADDER	MANDRAKE
MUSTARD	NASTURTIUM
NETTLE	PEONY
ROSEMARY	RUE
ST. JOHN'S WORT	SUNFLOWER
TARRAGON	WOODRUFF

PLANTS FOR WEST AND WATER

ACONITE	BELLADONNA
BURDOCK	CATNIP
CEREUS	CHAMOMILE
CHERVIL	CLEAVERS
CLOVER	COLTSFOOT
COLUMBINE	CORNFLOWER
DAISY	FEVERFEW
FORGET-ME-NOT	FOXGLOVE
FREESIA	GARDENIA
GERANIUM	HELLEBORE
HEMLOCK	HYACINTH
JASMINE	LADY'S MANTLE
LILY	MALLOW
MARSHMALLOW	MEADOWSWEET
MUGWORT	MULLEIN
NARCISSUS	ORRIS (IRIS)
OX-EYE DAISY	PERIWINKLE
PLUMARIA	POPPY (RED)
PURSLANE	ROSE
SKULLCAP	SNOWDROP
STEPHANOTIS	THYME
VALERIAN	VANILLA
VIOLET	YARROW

PLANTS FOR NORTH AND EARTH

FUMITORY	HOLLYHOCK
HONEYSUCKLE	LILAC
MIMOSA	PRIMROSE
RHUBARB	SAGE
SOAPWORT	SORREL
STRAWBERRY	TANSY
TULIP	VERVAIN
VETIVER	

Starting Out

Once the ground has been cleared, you need to determine what kind of soil you have. It will be obvious whether it is very stony, sandy, or heavy clay soil that sticks together.

Take time to know and understand the requirements of your herbs. Pennyroyal, violets, and thyme are quite happy to grow between cracks in paving slabs. Feverfew, pellitory, houseleeks, and wall germanders will grow next to a wall. Some plants like shade, including alexanders, angelica, chervil, and woodruff. A clay soil supports foxgloves, mint, and parsley, while broom, lavender, and thyme will be happier on a sandy soil. Some plants are easy to grow, like poppies and foxgloves, but some take a lot more effort and care. Start with some easy ones and work up to the more difficult customers as you gain confidence.

My coven blesses all our seeds at the Ostara ritual, and this gives them a good start. Remember that all plants want to grow just as much as you want them to grow; the trick is giving them the right conditions and not doing anything to hurt or overwhelm them. One of my friends planted a bean seed, surrounded it with crystals, and then wondered why it died—the poor thing was overwhelmed by the energy field. It just needed a nice comfy pot and some damp soil. I never put crystals in my garden—the wrong ones or too many can harm. If you wish, you can bless the water you nourish your plants with, and it all adds to the love and intent behind your gardening.

Though herbs generally prefer a poor soil, most flowers and vegetables need added nutrients. Soil usually needs to be improved with plenty of organic matter to enrich its nutrient content and help it to retain water. This is done by adding manure or compost. I get my manure from the dairy farm down the road. Manure needs to be well rotted before it goes on or it may be too "hot" and will burn young plants. I also add home compost.

Every garden, however small, should have its own compost heap. You can make a wooden box from palettes and throw in all your uncooked kitchen waste—eggshells, vegetable peelings, rotten fruit, non-seeding weeds, leaves, and other soft garden matter. Do not add meat, cheese, cooked food, seeding weeds, or perennial weeds. There are supposed to be all sorts of arcane secrets to good composting, but I just keep adding stuff on the top and getting nice crumbly compost out of the bottom.

The ash from my garden fires is rich in potash, and the fruit trees and bushes get a good dressing of this every spring.

Moon Gardening

Gardening by the moon can bring a very satisfying unity to your gardening and magical work. While the moon is a constant presence in the night sky, it is ever changing. As she waxes and wanes, pulling with her the tides of the sea, she influences all that is living. As the moon waxes, the energy flows upwards into the leaves and stalks of the plant; as it wanes, the virtue travels to the roots. Plants to be harvested for their roots should be planted and gathered at the waning moon, and plants required for their flowers, leaves, and fruits should be planted and gathered at the waxing moon.

WAXING MOON

The waxing moon is a time for beginnings—things that will grow to fullness in the future. As the earth breathes out, sap rises and growth above soil is favoured. A waxing moon is the best time to sow and plant anything that yields a harvest above the soil, including flowers and blooms. In the first week following the new moon, sow leafy vegetables and plants whose flowers and seeds are the edible part. Lawns also grow well when planted at the waxing moon. Do not prune during the waxing moon, as the sap is rising in plants and they will "bleed" heavily. Repot plants during the waxing moon, as they will recover and grow better than if done at the waning moon.

FULL MOON

The full moon is a good time for positive magic—healing, blessing, and so on. Growth above soil reaches its peak now. The concentration of active ingredients in herbs and plants is highest at the full moon, when they should be picked. Yule trees that are felled on the traditional day—the third day before the eleventh full moon of the year—will keep their needles for longer than those felled later.

WANING MOON

The waning moon is a time of winding down, relinquishing old relationships and situations. It is the time to perform purifications and cleansing magic. As Mother Earth breathes in with the waning moon, her receptivity increases. Strenuous physical work is easier now than during a waxing moon, and any injuries sustained by overdoing it will heal quicker. This is a good time to prune trees and shrubs—they will "bleed" less and recover more quickly. It is also a good time to weed and hoe to banish unwanted plants and pests.

The energies of the waning moon are good for root crops. Sow root vegetables such as carrots and turnips just after the full moon, along with lettuce, which seems to respond better to waning moon energies. Do not sow flowers at this time. Do not plant anything in the week before the new moon. Cleaning out the greenhouse and clearing beds is best done at the waning moon.

THE DARK MOON

The dark moon is the last three days of the lunar cycle, when the moon is absent from the sky for three days before the new moon appears. It brings to an end the lunar cycle of growth (new moon—beginning, full moon—growth, waning moon—diminishing). The three moonless nights are a fallow period associated with death goddesses and signify the death of the old before the start of the new. It is best to do no work in the garden at this time, if possible.

Indoor Gardening

If you don't have outside space, you can still grow herbs indoors. Bear in mind your herbs will need as much light as they can get, so put them on your sunniest windowsill. You can grow them in clay or plastic pots, and I recommend the biggest you can accommodate. I occasionally buy potted herbs from the supermarket, and most people don't realise that they are actually several plants in one pot, so I always pot them on into bigger containers where they will grow bigger and live longer.

Keep your herbs watered, but don't overdo it—they should be just slightly damp; nothing kills a plant faster than overwatering. Put a saucer under the pots to catch the excess water, but never let the plants sit in water for more than half an hour. If the water is not taken up, empty it out and don't imagine it's going to save you a job later on if you leave it. When the weather is hot, plants will need to be watered more often, and bigger plants need more water than smaller ones. I can't grow some windowsill herbs like basil in the winter, as it gets too cold at night for them; any leaves that touch cold glass may well get damaged.

Try these on your windowsill:

- Basil

- Chives

- Coriander leaf (cilantro)

- Lemon balm

- Marjoram

- Mint (all kinds)

- Oregano

- Parsley

- Rosemary (the restriction of the pot will prevent it getting too big)

- Sage (again, the pot will stop it getting too big)

- Thyme

Foraging

If you don't have a garden, you can still find lots of useful plants growing wild locally. I love foraging; it just seems like getting stuff for free! I go out into the countryside, the local park, or hedgerows to pick herbs, wildflowers, nuts, and fruits.

However, responsible foraging has some rules. Loss of habitat and overpicking has lowered stocks of many native plants.

- Don't take more than a few flowers or leaves from any plant.

- Cut them with a sharp knife.

- Never pick more than you need.

- Drop them into a flat basket or trug to avoid damaging what you do pick.

- Gather herbs on a dry day, preferably in full sun if you want the flowers to be open.

- Take flowers and foliage only from large patches of the plant.

- Be careful not to damage other vegetation when picking flowers.

- Research which plants are endangered in your locality, and do not pick them. As well as being irresponsible, it may be illegal.

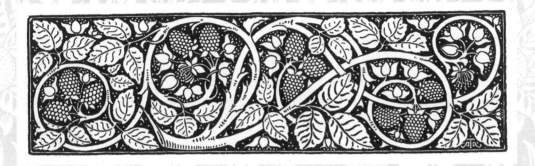

CHAPTER 9

Herbs for Healing

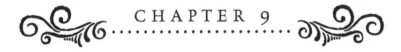

Herbs have been used since the dawn of time for healing ailments of the body. At one time all medicines were herb based; the word *drug* is derived from the Anglo Saxon *dregen*, which means "to dry" and refers to dried herbs. The wise woman often used herbs in conjunction with prayer, magic, and incantations, which no doubt helped the psychological aspect of the cure.

Though modern medicine still owes many of its cures to plant derivatives, Paracelsus's introduction of chemical drugs like sulphur, arsenic, and mercury eventually led to the preponderance of chemical remedies and the orthodox approach of the modern day in which large doses of active chemicals are used to treat the symptoms of a given disease. However, many people are increasingly unhappy with this approach and believe that there is more to curing a disease than suppressing or eliminating its symptoms.

All the chemical components of our blood and tissues are available from plants, which are natural chemical factories and energy powerhouses. From red plants we get iron; from sea plants, iodine; and so on. Some plants produce complex chemicals that appear to have no part in a plant's own metabolism but have a profound effect on the humans and animals that ingest them. This can be no accident but the reinforcing of Mother Nature's web, which links us all together in a complex, interdependent ecosystem.

The resurgence of interest in alternative medicine has led many people to be interested in herbs. They are all natural, aren't they? Well, that depends. The chemicals contained in plants can be synthesised or isolated and used in a conventional allopathic way. If you buy a jar of herbal tablets from the health food shop, read the label. If it says "standardised," it means that the active ingredient has been stripped away from the rest, leaving something akin to an allopathic drug. The scientific drive to quantify active ingredients in herbs creates herbal products that are analogous to pharmaceutical drugs. In a bid to be accepted by the medical profession, some herbalists seek to apply the scientific method and concentrate on a plant's so-called active ingredient. However, an article several years ago in JAMA on the use of ginkgo biloba to counter dementia explained that no active ingredient from among the several hundred constituents present had been determined; in fact, it was likely that the effect resulted from a complex synergistic interplay of the parts. In other words, the whole plant contains a range of chemicals that seem to work in concert.[31] This is true of all herbs: for example, a pharmaceutical diuretic normally robs the body of potassium, whereas dandelion is one of nature's best diuretics and is also a rich source of potassium.

For the hearth witch, the plant as a whole is the key; moreover, the life force or spirit of the plant is of as great an importance as any active ingredient. Hearth witches work with locally grown plants, honouring the earth and using the resources of their locality as their healing allies in an ecologically sustainable fashion.

The hearth witch recognises that health and illness are both part of life. We all suffer ill health at some time or another. The hearth witch does not see illness and disability as a personal failure to be whole.

Healing is not accomplished by the healer but by the patient and healer working together. The healer helps the patient seek their own cure and works to increase, not diminish, their personal power.

---

31 Susan Weed, www.susunweed.com

Simples

The easiest and often most effective way to use herbs for healing is as a simple, i.e., one herb at a time rather than a blend. In this way, you can, as wise woman Susun Weed puts it, match the uniqueness of the plant to the uniqueness of the patient.[32] Combining herbs with the same properties can be counterproductive. Remember, too, that when you use one plant at a time, it is much easier to discern the effect of that plant, so if someone has a bad reaction to the remedy, it is obvious what the source of the distress is and usually easy to rectify. The more herbs there are in a formula, the more likelihood there is of unwanted side effects.

Meeting the Plants

Only a few decades ago every child would have walked to school picking rose hips to make itching powder, nibbling "bread and cheese" (the hawthorn buds before they unfold in the spring), telling the time with dandelion clocks, throwing sticky buds, and playing pooh sticks. Not too long ago children knew most of their local plants and played in the open fields and parks. However, whenever I gave talks on herbalism at Pagan camps, I am always shocked to discover that two out of three people cannot even recognise an oak tree.

Begin by getting to know the plants that grow in your local area—those vegetation spirits that live with you, along your local hedgerow, meadow, park, road, or in your garden. Don't assume that medicinal plants are hard to find; dandelion, plantain, and nettles (to name just a few) are as common in cities and suburbs as in the country. Get a good field guide to help you identify them and a reputable modern herbal to tell you what they may be used for. You will need to refer to the botanical name since these names are specific, while the same common name can refer to several very different plants.

---

32   Ibid.

Safety First

Use some common sense and follow safety procedures.

- Just because something is natural does not mean that it is safe. The whole reason we use herbs is that they are little chemical factories, and many are very dangerous. Remember that anyone can be allergic to anything.

- Many herbs are incompatible with prescription medicines, so always check with your health care professional before using any herbal remedy.

- Always consult a medical practitioner if you have any acute or persistent health concerns.

- Make sure that you have looked up the method of preparation and the safe dosages.

- Pick your herbs from unpolluted locations.

- This is not a job for an amateur: do not dose people with potions until you have had proper training and know what you are doing.

- Never use herbs that can harm as well as heal.

- First make sure that you identify your herb correctly—if in any doubt at all, leave it alone.

- Do not take any herb for an extended period.

Using Your Plant

How do you extract the goodness from the plant and put it to use? You can't just eat all the herbs you want to employ, and strangely enough, some dried herbs have more medicinally active constituents than fresh ones. Herbs may be prepared in a variety of ways for internal and external use, so let's look at the basic methods.

Internal Remedies

DRIED HERBS IN CAPSULES

This is usually the way you purchase herbs from a shop, and it is the worst way to take them and the least effective. They are poorly digested, poorly utilized, often stale or ineffective, usually "standardised" (see above), and quite expensive.

HOT INFUSION

Infusions can be made from the soft green and flowering parts of an herb. Many of an herb's components—such as its minerals, vitamins, sugars, starches, hormones, tannins, volatile oils, and some alkaloids—dissolve well in water, and for this reason herbs are often taken as infusions or tisanes (which you might know as an herb tea). Generally the difference between the two is simply of strength—a standard infusion is a medicinal dose, whereas a tea, or tisane, is weaker. A "strong infusion" indicates a greater measure of herbs to water.

. . . .
STANDARD HOT INFUSION

1 OUNCE DRIED HERB OR 2 OUNCES CHOPPED FRESH HERB

1 PINT BOILING WATER

Put the herbs in a ceramic heatproof pot and pour on the boiling water. Cover (or put the lid on the teapot) and infuse for 20 minutes. Strain before use.

COLD INFUSION

Some herbs have properties, such as mucilage and bitter principles, which are destroyed by heat, so a cold infusion is made.

. . . .
STANDARD COLD INFUSION

1 OUNCE OF THE HERB

1 PINT COLD WATER

Use a non-metal container and put in the herb and water. Close the lid or cover with cling film (plastic wrap) and leave overnight. Strain before use.

DECOCTION

Some of the harder, woodier parts of a plant, such as the seeds, roots, buds, and barks, need to be boiled in water for a while. This is called a decoction. Never use an aluminium pan. If the herbs are dried, they should be pounded into a powder first.

STANDARD DECOCTION

½ OUNCE DRIED HERB OR 1 OUNCE FRESH HERB

1 PINT COLD WATER

Put the herbs in a pan and pour on the water. Cover and let the herbs macerate in the cold water for a few hours. Put the pan on the heat and bring to a boil. Simmer gently 15–20 minutes. Strain.

TINCTURES

Plant constituents are generally more soluble in alcohol than water, so tinctures are made. Alcohol will dissolve and extract resins, oils, alkaloids, sugars, starches, and hormones, though it does not extract nutrients such as vitamins or minerals. Brandy or vodka is usually used. Because a tincture is much stronger than an infusion or decoction, you only need a few drops in a glass of water as a medicinal dose. Alternatively, a few drops may be added to a salve or bath.

STANDARD TINCTURE

To make a tincture, put 4 ounces of dried herbs or 8 ounces fresh herbs into a clean jar and pour on 1 pint of vodka or brandy. Seal and keep in a warm place for 2 weeks, shaking daily. Strain and store in a dark bottle.

SYRUPS

Some bitter-tasting herbs are more palatable when taken in the form of syrup, particularly for children.

STANDARD SYRUP

To make syrup, for every 1 pint of infusion or decoction, add 1 pound of sugar and heat gently until the sugar is dissolved. This will need to be kept in the fridge. If you wish, you can use honey instead of sugar.

HERBAL VINEGARS

By placing a few springs of herbs in vinegar, you can make an herbal vinegar that is not only pleasant tasting, but also therapeutic. Try garlic cloves, tarragon, thyme, rosemary, or dill, alone or in any combination that appeals to you.

External Remedies

BATHS

Add 1 pint of herbal infusion or decoction to the bathwater and soak.

STEAM INHALATIONS

Steam inhalations of herbs may be used to relieve cold symptoms (peppermint, thyme, and ginger, for example) and hay fever (yarrow).

· · · · · · · · · · · · · · · · · ·

STANDARD STEAM INHALATION

2 PINTS BOILING WATER

2 TEASPOONS HERB

Pour the boiling water over the herb, and with a towel over your head, inhale the vapour for about 5 minutes.

SALVES

Herbs can be made into salves or ointments, which can then be applied to the affected area.

· · · · · · · · · · · · · · ·

BASIC SALVE METHOD 1

8 OUNCES PETROLEUM JELLY OR UN-PATROLEUM JELLY

2 TABLESPOONS HERB

Place the jelly and the herb in a double boiler. Simmer for 20 minutes. Strain into warm glass jars.

BASIC SALVE METHOD 2

8 FLUID OUNCES OLIVE OIL

2 TABLESPOONS HERB

5-6 OUNCES BEESWAX, GRATED

In a double boiler simmer the herb in the oil for 20 minutes. Strain and return the oil to the pan, add the beeswax, and melt. Pour into warm glass jars. This is my preferred method.

COMPRESSES

Prepare a clean cotton cloth and soak it in a hot infusion or decoction. Use this as hot as possible on the affected area (take care and do not burn yourself). Change the compress as it cools down and apply it up to four or five times in one session.

POULTICE

Bruise fresh herbs, apply directly to the skin, and cover with a cloth.

COLD INFUSED OIL

Fats and oils extract the oily and resinous properties of an herb, which are often the antibacterial, antifungal, and wound-healing components.

STANDARD COLD INFUSED OIL

To make a cold infused oil, cut up the herb and cover with vegetable oil (olive, sunflower, etc.) in a glass bottle or jar. Leave on a sunny windowsill for 2 weeks, shaking daily. Strain into a clean jar. Infused herbal oils may be used as they are or thickened into salves with beeswax. Unlike essential oils, they do not need to be diluted for use.

HEAT-MACERATED OILS

Using a hot maceration gives you a quicker result than a cold oil infusion.

STANDARD HEAT-MACERATED OIL

Put the chopped herb in a double boiler and cover with a vegetable oil (sunflower, olive, etc.). Simmer very gently, covered, for 2 hours. Turn off the heat and allow the oil to cool before straining.

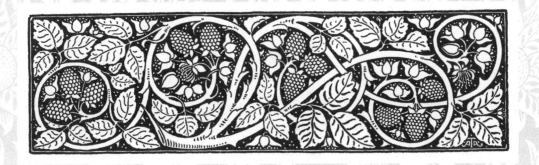

CHAPTER 10

Home Remedies

I f you have any health problems, always consult your doctor to get them checked out in the first instance. You can use herbs to treat some common complaints such as coughs and colds at home, but please bear in mind that although many herbal remedies are safe when used correctly, they may also have side effects, just like any prescription medication. Many herbs can be dangerous or even deadly when misused. Some herbs can interact with other medicines such as oral contraceptives or heart medications, so please do read through all the cautionary notices and discuss your intended use of herbs with your medical practitioner.

Anxiety

. . . .

CHAMOMILE TEA

Chamomile contains two chemicals that promote relaxation, apigenin and luteolin.

1 CUP BOILING WATER

A HANDFUL OF CHAMOMILE FLOWERS

Pour the water over the flowers, infuse 10 minutes, strain, and drink. Sweeten with honey if you wish.

Caution: Chamomile is generally considered a safe herb, but it should not be taken by people who are allergic to it or any of the daisy and chrysanthemum family. It is advisable to avoid chamomile if you are on blood-thinning medication, sedatives, aspirin, or NSAIDS and if you are pregnant or breastfeeding. It may interact with ginkgo biloba, garlic, saw palmetto, St. John's wort, and valerian.

. . . .

EPSOM AND LAVENDER BATH

A warm bath is very soothing, and lavender, chamomile, and the magnesium in Epsom salts have all been shown to reduce anxiety.

½ CUP EPSOM SALTS

A FEW DROPS OF LAVENDER ESSENTIAL OIL

A FEW DROPS OF CHAMOMILE ESSENTIAL OIL

Mix the oils into the salts with the back of a metal spoon. Pour into the bath after it has run and swirl it around.

Caution: The use of Epsom salts should be avoided by diabetics.

CALMING TEA

1 OUNCE DRIED PEPPERMINT

½ OUNCE DRIED LEMONGRASS

1 OUNCE DRIED LEMON BALM

½ OUNCE DRIED CATNIP

1 OUNCE DRIED CHAMOMILE FLOWERS

¼ OUNCE DRIED LAVENDER FLOWERS

Combine the ingredients and store in an airtight tin. To use, put 2 teaspoons in a teapot and pour on a cup of boiling water. Infuse for 10 minutes, strain, and drink with a spoonful of honey (optional).

Caution: Avoid if you are on blood-thinning medication, pregnant, or breastfeeding.

VALERIAN AND LEMON BALM TEA

Several studies have shown that valerian reduces anxiety and stress. Preliminary research shows lemon balm can reduce some symptoms osf anxiety such as nervousness and excitability.

1 OUNCE DRIED LEMON BALM LEAVES

½ OUNCE DRIED VALERIAN ROOT

Powder the ingredients in a coffee grinder or by hand in a pestle and mortar, and store in an airtight tin. To use, put 2 teaspoons in a teapot and add a cup of boiling water. Infuse for 10 minutes, strain, and drink with a spoonful of honey (optional).

Caution: Valerian is generally considered safe at recommended doses, but don't take it for more than a few weeks at a time. In some people it can cause mild side effects such as headaches and drowsiness, so it is best taken at bedtime. Lemon balm is generally well-tolerated and considered safe for short-term use, but excessive use can cause nausea and abdominal pain. It should be avoided if you have an underactive thyroid.

Arthritis and Rheumatism

Arthritis is an umbrella term that encompasses over 120 diseases and conditions that affect joints, surrounding tissues, and connective tissues. Osteoarthritis is thought to be due to the wear and tear on the cartilage that protects the joint, while rheumatoid arthritis is an autoimmune disorder where the tissues surrounding the joint are attacked by the body's own immune system. Arthritis is a chronic condition that conventional medicine finds hard to treat and impossible to cure. Studies have found that a meat-free diet is beneficial, and many have found relief by avoiding certain foods such as wheat, sugar, fats, salt, caffeine, and nightshade plants (such as tomatoes, potatoes, peppers, and aubergines/eggplants). There are several herbs with anti-inflammatory properties, some of which have been shown to be as effective as non-steroidal anti-inflammatory drugs (NSAIDs).

. . . .

GINGER AND NETTLE TEA

Ginger contains an anti-inflammatory compound called gingerol. This and other components in ginger have been found to reduce inflammation. It has properties similar to those of non-steroidal anti-inflammatory drugs (NSAIDs), including interfering with the pathway that leads to chronic inflammation.

1 OUNCE GROUND DRIED NETTLE LEAVES

½ OUNCE POWDERED GINGER

Powder the nettle leaves and combine with the ginger powder. To use, put 2 teaspoons in a teapot and add a cup of boiling water. Infuse for 10 minutes, strain, and drink with a spoonful of honey (optional).

You can also use the ingredients fresh: put a small handful of fresh nettle leaves and half-inch of peeled and grated fresh ginger in a teapot and pour on the boiling water. Infuse 15 minutes, strain, and drink with a little honey (optional).

. . . .

NETTLE TEA

Rich in minerals and anti-inflammatory properties, a cup of nettle tea a day can help reduce inflammation, prevent water retention, and support the kidneys and adrenal glands.

STINGING NETTLE (*URTICA DIOICA*) LEAVES, DRIED OR FRESH

Powder the nettle leaves. To use, put 2 teaspoons in a teapot and add a cup of boiling water. Infuse for 10 minutes, strain, and drink with a spoonful of honey (optional). You can also use the leaves fresh by putting a small handful in a teapot and pouring on the boiling water and infusing for 10 minutes. Nettle tea bags are also commercially available.

Caution: Stinging nettle is considered safe for most people, but it should be avoided if pregnant or breastfeeding. It can lower blood sugar and blood pressure, so if you are diabetic or have low blood pressure, you should monitor your levels. Do not take if you have kidney problems.

. . . .

NETTLE SYRUP

1 POUND YOUNG NETTLE TOPS

2 PINTS WATER

SUGAR

Boil for 1½ hours, then strain the liquid into a clean pan and add 1 pound of sugar for every pint of water. Boil for 30 minutes and bottle in sterilised bottles. Keep refrigerated. Use within 2 weeks after opening. Take 1 teaspoon 3 times a day.

Caution: Stinging nettle is considered safe for most people, but it should be avoided if pregnant or breastfeeding. It can lower blood sugar and blood pressure, so if you are diabetic or have low blood pressure, you should monitor your levels. Do not take if you have kidney problems.

. . . . .

Meadowsweet Compress

Like willow bark, meadowsweet contains salicylic acid, the painkilling substance from which aspirin was developed. When applied as a compress, it has an anti-inflammatory effect and helps to relieve pain in joints.

Prepare a clean cotton cloth and soak it in a hot infusion of meadowsweet. Use this as hot as possible on the affected area (do take care and do not burn yourself). Change the compress as it cools down by resoaking it in the hot infusion and reapplying it. You can do this up to four or five times per session.

Celery Water

Celery contains over twenty-five anti-inflammatory compounds, as well as providing potassium (potassium deficiency may be a culprit of arthritic pain). Celery also promotes sleep, increases urine flow, promotes muscle relaxation, decreases blood sugar, and lowers blood pressure.

1 STICK CHOPPED CELERY

½ PINT WATER

Boil the celery in the water for 4 minutes. Turn off the heat and leave for 10 minutes. Strain and drink a cup daily.

Caution: Avoid celery supplements if you have kidney problems, low blood pressure, a bleeding disorder, or if you are taking Levothyroxine, lithium, or sedatives.

Coconut Oil Rub

One study found that the unique coconut oil antioxidants reduced the inflammation associated with arthritis more effectively than current pharmaceutical drugs.[33] Coconut oil has anti-inflammatory properties that can reduce swelling and pain when applied topically or taken internally. Be sure to use virgin coconut oil though, as the refined ones have little of the active ingredients necessary to be effective.

---

33 "Polyphenolics Isolated from Virgin Coconut Oil Inhibits Adjuvant Induced Arthritis in Rats Through Antioxidant and Anti-inflammatory Action," http://www.ncbi.nlm.nih.gov /pubmed/24613207?dopt=.

Just heat some virgin coconut oil till it gets lukewarm and massage it into your painful joints two or three times a day. Heating the oil increases blood supply to the area and increases absorption of the oil.

CASTOR OIL AND JUNIPER RUB

Warm some castor oil slightly, add a few drops of juniper essential oil, and massage into the affected parts to help reduce pain.

OLIVE OIL AND EUCALYPTUS RUB

Eucalyptus oil has natural anti-inflammatory properties and helps reduce stiffness. Olive oil is also beneficial for arthritis.

30 MILLILITRES OLIVE OIL

10 DROPS EUCALYPTUS ESSENTIAL OIL

Put the olive oil into a dropper bottle and add the eucalyptus oil. Massage into affected areas to reduce pain.

TURMERIC AND GINGER TEA

Like turmeric, ginger contains anti-inflammatory properties.

1 PINT WATER

½ TEASPOON TURMERIC POWDER

1 INCH FRESH GINGER ROOT, PEELED AND GRATED

Bring water to boil, add the turmeric and ginger, and simmer for about 10 minutes. Strain and drink sweetened with a little honey (optional).

Caution: Avoid if you are a diabetic or on blood-thinning medication and for two weeks before surgery.

. . . .

COCONUT AND TURMERIC BEDTIME DRINK

Turmeric (Curcuma longa), a plant of the ginger family, is known to have many health benefits. It contains curcumin, a powerful antioxidant and anti-inflammatory; curcumin downregulates the production of chemicals that play a vital role in the spread of inflammation. Some studies have found turmeric to be as effective as non-steroidal anti-inflammatory drugs and without their side effects such as damage to the gastrointestinal system and kidneys. This drink is soothing, calming, and will help you sleep.

1 CUP COCONUT MILK

1 TEASPOON TURMERIC

½ INCH GINGER ROOT, PEELED AND GRATED

1 TEASPOON HONEY

Warm the milk, ginger, and turmeric in a pan, strain, add the honey, and drink before bed.

Caution: The use of turmeric as a spice is considered safe for adults and children alike—people have been eating it on a daily basis in India for thousands of years. As a supplement, for adults 1200–2100 mg of curcumin a day for 2–6 weeks is considered safe. However, turmeric is known to lower blood sugar and is a blood-thinning agent, so it should be avoided by diabetics, if you are on blood-thinning medication, and for two weeks before surgery.

. . . .

TURMERIC TEA

1 PINT WATER

1 TABLESPOON TURMERIC POWDER

Bring the water to a boil, add the turmeric, and boil for 10 minutes. Remove from the heat and allow to cool. Drink within 4 hours.

Caution: See caution for coconut and turmeric bedtime drink, above.

. . . .

Chilli Salve

Cayenne contains a substance called capsaicin, which helps reduce pain by blocking pain signals to the brain.

4 FRESH CHILLIES (CAYENNE), CHOPPED

½ CUP SUNFLOWER OIL

1 TABLESPOON BEESWAX

Put the chillies and oil in a double boiler and simmer for 40–50 minutes. Strain out the chillies and return the oil to the pan. Add the beeswax and stir until it has melted. Pour into warmed, sterilised glass jars. Apply directly to your joints.

Caution: Wash your hands after handling the chillies, and avoid touching the eye area.

. . . .

Chilli Oil

1 OUNCE CHILLI POWDER OR 3 CHOPPED CHILLIES

1 PINT SUNFLOWER OIL

Heat chillies and oil in a double boiler for 2 hours. Strain and massage into the affected areas.

Caution: Do not exceed the recommended amount, as it can cause skin irritation. Avoid touching the eyes or cuts after handling chillies.

. . . .

Apple Cider Vinegar

1 TABLESPOON APPLE CIDER VINEGAR

¼–½ PINT WATER

HONEY (OPTIONAL)

Mix apple cider vinegar in a glass of warm water and add honey if desired. Take 3 times a day.

Athlete's Foot

Athlete's foot is a fungal infection that grows between the toes or fingers and on nails, causing white or scaly patches, redness, and itching. It proliferates on damp feet, especially those inclined to be sweaty, so make sure that you wash and, more importantly, dry your feet and hands well.

. . . .

TEA TREE RUB

20 DROPS TEA TREE ESSENTIAL OIL

30 MILLILITRES CARRIER OIL

Combine the tea tree essential oil and carrier oil (you can use sunflower oil, almond oil, etc.). Use to massage into the feet twice a day.

. . . .

CIDER VINEGAR FOOT SOAK

½ PINT CIDER VINEGAR

2 TABLESPOONS SALT

2 PINTS WARM WATER

Combine the cider vinegar, salt, and water in a foot bath or large bowl and soak your feet for 15–20 minutes. Dry your feet thoroughly and follow with a tea tree rub (see above).

. . . .

COMFREY FOOT SALVE

A SMALL HANDFUL OF ROSEMARY LEAVES, CHOPPED

A HANDFUL OF COMFREY ROOT, CHOPPED

OLIVE OIL

BEESWAX

Put the rosemary and comfrey in a double boiler and cover with the oil. Simmer very gently for 30 minutes and strain. Return the herb-infused oil to the clean pan and add some beeswax—the more you add, the harder the set. When the wax has melted, put the salve into clean jars, put on the lids, and label. Rub into the feet once or twice a day.

. . . . .

ANTIFUNGAL FOOT POWDER

Cloves contain eugenol, which is an antifungal agent, while oregano contains two powerful compounds, carvacrol and thymol, which fight fungal and bacterial infections. Calendula is also a very powerful fungus fighter, and tea tree oil is one of the best antifungal herbal helpers there is.

4 TABLESPOONS DRIED AND POWDERED OREGANO LEAVES

4 TABLESPOONS DRIED AND POWDERED CALENDULA FLOWERS

½ TEASPOON POWDERED CLOVES

7 TABLESPOONS CORNFLOUR (CORNSTARCH)

7 TABLESPOONS BICARBONATE OF SODA (BAKING SODA)

20 DROPS TEA TREE ESSENTIAL OIL

Grind up the herbs in a pestle and mortar and mix in the cornflour and soda. Add the tea tree oil and mix in with the back of a metal spoon. You can put the mixture in an old talcum powder tin or a salt shaker. Apply to the feet morning, evening, and night.

Bloating

· · · · · · · · · ·

CARAWAY TEA

½ OUNCE CARAWAY SEEDS

½ OUNCE FENNEL SEEDS

½ OUNCE ANISEED

Crush the seeds in a pestle and mortar. They can be stored for later use in an airtight jar or tin. To use, place 2 teaspoons of the seeds in a teapot, add a cup of boiling water, and infuse for 10 minutes. Pour through a strainer into a cup and drink after meals if you have a tendency to bloat after eating.

· · · · · · · · · ·

PMT BLOAT TEA

If you bloat and retain water before your period, dandelion can help your premenstrual tension. It is a diuretic, but unlike pharmaceutical diuretics, it doesn't rob the body of potassium. The leaves are also very rich in vitamin A, vitamin C, and iron.

2 DANDELION LEAVES

½ PINT BOILING WATER

HONEY TO TASTE (OPTIONAL)

Infuse the leaves in the boiling water. Strain, add the honey, and drink up to 2 cups a day.

Blocked Sinuses

CHAMOMILE AND PEPPERMINT STEAM

Add a small handful of chamomile flowers and peppermint leaves (or a few drops of chamomile and peppermint essential oils) to a bowl of boiling water. Put a towel over your head and inhale the steam for a few minutes. An alternative is to use eucalyptus essential oil.

Caution: Avoid the use of peppermint and chamomile essential oils if you are pregnant. Chamomile helps relieve inflammation in the sinuses and loosens phlegm.

GINGER COMPRESS

You may also find this compress beneficial for arthritis pain when applied to the inflamed joint.

1 TABLESPOON GRATED FRESH GINGER ROOT

½ PINT WATER

Tie the ginger in a piece of muslin and put in a pan. Add the water, bring to a boil, and then allow to cool to just warm. Remove the ginger piece and discard. Soak a clean cloth or piece of flannel in the water and place over your forehead and nose (avoid the eyes). As it cools, soak it in the water again and reapply. Keep repeating this process for four or five times per session. If the skin becomes irritated, discontinue.

Boils

. . . .

HORSETAIL COMPRESS

The antimicrobial and anti-inflammatory activity of horsetail may help with the inflammation and infection caused by boils and carbuncles.

DRIED HORSETAIL HERB

WARM WATER

Infuse the herb in the warm water for 15 minutes. Strain. Soak a clean cloth in the liquid and apply to the boil 2 or 3 times a day to reduce the inflammation and draw out the pus.

. . . .

MARSHMALLOW PASTE

Mix 1 teaspoon of powdered marshmallow root with a little water and apply to the affected area. Cover with a warm cloth.

. . . .

SLIPPERY ELM POULTICE

Make a paste with warm water and powdered slippery elm and apply to the affected area. Cover with a warm cloth. Repeat daily for several days.

Bruises

COMFREY COMPRESS

Use a cold compress made from a clean cloth soaked in a comfrey infusion and apply to the affected area.

COMFREY SALVE

1 OUNCE COMFREY LEAVES

¼ PINT OLIVE OIL

1 TABLESPOON BEESWAX

Put the comfrey leaves and olive oil in a double boiler and warm over low heat for 30 minutes. Strain. Return to the pan and add the beeswax. Allow the wax to melt, then pour into clean jars.

Burns

. . . .

MARIGOLD OINTMENT

This is good for burns and as an antiseptic cream.

½ PINT OLIVE OIL

½ POUND FRESH MARIGOLD FLOWERS

2 OUNCES BEESWAX

Warm the oil (do not boil) and add the petals, trying to avoid the green parts. Simmer very gently for 30 minutes and strain out the flowers. Add the wax and melt in. Remove from the heat and stir continually while it cools. Spoon into clean jars and label.

. . . .

ALOE VERA

Break open the stem of an aloe vera leaf and apply to the affected area.

Cold Sores

. . . .

LEMON BALM TINCTURE

Several studies support lemon herbal extract as an effective cold sore remedy. One study found that lemon balm used as lip cream decreased symptoms of cold sores after two days. In most studies lemon balm was applied two to four times a day for five days or more to promote healing.

FRESH LEMON BALM LEAVES

VODKA

Pack the lemon balm leaves into a clear glass jar and top up with vodka. Leave on a sunny windowsill for 2 weeks, shaking daily. Strain the liquid into dropper bottles. Use a cotton bud to dab onto the affected area 4–5 times a day.

. . . .

LEMON BALM LIP SALVE

FRESH LEMON BALM LEAVES

VEGETABLE OIL (SUNFLOWER, RAPESEED, OLIVE, ETC.)

BEESWAX

Put the lemon balm leaves in a clear glass jar, cover them with the oil, and put on the lid. Leave on a sunny windowsill for 2 weeks, shaking daily. Strain off the oil into a double boiler and warm gently. Add some beeswax (the more you add, the harder the set) and pour into small wide-necked jars or little tins.

Colds and Flu

. . . .

HONEY AND LEMON TEA

Put the juice from one lemon (rich in vitamin C) into a cup and top up with boiling water. Add a couple of teaspoons of honey (which has antiviral properties).

. . . .

PEPPERMINT AND EUCALYPTUS STEAM

Steam treatments help soothe mucus membranes and moisturise the respiratory tract. The menthol in peppermint oil soothes the throat and acts as a decongestant. Eucalyptus helps expel phlegm, decongest the airways, and boost the immune system.

BOILING WATER

6 DROPS PEPPERMINT ESSENTIAL OIL

6 DROPS EUCALYPTUS ESSENTIAL OIL

Put a heatproof bowl on a heatproof mat and pour in the boiling water. Add the essential oils. Lean over the bowl, put a towel over your head, and inhale the steam.

Caution: Avoid the use of peppermint oil if you are pregnant.

. . . .

ELDERBERRY ROB

2½ POUNDS ELDERBERRIES

½ POUND SUGAR

Simmer together in a saucepan until it thickens to the consistency of runny honey. Strain and bottle. Take a couple of tablespoons in warm water for colds, fevers, and coughs. If you like, you can add a little whiskey. Once opened, store in the fridge for up to 2 months.

. . . .

ROSEHIP TEA

Rosehips contain twenty times more vitamin C than oranges, so they are an excellent immune system booster to prevent or treat a cold.

1 OUNCE FRESH ROSEHIPS (*ROSA CANINA*, WILD OR DOG ROSE)

½ PINT WATER

A DASH OF LEMON JUICE

Cut the rosehips open, put them in a pan with the water, and bring to a boil. Turn off the heat and allow the rosehips to infuse for 15 minutes. Strain the liquid through a very fine sieve or a coffee filter (rosehips contain irritant hairs). Add the lemon juice.

. . . .

ROSEHIP SYRUP

Rosehip syrup is a well-known childhood remedy for boosting vitamin C levels and keeping winter infections away.

ROSEHIPS (*ROSA CANINA*, WILD OR DOG ROSE)

WATER

SUGAR

Crush the rosehips (or preferably chop them up in a food processor) and put them in a pan. Cover with water, bring to a boil, and then turn down the heat and simmer for 20 minutes, uncovered. Strain through fine muslin (rosehips contain very fine irritant hairs, so don't be tempted to squeeze it through the bag) and measure the liquid.

For each pint, you will need 11 ounces of sugar. Put the liquid and sugar in a large pan and heat slowly, stirring, until the sugar has dissolved. Turn up the heat and bring to a boil for 3 minutes, skimming off any scum that appears. Pour into warmed and sterilised bottles and seal. Allow the bottles to cool. Label. This will keep unopened for 3–4 months, but refrigerate after opening.

· · · · · · · · · · · ·

ANTIVIRAL TINCTURE

Make this in advance of the winter, and take 2 teaspoons up to 5 times a day when you have an infection.

4 CLOVES GARLIC

1 ONION

4 TEASPOONS FRESH CHILLIES

2 TABLESPOONS GRATED FRESH GINGER ROOT

CIDER VINEGAR

Chop the garlic, onion, and chillies, add the ginger, and pack into a jar. Cover with cider vinegar and put on a sunny windowsill for 2 weeks, shaking daily. Strain through a fine cloth into a clean jar and label.

Constipation

. . . .

SYRUP OF FIGS

Senna is a natural herbal laxative, and the figs and prunes contain fibre that helps the whole process along.

8 OUNCES FIGS

8 OUNCES PRUNES

8 FLUID OUNCES HONEY

4 OUNCES POWDERED SENNA

Mash the figs and prunes together (you can put them in a food processor). Slightly warm the honey and stir in the senna powder, then combine with the fig and prune mixture. Spoon into a clean glass jar and secure with an airtight lid. When you are constipated, take ¼–½ teaspoon before bed.

Note: Do not exceed the stated dose, and do not take for more than 4 days.

Caution: Do not use senna if you have abdominal pain or diarrhoea or if you are pregnant, breastfeeding, have heart disease, a potassium deficiency, Crohn's disease, or if you are taking heart medication, blood-thinning, or diuretic drugs.

Corns

If badly fitting shoes keep rubbing on the same spot, the skin builds up a callus to protect itself, and this can develop into a corn, which is a callus with a hard core. These are usually painless, if unsightly, but if they press on a nerve or bone they can be very uncomfortable.

EPSOM SALT FOOTBATH

Rub the corns gently with a pumice stone (available from pharmacies), but don't go too deep. Soak your feet for 20 minutes in a basin of warm water with Epsom salts dissolved in it. Apply castor oil afterwards to keep the corns moisturised.

Caution: Avoid Epsom salts if you are diabetic.

Coughs

Coughing is a reaction to irritation of the throat or lungs caused by viruses, bacteria, dust, pollen, etc. Many of the so-called active ingredients of over-the-counter cough medicines have been proven to be ineffective, but there are many natural ways to treat your cough.

Do remember that while most coughs are the result of a short-term illness or irritation, a persistent cough can indicate an ongoing health problem. If you have a cough for more than two weeks, you should see your doctor.

. . . .

GARLIC HONEY

Honey has been used for centuries as a remedy for sore throats, coughs, and colds. It has been found to relieve coughs more effectively than many over-the-counter medicines.[34] *Both honey and garlic have antibacterial and antiviral properties.*

Peel and crush 2 whole heads of garlic. Mix into a cup of honey. Take 1 teaspoon for coughs, colds, and sore throats as needed.

. . . .

THYME AND LEMON TEA

In Germany thyme is an officially approved treatment for coughs, bronchitis, and upper respiratory infections. It contains compounds that help relax the tracheal and ileal muscles and reduce inflammation.

2 TEASPOONS FRESH THYME LEAVES

½ PINT BOILING WATER

2 TEASPOONS HONEY

2 TEASPOONS LEMON JUICE

Pour the boiling water over the crushed thyme leaves and steep for 10 minutes. Strain and stir in the honey and lemon.

Caution: Thyme is considered safe when consumed in normal food amounts or taken as a medicine for a short period of time. However, avoid medicinal amounts if you are pregnant or breastfeeding, on blood-thinning medication, before surgery, or if you have a condition made worse by exposure to oestrogen.

---

34 "Effect of Honey, Dextromethorphan, and No Treatment on Nocturnal Cough and Sleep Quality for Coughing Children and Their Parents," http://www.ncbi.nlm.nih.gov/pubmed/18056558.

. . . .

Ginger and Lemon Tea

Ginger has antihistamine and decongestant capabilities that help ease colds and flu.

2-INCH PIECE OF GINGER ROOT, PEELED AND GRATED

1 PINT WATER

JUICE OF HALF A LEMON

1 TABLESPOON HONEY (OPTIONAL)

Put the ginger and water in a pan. Simmer for 20 minutes. Strain the liquid into a jug and add the lemon and honey. Drink a cup up to 3 times daily.

. . . .

Herbal Cough Drops

Aniseed and elecampane are good for relieving coughs. Hyssop soothes and moistens sore throats. Ginger reduces inflammation and boosts your immune system. The mucilage in marshmallow is wonderful for inflamed throats and soothes coughs. Thyme is antibacterial and antiviral, while honey is soothing, antibacterial, and antiviral.

If you don't have all these herbs, you can just use some of them or substitute anti-inflammatory chamomile, decongestant cinnamon, antiseptic cloves, immune-boosting echinacea, soothing liquorice, cough-relieving mullein leaf, or sage, which is a great all-rounder for sore throats, coughs, and inflammation.

½ TEASPOON CRUSHED ANISEED

2 TABLESPOONS ELECAMPANE

3 TEASPOONS GRATED FRESH GINGER ROOT

2 TABLESPOONS HYSSOP

1 TABLESPOON CHOPPED MARSHMALLOW ROOT

1 TABLESPOON THYME

1 PINT BOILING WATER

12 FLUID OUNCES HONEY

Cover the herbs with boiling water and allow to infuse for 20 minutes. Strain. Use ½ pint of the resulting infusion and put it in a pan with the honey. Cook over medium heat until the mixture reaches setting point—drop a bit of the

. . . . .

mixture in very cold water and see if it sets to a hard lump. Remove the pan from the heat and pour the syrup into a greased baking tray. When it has cooled, you can break it into pieces.

. . . .
GINGER SYRUP

4 OUNCES FRESH GINGER ROOT

2 PINTS WATER

RIND OF 1 LEMON

SUGAR

Put the ginger and lemon in a pan, bring to a boil, and simmer for 45 minutes. Strain. To every pint of liquid, add 1 pound sugar and the juice of 1 lemon. Put in a clean pan and boil 10 minutes. Cool and bottle. For coughs and colds, take 1 tablespoon in hot water. Keep refrigerated and use within 2 months after opening.

. . . .
QUEEN ELIZABETH'S ELECTUARY

This is good for coughs, colds, and indigestion.

1 PINT HONEY

BUNCH OF HYSSOP, BRUISED

¼ OUNCE LIQUORICE ROOT

¼ OUNCE ANISEED

⅛ OUNCE ELECAMPANE ROOT

⅛ OUNCE ANGELICA ROOT

A PINCH OF PEPPER

¼ OUNCE FRESH GINGER ROOT

Boil the honey and skim off the scum. Add the hyssop and simmer for 30–40 minutes. Strain off the honey and add the other ingredients. Simmer 10 minutes, then strain off and bottle.

Caution: Not suitable if you are diabetic or have high blood pressure.

. . . . .

. . . .

Horehound Cough Sweets

2 PINTS BOILING WATER

1 OUNCE DRIED HOREHOUND (*MARRUBIUM VULGARE*)

DEMERARA SUGAR

CREAM OF TARTAR

Pour the boiling water over the herb. Cover and infuse 30 minutes. Strain through muslin and squeeze out all the juice. For every 2 cups of infusion you have, add 2 cups of demerara sugar and 1 teaspoon cream of tartar. When the sugar has melted, bring to a boil and continue boiling until setting point is reached (drop a little of the mixture into cold water and see if it hardens). Pour into a buttered Swiss roll tin. When slightly cool, mark into squares and allow to set.

. . . .

Honey and Lemon Cough Syrup

2 LEMONS

¼ PINT RUNNY HONEY

2 FLUID OUNCES GLYCERINE

Juice the lemons and strain through muslin to get a clear liquid. Add the honey and glycerine and mix together well. Bottle and refrigerate. Use within 2 months after opening. Take a tablespoonful as required.

. . . .

Cough Drops

2 TABLESPOONS ROSE WATER

2 TEASPOONS GUM ARABIC

CINNAMON POWDER

CASTER SUGAR

Warm the rose water and dissolve the gum arabic in it. Mix together equal amounts of cinnamon and sugar and work this into the gum paste, adding until it becomes quite solid. You can shape this into little pastilles.

. . . . .

Earache

MULLEIN OIL

Pack a jar with mullein flowers and pour on a vegetable oil (such as olive or sunflower). Put on the lid and leave on a sunny windowsill for 2 weeks, shaking daily. Strain well. Use to treat earache, ear infections, or wax buildup by dripping in 2–3 drops daily.

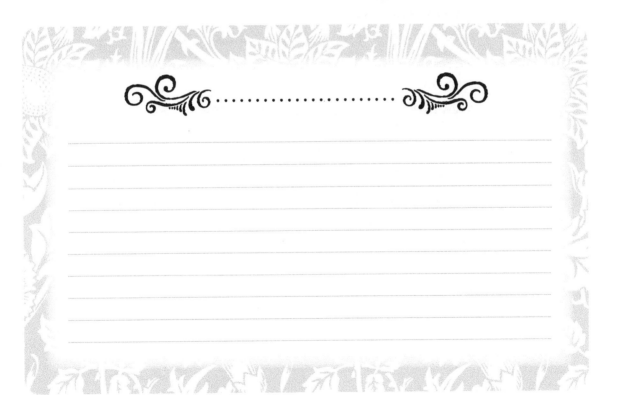

Eczema

The term *eczema*, from a Greek word meaning "to boil over," is applied to a wide range of persistent skin conditions. Also called dermatitis, it is a chronic inflammation of the skin, with symptoms including dryness, rashes, swelling, itching, cracking, flaking, and oozing. It may be caused by an allergy, but it is often related to stress. The most important thing is to keep the skin soft and supple, so use an emollient to keep the moisture in and allergens out while avoiding anything that might dry the skin out, such as soaps and shower gels.

. . . .

CHAMOMILE AND CHICKWEED SALVE

Chamomile is antibacterial, antifungal, anti-inflammatory, antiseptic, and helps neutralise skin irritants. One clinical trial in Germany found chamomile to be 60 percent as active as 0.25 percent hydrocortisone when applied topically. Chickweed is used by herbalists for skin diseases for its anti-inflammatory and antiviral activity. Calendula reduces inflammation, eliminates bacteria, and helps the skin heal.

- A HANDFUL OF CHAMOMILE FLOWERS (*ANTHEMIS NOBILIS* OR *MATRICARIA RECUTITA*)

- A HANDFUL OF CHICKWEED (*STELLARIA MEDIA*) AERIAL PARTS

- OLIVE OIL

- BEESWAX

- A FEW DROPS OF CALENDULA (*CALENDULA OFFICINALIS*) ESSENTIAL OIL (OPTIONAL)

Pack the plant material into a clear glass jar and top up with oil so that they are fully covered. Put a lid on the jar and put on a sunny windowsill for 2 weeks, shaking daily. Strain the oil into a double boiler and heat gently until warm—do not boil. Add some grated beeswax (the more you add, the harder the set) and when the wax has melted, pour into small jars, add a few drops of calendula oil, stir, put on the lids, and label. This salve will keep indefinitely and does not need to be refrigerated.

. . . .
Oat Bath Sachet

Oats contain anti-inflammatory and antioxidant compounds, which many studies have found reduce the redness, dryness, scaliness, and itching of eczema.

Tie a handful of oatmeal (*Avena sativa*) into a square of muslin and hang from the bath tap as you run the hot water. Alternatively, just drop the sachet into the bath.

. . . .
Horsetail Bath Infusion

Horsetail is rich in silicon, which is needed for the normal regeneration of healthy skin tissues. It is anti-inflammatory and helps to relieve the itching, irritation, and inflammation of eczema.

A HANDFUL OF HORSETAIL (*EQUISETUM ARVENSE*) AERIAL PARTS

1 PINT BOILING WATER

Pound up the horsetail in a pestle and mortar. Put into a heatproof jug and pour on the boiling water. Strain into a clean jug and add this infusion to your bath (don't use bubble bath or bath salts).

Gout

Gout is a form of arthritis caused by excessive uric acid in the blood, which forms crystals in and around the joints, especially the hands, wrists, feet, knees, and ankles, causing pain, inflammation, redness, stiffness, and itching. Gout can be the result of a diet too rich in meat and dairy products, excessive alcohol consumption, the use of diuretics, niacin (vitamin B3) or aspirin consumption, as well as a variety of medical conditions such as high blood pressure, hypothyroidism, or trauma.

· · · · · · · · · ·

ANTI-GOUT TEA

½ OUNCE DRIED HORSETAIL (*EQUISETUM ARVENSE*) AERIAL PARTS

2 TEASPOONS DRIED STINGING NETTLES

1 TEASPOON GRATED GINGER

½ PINT BOILING WATER

Pour the boiling water over the herbs and infuse for 15 minutes. Strain and drink.

· · · · · · ·

GET JUICING!

Various fruits have been found useful in relieving the symptoms of gout, notably cherries, apples, and grapes. Include some in your diet or make use of your juicer. If you have gout, you should drink plenty of fluids to help eliminate the waste products that cause it.

Epsom Salt Bath

Bathing in warm water mixed with 2 cups Epsom salts can reduce the pain and discomfort of gout.

Caution: Epsom salts should be avoided by diabetics.

Cider Vinegar, Honey, and Lemon Tea

1 TABLESPOON RAW CIDER VINEGAR

1 TEASPOON LEMON JUICE

1 TEASPOON HONEY

½ PINT HOT WATER

Combine and drink one cup a day to reduce the symptoms of gout.

Haemorrhoids

Haemorrhoids (or "piles") are swollen veins around the anus thought to be caused by excessive straining during bowel movements. They are very common, with about half of adults being afflicted at some time or another. Haemorrhoids can be itchy and painful, but you can help ameliorate this by keeping the area clean (don't use soap though) and trying one of these soothing remedies.

CHAMOMILE OIL SOOTHER

30 MILLILITRES CARRIER OIL (SUCH AS SUNFLOWER)

10 DROPS CHAMOMILE ESSENTIAL OIL

5 DROPS VITAMIN E OIL

Combine and store in a dark bottle. Dab a few drops onto the affected area to reduce pain, itching, and discomfort.

CALENDULA AND CHAMOMILE GEL

1 PART CHAMOMILE FLOWERS

1 PART ST. JOHN'S WORT FLOWERS

2 PARTS CALENDULA (*CALENDULA OFFICINALIS*) FLOWERS

VEGETABLE OIL (OLIVE, SUNFLOWER, ETC.)

WHITE PETROLEUM JELLY (OR UN-PETROLEUM JELLY)

Put the flowers in a clear glass jar, cover with the oil, and leave on a sunny windowsill for 2 weeks, shaking daily. Strain through muslin or a coffee filter and measure the quantity of the resulting herb-infused oil. Add one part of the oil to two parts of petroleum jelly in a double boiler, heat very gently until they are combined, and pour into clean glass jars. Dab a little onto the affected area when needed.

Headaches

Most of us suffer from the occasional tension headache, and many experience debilitating migraines. Both types of headaches benefit from using relaxation techniques, and there are some natural remedies you can try.

. . . .

MIGRAINE TEA

Feverfew has been used for migraines for centuries, and many find that skullcap is helpful in reducing headaches and migraines. Ginger root may help with the nausea and vomiting that sometimes accompany migraine headaches, as well as having anti-inflammatory and pain relief properties. Chamomile is generally relaxing and helps to ease pain.

4 OUNCES DRIED CHAMOMILE FLOWERS

3 OUNCES DRIED LEMON BALM (MELISSA OFFICINALIS) LEAVES

2 OUNCES DRIED FEVERFEW (TANACETUM PARTHENIUM)

1 OUNCE DRIED SKULLCAP (SCUTELLARIA SP.)

1 OUNCE DRIED PASSIONFLOWER (PASSIFLORA INCARNATE)

¼ OUNCE GINGER ROOT POWDER

Powder the ingredients and combine well. Store in an airtight tin. To use, put 2 teaspoons in a teapot and add a cup of boiling water. Infuse 10 minutes, strain, and drink sweetened with honey (optional).

Caution: Avoid if you are allergic to any of the ingredients, if you are pregnant or breastfeeding, or if you are taking blood-thinning medications, including aspirin.

. . . .

ROSEMARY AND THYME OIL RUB

Thyme and rosemary oils both contain carvacrol, which acts as a COX-II inhibitor,
much like non-steroidal anti-inflammatory drugs such as ibuprofen.

30 MILLILITRES VEGETABLE CARRIER OIL, SUCH AS OLIVE OR SUNFLOWER

10 DROPS ROSEMARY ESSENTIAL OIL

10 DROPS THYME ESSENTIAL OIL

5 DROPS VITAMIN E OIL (OPTIONAL, BUT THIS HELPS PRESERVE THE OIL)

Combine and put into a dropper bottle. When you have a headache, rub some
of the oil on your forehead.

Caution: Avoid if you are pregnant or breastfeeding.

. . . .

PEPPERMINT AND LAVENDER FOOTBATH

Footbaths can help relieve headaches, as it is believed that the warm water draws
blood to the feet, easing pressure on the head.

Fill a basin with warm water and add 5 drops of lavender essential oil and 5
drops of peppermint essential oil. Soak your feet for 20 minutes.

Caution: Avoid if you are pregnant or breastfeeding.

. . . .

PEPPERMINT OIL RUB

A 2010 study published in the International Journal of Clinical Practice found that
menthol was effective at stopping migraine pain and easing nausea when applied to
the forehead and temples.

30 MILLILITRES VEGETABLE CARRIER OIL SUCH AS OLIVE OR SUNFLOWER

30 DROPS PEPPERMINT ESSENTIAL OIL

5 DROPS VITAMIN E OIL (OPTIONAL, BUT THIS HELPS PRESERVE THE OIL)

Combine in a dropper bottle. When you have a headache, rub some of the oil
on your forehead.

Caution: Avoid if you are pregnant or breastfeeding.

. . . . .

LINDEN AND HOP TEA

Linden is an old remedy for calming nerves and anxiety as well as tension and inflammatory problems. Hops are calming and slightly sedative. Note: Use only young, fresh linden flowers or dried flowers that have not been stored for too long.

A SMALL HANDFUL OF LINDEN BLOSSOMS (*TILIA CORDATA*)

A SMALL HANDFUL OF HOP FLOWERS (*HUMULUS LUPULUS*)

1 PINT BOILING WATER

Pour the water over the flowers and infuse 15 minutes. Strain and drink sweetened with a little honey if you like.

ROSE PETAL VINEGAR

ROSE PETALS (RED OR PINK)

WHITE VINEGAR

Fill a glass jar with the rose petals. Cover with the vinegar and leave on a sunny windowsill for 2 weeks until the vinegar has turned a good red. Strain into a clean dark bottle and seal. When you have a headache, pour some of the vinegar into a bowl and soak a clean flannel in it, wring out, and apply to the forehead. Repeat as necessary. (You can also chill the bowl of vinegar in the fridge, which will help if your headaches are relieved by cold.)

Indigestion

. . . .

PEPPERMINT TEA

1 TABLESPOON PEPPERMINT LEAVES

½ PINT BOILING WATER

Infuse the leaves in the water for 10 minutes, strain, and drink to help relieve indigestion, heartburn, and wind.

Caution: Avoid if you are pregnant or breastfeeding.

. . . .

ELDERBERRY HEARTBURN TEA

1 TEASPOON RIPE ELDERBERRIES

½ PINT BOILING WATER

Crush the elderberries. Add the boiling water and infuse for 10 minutes. Strain and drink sweetened with a little honey (optional).

Insect Bites

PLANTAIN LEAF

A fresh plantain leaf (*Plantago major*) can be crushed between the fingers and applied directly to insect bites to help soothe them.

YARROW TINCTURE INSECT REPELLENT

YARROW (*ALCHELLIA MILLEFOLIUM*) FLOWERS

VODKA

Pack the flowers into a clear glass jar and cover with vodka. Put on the lid and leave on a sunny windowsill for 2 weeks, shaking daily. Strain into a clean jar. To use, dilute with a little water and apply to the skin to repel ticks, mosquitoes, and flies.

Insomnia

· · · · · · · · ·

SLEEPY TEA

½ OUNCE LEMON BALM LEAVES, DRIED

½ OUNCE HOP FLOWERS, DRIED

½ OUNCE VALERIAN ROOT, DRIED

1 OUNCE PASSIONFLOWER LEAVES, DRIED

Crush the herbs in a pestle and mortar and store in an airtight tin. To make a bedtime tea that will aid restful sleep, put 2 teaspoons of the herb mixture in a teapot, add boiling water, and infuse for 15 minutes. Pour through a tea strainer into a cup and drink half an hour before bed. You can sweeten the tea with a little honey (optional).

Caution: Avoid if you are pregnant or breastfeeding.

· · · · · · · · · · ·

SLEEP PILLOW

1 OUNCE DRIED CHAMOMILE

2 OUNCES DRIED HOP FLOWERS

½ OUNCE DRIED LAVENDER FLOWERS

AN OBLONG OF COTTON FABRIC

Sew the herbs into the cotton cloth to make a small pillow or bag. Use at the side of your regular pillow to promote restful sleep and a clear head.

BEDTIME TEA

1 OUNCE LEMON VERBENA LEAVES, DRIED

1 OUNCE PASSIONFLOWER, DRIED

1 OUNCE HOPS, DRIED

1 OUNCE SKULLCAP, DRIED

2 OUNCES PEPPERMINT, DRIED

1 OUNCE CATMINT, DRIED

Crush the herbs in a pestle and mortar and store in an airtight tin. To make a bedtime tea that will aid restful sleep, put 2 teaspoons of the herb mixture in a teapot, pour on boiling water, and infuse for 15 minutes. Pour through a tea strainer into a cup and drink half an hour before bed. You can sweeten the tea with a little honey (optional).

Caution: Avoid if you are pregnant, breastfeeding, or taking sedatives.

HOP AND LAVENDER BATH

Lavender relaxes while hops have a mild sedative effect and calm the nerves.

A HANDFUL OF HOP FLOWERS

A FEW LAVENDER FLOWERS

PIECE OF MUSLIN ABOUT 8 INCHES SQUARE

STRING

Gather up the hops and lavender in the muslin and secure the top with the string. Tie beneath the hot tap as the bath runs and take a warm, relaxing bath just before bedtime that will help you drop off to sleep.

Menopause

· · · · · · · · · ·

HOT FLUSH TEA

Sage is known to reduce sweating, and raspberry balances female hormones.

1 TABLESPOON DRIED SAGE LEAVES

1 TABLESPOON DRIED RASPBERRY LEAVES

Crush the herbs in a pestle and mortar and store in an airtight tin. To use, put 2 teaspoons into a teapot and add boiling water. Infuse 10 minutes. Pour through a strainer into a cup and sip. You can also make up the tea and then chill in the fridge to sip throughout the day and drink whenever you feel a hot flash coming on.

Caution: Avoid if you are pregnant or breastfeeding.

Muscle Cramps

Muscle Cramp Oil

30 MILLILITRES CARRIER OIL

5 DROPS BASIL ESSENTIAL OIL

4 DROPS ROSEMARY ESSENTIAL OIL

4 DROPS MARJORAM OIL

5 DROPS VITAMIN E OIL

Combine and store in a dark bottle. Rub onto painful cramped muscles or add a few drops to a warm bath.

Caution: Avoid rosemary oil if you are pregnant.

Nausea

GINGER TEA

Ginger is a safe and age-old remedy for nausea, travel sickness, and morning sickness. You can nibble on a piece of crystallised ginger instead of drinking the tea.

½ PINT BOILING WATER

½ INCH PIECE OF FRESH GINGER ROOT, CHOPPED

Pour the water over the ginger and infuse 10 minutes. Strain and drink. You can add a spoon of honey or a squeeze of lemon if you wish.

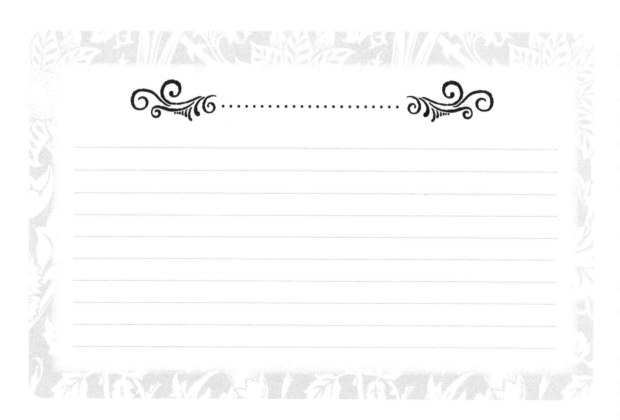

Poor Circulation

People who suffer from cold hands and feet usually describe themselves as having "poor circulation." These recipes will get the blood rushing to your extremities!

ROSEMARY AND HORSE CHESTNUT FOOTBATH

Horse chestnuts help strengthen blood vessels, and rosemary stimulates circulation.

½ PINT BOILING WATER

½ OUNCE DRIED HORSE CHESTNUTS, CHOPPED

A HANDFUL OF FRESH ROSEMARY LEAVES

Pour boiling water over the horse chestnuts and rosemary and infuse for 15–20 minutes. Strain and add to warm water in a footbath or large bowl. Soak your feet for 10–15 minutes. Rinse with cold water and dry vigorously on a warm towel.

Caution: Horse chestnuts are poisonous and should not be taken internally. They may irritate some skins, so do a patch test first.

MUSTARD FOOT OIL

1 PINT VEGETABLE OIL

3 FRESH HOT RED CHILLIES

2 OUNCES MUSTARD POWDER

Put the ingredients into a double boiler and simmer very gently for 40 minutes. Strain through a fine sieve into clean glass jars. This oil can be rubbed into the feet at bedtime, but do wash your hands very well afterwards and be careful not to get any near your eyes.

Sore Eyes

· · · · · · · · · · · · · · · · · ·

CORNFLOWER COMPRESS

1 PINT BOILING WATER

1 OUNCE CORNFLOWERS

Pour the water over the flowers and infuse for 10 minutes. Strain and cool. Dip cotton balls or cotton pads into the liquid and place them over your closed eyes, lie back, and relax for half an hour.

Sprains

COMFREY COMPRESS

3 OUNCES FRESH COMFREY ROOT, CHOPPED

1½ PINTS WATER

Put the fresh, chopped comfrey root in a pan with the water and boil for 15 minutes. Strain and soak a clean cloth or flannel in the resulting decoction. Place this on the affected part. Refresh when it cools.

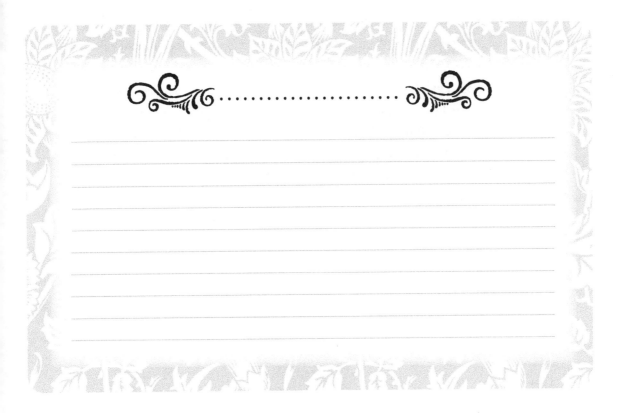

Varicose Veins

· · · · · · · · · ·

Horsetail Tea

2 TEASPOONS FRESH AERIAL PARTS OF HORSETAIL, CHOPPED

½ PINT WATER

Chop the horsetail and put two teaspoons into a jug and add ½ pint cold water. Leave overnight. The next day, put into a pan and bring to a boil. Strain. Drink 2 cups a day for up to 4 weeks.

· · · · · · · · · · · ·

Horse Chestnut Gel

15 HORSE CHESTNUTS (*AESCULUS HIPPOCASTANUM*), OR CONKERS

½ PINT VODKA

1 SACHET VEGETABLE GELATINE

2 FLUID OUNCES WATER

Put the horse chestnuts and vodka in a food processor and whizz up. Put into a jar and keep for 2 weeks, shaking daily. Strain through a fine sieve. Measure out 2 fluid ounces of this tincture to make the gel. Put the water and gelatine into a pan and heat gently, whisking continually until the gelatine has dissolved. As it starts to thicken, add the 2 fluid ounces of horse chestnut tincture a drop at a time. Pour into a clean jar and label. Apply twice daily to the affected area.

Caution: Horse chestnuts are poisonous and should not be taken internally. They may irritate some skins, so do a patch test first.

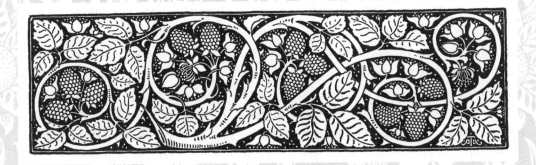

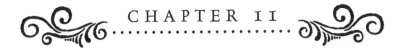

CHAPTER 11

Essential Oils

I've already mentioned essential oils many times throughout the course of this book. They form a valuable part of the hearth witch's tool kit, both for healing and magic, but it is important that we look at them in a bit more detail so that you know how to use them properly and safely.

Breathe in the fresh, sharp scent of lemon zest or the velvety perfume of a red rose: you are inhaling the characteristic essence of that plant's fragrance, and this is what is extracted to make an essential oil. The volatile oils that give a plant its distinguishing perfume are located in tiny secretory structures found in different parts of different plants: the flowers of lavender, the leaves of eucalyptus, the petals of a rose, the peel of an orange, and so on. To make the essential oils that we can buy and use, these volatile oils are extracted from the peels, petals, leaves, barks, seeds, and resins of various plants by methods such as distillation, expression, and cold pressing.

Essential oils are complex chemical structures often containing more than 100 compounds such as alcohols, aldehydes, esters, ketones, lactones, phenols, and terpenes, which are not only essential nutritionally for the plant but also help it adapt to its environment, attract pollinating insects, defend it from predators, or release antifungal or antimicrobial agents to protect it. They also interact with our own physiology, and many studies now bear this out. One concluded that the essential oil of *Melaleuca alternifolia* (tea tree) has broad-spectrum antimicrobial activity.[35] Another showed that menopausal women who received an aromatherapy massage once a week for eight weeks showed a greater reduction in menopausal symptoms such as hot flushes, depression, and pain than those in a control group.[36] A 2007 study showed that peppermint, caraway seed, pennyroyal, and fennel oils were effective against *Staphylococcus aureus* and *Escherichia coli*,[37] while a 2013 investigation demonstrated the potential of Carum and Ferula oil as natural antioxidants and antimicrobial agents.[38]

As I am writing this, Prof. Mark Moss and his team at Northumbria University in the UK are in the news for demonstrating that rosemary essential oil improves the memory. They recruited sixty senior volunteers and put them in a room infused with either rosemary essential oil, lavender essential oil, or no aroma, and told the subjects that they were testing the effects of a vitamin drink, dismissing the aromas as being left over from the room's previous occupants. Their memories were then tested, and results showed that those who inhaled the rosemary did significantly better than those in the control group, but that lavender caused a significant decrease in performance; lavender is associated with sleep and sedation. But can just inhaling a compound do this? Absolutely. Some prescription drugs are inhaled. When you ingest a drug it may be broken down in the liver, but with inhalation small molecules can pass directly into the bloodstream and from there to

---

35   Christine F. Carson, Brian J. Mee, and Thomas V. Riley, "Mechanism of Action of *Melaleuca alternifolia* (Tea Tree) Oil on *Staphylococcus aureus* Determined by Time-Kill, Lysis, Leakage, and Salt Tolerance Assays and Electron Microscopy," *Antimicrobial Agents and Chemotherapy* (June 2002): 1914–1920.

36   Myung-Haeng Hur, Yun Seok Yang, and Myeong Soo Lee, "Aromatherapy Massage Affects Menopausal Symptoms in Korean Climacteric Women: A Pilot-Controlled Clinical Trial," *Advance Access Publication* (23 April 2007).

37   "Evaluation of Antibacterial Activity of Selected Iranian Essential Oils against *Staphylococcus aureus* and *Escherichia coli* in Nutrient Broth Medium," Department of Food Hygiene and Public Health, Ferdowsi University of Mashhad, Iran. http://www.ncbi.nlm.nih.gov/pubmed/19093484.

38   G. Kavoosi, A. Tafsiry, A. A. Ebdam, and V. Rowshan, "Evaluation of Antioxidant and Antimicrobial Activities of Essential Oils from *Carum copticum* Seed and *Ferula assafoetida* Latex," *J Food Sci* 78, no. 2 (February 2013): T356–61, doi: 10.1111/1750-3841.12020, http://www.ncbi.nlm.nih.gov/pubmed/23320824.

the brain without being broken down. When Mark and his team analysed blood samples from the volunteers, they found traces of the chemicals in rosemary oil in their blood and concluded that "volatile compounds (e.g., terpenes) may enter the bloodstream by way of the nasal or lung mucosa. Terpenes are small organic molecules which can easily cross the blood-brain barrier and therefore may have direct effects in the brain by acting on receptor sites or enzyme systems."[39] One of the compounds in rosemary oil is 1,8-cineole, and it is thought that it may act in the same way as the drugs licensed to treat dementia, causing an increase in a neurotransmitter called acetylcholine by preventing the breakdown of the neurotransmitter by an enzyme.[40]

This illustrates the fact that different essential oils may have drastically different composition and effects.

Is It Really an Essential Oil?

Perfume oils, which are made from synthetic chemicals blended to smell like a particular plant, are useless for healing and magical purposes alike. In order to get the benefit of an essential oil, you need to be sure that what you are buying is really a pure and natural essential oil with nothing added and nothing taken away. If it just says "lavender oil" on the bottle, it is most likely a synthetic perfume; even if it says "essential oil," all may not be as it appears, as sometimes essential oils are reprocessed to fit standardised fragrance profiles and have synthetic chemicals added to achieve this. Make sure the plant's botanical name is listed on the label or website; if it just says "lavender essential oil," the chances are that it is adulterated. Look out for a product that says "therapeutic grade." Furthermore, try to make sure that your essential oil is organically produced to avoid pesticide residues.

Despite what you may read on some websites, it is impossible to make an essential oil at home—you can make an infused oil, but this is an infinitely weaker infusion in a carrier oil.

39   M. Moss and L. Oliver, "Plasma 1,8-cineole Correlates with Cognitive Performance Following Exposure to Rosemary Essential Oil Aroma," *Therapeutic Advances in Psychopharmacology* 2, no. 3 (2012): 103–113, doi:10.1177/2045125312436573.

40   Ibid.

Safety First

As always, just because something is 100 percent natural doesn't mean it is 100 percent safe. Each essential oil is different and some are more toxic than others, so please see the safety guidelines for each oil.

- Any oil can cause contact dermatitis or an allergic reaction in sensitive individuals, so always do a patch test forty-eight hours before using any oil to check for reactions.

- The long-term use of some oils can induce sensitivity to them or even cause liver and kidney damage.

- Specific oils should be avoided if you are suffering from particular health conditions.

- You should not use essential oils if you are pregnant or breastfeeding or on children under six, except under the guidance of a qualified practitioner.

- Do not use vaporizers in a house where someone lives with a respiratory disease.

- The internal use of essential oils is not recommended here, and never use an oil undiluted.

- Despite what you might read on some websites, never, ever use essential oils on a pet, as some oils that are safe for humans are extremely toxic to animals, cats in particular.

- Be careful how you store your oils, as they are highly flammable.

How to Use the Oils

Pure essential oils can be used in several ways for healing; we'll look at their magical virtues later in this chapter. The usual therapeutic methods are:

MASSAGE. Most oils (diluted with a carrier oil) may safely be applied to the skin. An aromatherapy massage is a relaxing experience designed to free the body from tension, increase the circulation of the blood and lymph flow, and help clear toxins as well as apply healing oils to the skin. The skin is partly permeable, and through it small molecules can be absorbed into the bloodstream (this is how hormone and nicotine patches work). Warming or massaging the skin increases absorbency.

For example, for headaches and migraines, a suitable oil could be massaged just into the temples and neck. For arthritic knees, a different blend can be applied directly to the knees.

To make a massage oil, add 10 drops of essential oil to 20 millilitres of carrier oil, though for the elderly and children under six you would reduce this to 5 drops of essential oil. Consult a qualified practitioner before using essential oils on children under six.

IN THE BATH. Blend 20 drops of essential oil with 30 millilitres of vegetable oil and add 2 teaspoons to the bath after it has run. Swirl it about in the water to ensure dispersion over the surface. As you get into the bath, the oil will coat your skin and the heat of the water will help its absorption. You will also breathe in the vapours. For an aromatherapy bath, do not use soap—treat the bath as a therapy, not a wash.

IN CREAMS AND LOTIONS. You can add essential oils to your regular skin cream or lotion (20 drops to 100 millilitres of lotion) to get the benefit of their skincare or therapeutic actions.

IN A SHAMPOO. Some essential oils are good for your hair, and you can add a few drops to your regular shampoo. Add 20 drops of essential oil per 100 millilitres of shampoo, but reduce this by half for the elderly and children.

IN A COMPRESS. In the same way that you would use a compress made with an herbal infusion, you can make a compress with essential oils. Drip a few drops of essential oil into water, dip a cloth into it, and apply it to the affected part. Use hot water to make a hot compress for muscular aches and pains, rheumatism, arthritis, and cramps, including menstrual cramps. Use chilled or iced water to make a cold compress for migraines, headaches, sprains, bruising, fever, and inflammation. Dip the cloth or towel into the water, wring it out, and apply directly to the affected area.

VAPORISATION. All essential oils readily evaporate, and when they are inhaled, the minute molecules are readily absorbed into the bloodstream. The aroma sends a signal directly to the limbic system in the brain, which is the centre of emotions, memory, and sexual arousal. You can simply put essential oil onto a tissue and smell it, put a few drops into a dish of boiling water, or put a dish of water with some oil in it on a radiator. Alternatively, you can buy a purpose-made oil burner, which consists of a dish in which water and oil is evaporated by a tealight candle underneath. You can also get lightbulb rings, but be sure to follow the manufacturer's instructions with these.

Carrier Oils

Generally speaking, essential oils are diluted with a carrier oil. These are natural vegetable oils such as:

ALMOND, SWEET. Obtained from the dried kernels of the almond tree, sweet almond oil is non-greasy, moisturising, softening, and soothing to the skin. It is one of the most popular carrier oils, as it is not absorbed too fast, so it gives you time to complete a massage. It has a shelf life of twelve months.

APRICOT KERNEL. Easily absorbed, apricot oil is great in facial treatments for dry and mature skin. This has a shelf life of twelve months.

AVOCADO. A rich, heavy oil full of vitamins, avocado oil is great for dry and mature skin, eczema, or psoriasis. This has a shelf life of twelve months.

GRAPE SEED. A light oil easily absorbed by the skin, mildly astringent, and with good moisturizing properties. It has a shelf life of six months.

HAZELNUT. Highly penetrative, hazelnut oil tightens the skin and helps in cell regeneration. Avoid if you have a nut allergy. It has a shelf life of up to three years.

JOJOBA. An excellent moisturiser for all skin types, easily absorbed, with anti-inflammatory and antioxidant actions that make it suitable for use on acne-prone skin. It has a long shelf life and can last for several years before going rancid.

OLIVE. Soothing and healing, great for sore, inflamed, and dry skin. Olive oil has a shelf life of up to two years.

MACADAMIA. Great for dry and aging skin. It has a shelf life of up to twelve months.

SESAME SEED. A thick oil full of vitamins and minerals, sesame oil is good for dry and mature skin, as well as eczema and psoriasis. It has a shelf life of up to twelve months.

It is best to buy carrier oils in small amounts, as they can go rancid within six to twelve months owing to the presence of unsaturated fatty acids that tend to oxidise quickly if not stored properly. Store in dark bottles in a cool, dark place.

A–Z of Essential Oils

AJWAIN (*Carum copticum* syn. *Trachyspermum ammi/Trachyspermum copticum*) Steam distilled from the seeds, the oil appears brownish in colour and has a peppery thyme scent. It has strong antioxidant and anti-inflammatory properties, as well as being antibacterial and antifungal, good for relieving stuffy noses, sinus congestion, colds, coughs, and skin problems such as acne and spots. Blends well with thyme, parsley, and sage.

Caution: Do not use for more than two weeks. Use double diluted as it may irritate the skin. Avoid completely during pregnancy. Should not be used by children.

ALLSPICE (*Pimenta dioica* or *Pimenta officinalis*) Steam distilled from the berries or leaves, allspice has a middle note spicy-sweet aroma. Used externally, it has warming effects that are good for arthritis and rheumatism, as well as muscular aches and pains. Allspice blends well with bay, black pepper, geranium, ginger, lavender, orange, patchouli, and ylang-ylang.

Caution: Use double diluted; may irritate the skin.

ANGELICA (*Angelica archangelica* or A. *officinalis*) This yellowish-brown, richly scented oil is extracted by steam distillation of the root, seeds, and the whole herb. Angelica oil can be used in the treatment of dull or irritated skin, psoriasis, water retention, bronchitis, coughs, anaemia, anorexia, flatulence, indigestion, fatigue, migraine, anorexia, chronic fatigue syndrome (also called ME, or myalgic encephalomyelitis), nervous tension, and stress-related disorders. It makes a good topical oil for arthritis, gout, and rheumatism. Angelica blends well with chamomile, geranium, grapefruit, lavender, lemon, and mandarin.

Caution: Phototoxic—do not expose the skin to sun after use, as it may cause pigmentation. Avoid completely during pregnancy or if you are diabetic. Overuse can cause hyperactivity of the nervous system.

MAGICAL VIRTUES: Aligning and anointing the heart chakra, purification, exorcism, protection, divination and visions, healing, wards off negativity

DEITIES: Sun gods, Venus

PLANET: Sun

ELEMENT: Fire

SIGN: Leo

ANISEED (*Pimpinella anisum* syn. P. *officinale*/P. *vulgare*) Extracted by steam distillation of the dried fruits, this is a medium-thin and clear oil with a warm, spicy perfume. It is good for nervous and anxious people, as it has a sedative, calming effect. It is also helpful for migraines and headaches. It relieves rheumatic and arthritic pains by stimulating blood circulation, helps heal wounds, and can be used as an insecticide against head lice and mites. Aniseed blends well with cardamom, caraway, cedarwood, coriander, dill, and fennel.

Caution: Do not use for more than two weeks. Avoid during pregnancy.

MAGICAL VIRTUES: Prosperity, courage, healing, luck, determination, magical power, energy, strength, aligning and anointing the root chakra

DEITIES: Aphrodite, Ares, Mars, Venus

PLANET: Mars

ELEMENT: Fire

SIGN: Aries/Scorpio

BASIL (*Ocimum basilicum*) A thin, greenish-yellow, fresh-smelling oil extracted by steam distillation of the leaves and the flowering tops, basil is an uplifting oil that can help nervous disorders, stress headaches, migraines, and allergies. It is often used for asthma, bronchitis, and sinus infections, as well as helping in cases of scanty or irregular periods. It is useful for arthritis and gout, helping to minimise uric acid in the blood. Basil also may be used for acne and insect bites. It blends well with bergamot, cedarwood, geranium, lemon, and verbena.

Caution: Use double diluted as it may irritate the skin. Avoid completely during pregnancy or on children under sixteen.

MAGICAL VIRTUES: Cleansing, protection, exorcism, banishing negativity, aligning and anointing the root (sacral) chakra

DEITIES: Erzulie, Lakshmi, Krishna, Vishnu

PLANET: Mars

ELEMENT: Fire

SIGN: Scorpio

BAY (*Laurus nobilis*)—The leaves from mature trees are subjected to steam distillation to create this deep-yellow, medium-thickness oil with a sweet, spicy scent. It is a warming and calming oil used for rheumatism, neuralgia, muscular pain, circulation problems, colds, flu, skin infections, and sprains. Bay is also helpful for hair loss. It blends well with cedarwood, coriander, geranium, juniper, lavender, lemon, rose, rosemary, and thyme.

Caution: Do not use more than two weeks. It may irritate the skin and mucus membranes. Avoid completely during pregnancy.

MAGICAL VIRTUES: Divination, psychic awareness, protection, anointing and aligning the sacral and heart chakras

DEITIES: Adonis, Apollo, Aesculapius, Ceres, Ceridwen, Cupid, Daphne, Eros, Faunus, Ra, Vishnu

PLANET: Sun

ELEMENT: Fire

SIGN: Leo

BENZOIN (*Styrax benzoin*) Benzoin oil is very thick and brown in appearance, with a sweet, warm perfume. It has a relaxing, calming effect in cases of nervous tension and stress and is also used for bronchitis, coughs, colds, and skin conditions such as wounds, acne, and scar tissue. It reduces redness and itching in eczema, psoriasis, and rashes. It eases rheumatism, arthritis, and muscle pains.

MAGICAL VIRTUES: Cleansing, purification, consecration, astral projection, anointing and balancing the solar plexus chakra

DEITIES: Aphrodite, Ares, Freya, Hathor, Khephera, Mut, Nike, Sol, Typhon, Venus

PLANET: Sun

ELEMENT: Air

SIGN: Leo/Aquarius

BERGAMOT (*Citrus aurantium* var. *bergamia* syn. *C. bergamia*)—A thin, greenish-yellow, citrus-scented oil extracted by expression from the ripe and unripe fruit, bergamot is strongly antiseptic and used for cystitis, vaginal thrush, urinary infections, and wounds. It eases stress, depression, and stress-related eczema and psoriasis. It blends well with cypress, frankincense, geranium, jasmine, lavender, mandarin, neroli, nutmeg, and orange.

Caution: Phototoxic—do not expose the skin to sun after use, as it may cause pigmentation.

MAGICAL VIRTUES: Money-drawing, protection, anointing
and aligning the solar plexus and heart chakras

DEITIES: Hermes, Mercury

PLANET: Mercury

ELEMENT: Air

SIGN: Gemini, Virgo

BLACK PEPPER (*Piper nigrum*)—This thin, amber-coloured spicy oil is extracted from unripe peppercorns by steam distillation. Black pepper is warming and stimulating, particularly good for muscular aches and pains, strains, arthritis, and rheumatism, as well as for stimulating blood circulation.

Caution: Use double diluted; may irritate the skin. Not compatible with homeopathic treatments. Avoid during pregnancy.

MAGICAL VIRTUES: Purification, protection, exorcism,
anointing and aligning the root chakra

DEITIES: Ares, Mars

PLANET: Mars

ELEMENT: Fire

SIGN: Cancer

BIRCH (*Betula alba*)—This pale yellow oil has a balsamic scent and is extracted from the leaf buds by steam distillation. Birch oil is good for dermatitis, dull skin, eczema, and psoriasis, and it also eases the pain of arthritis, rheumatism, and muscle aches. Birch oil blends well with benzoin, sandalwood, and rosemary.

Caution: Avoid during pregnancy.

MAGICAL VIRTUES: Protection, purification, wards
negativity, love, new beginnings, changes, Beltane

DEITIES: Aphrodite, Freya, Brigantia, Brighid, Earth Mother,
Thor, Frigga, Idunna, Nethus, Persephone, Sif, Venus

PLANET: Venus

ELEMENT: Water

SIGN: Cancer

CAJEPUT (*Melaleuca cajuputi*) This sweet-scented oil is extracted from the fresh leaves and twigs by steam distillation. It is antiseptic and pain relieving, helpful for infections of the respiratory tract and the urinary system as well as for colds, bronchitis, headaches, gout, muscle pains, and rheumatism. It can also be used as an insect repellent. Cajeput blends well with bergamot, cloves, geranium, and lavender.

CALAMUS (*Acorus calamus* var. *angustatus*) This warm, spicy oil is extracted from the roots by steam distillation. Calamus is soothing for headaches, nervous complaints, neuralgia, and panic attacks. It is also a pain reliever and reduces swelling in the joints. It blends well with cinnamon, cedarwood, lavender, patchouli, and ylang-ylang.

Caution: Use at double dilution. Avoid during pregnancy.

CAMPHOR, WHITE (*Cinnamomum camphora* syn. *Laurus camphora*) Extracted by steam from the chipped wood, root, and branches of the tree, this oil is rarely used in aromatherapy but may be useful for nervous conditions, depression, colds, coughs, fever, rheumatism, and arthritis. Camphor blends well with cajuput, chamomile, lavender, and melissa.

Caution: Use only under the direction of a qualified therapist. It should be avoided by people with epilepsy and by pregnant women. It is not compatible with homeopathic treatments.

MAGICAL VIRTUES: Divination, prophetic dreams, psychic awareness,
purification, anointing and balancing the brow chakra

DEITIES: Artemis, Chandra, moon deities

PLANET: Moon

ELEMENT: Water

SIGN: Cancer

CARAWAY (*Carum carvi* syn. *Apium carvi*) This sweet, spicy oil is extracted by steam distillation from the dried ripe seeds of the plant. Caraway is a detoxifying, warming, soothing oil that calms the nerves and aids nervous indigestion. It has a regenerative effect on the skin, helping infected wounds, boils, bruises, oily skin, acne, and itching. It may also be helpful in cases of respiratory problems, bronchitis, and coughs. Caraway blends well with coriander, frankincense, lavender, and orange.

Caution: Use double diluted; may irritate the skin.

MAGICAL VIRTUES: Love, fidelity, handfastings

PLANET: Sun, Mercury

ELEMENT: Air, fire

SIGN: Gemini

CARDAMOM (*Elettaria cardomomum*) This thin, pale yellow oil has a sweet, spicy fragrance and is extracted by steam distillation from the seeds of the fruit. Cardamom is helpful for the digestive system, colic, wind, dyspepsia, heartburn, and nausea. It is refreshing, stimulating, and uplifting in cases of mental and physical fatigue, and it has the reputation of being an aphrodisiac. It blends well with rose, orange, cinnamon, cloves, and caraway.

> MAGICAL VIRTUES: Love, handfastings, anointing
>   and balancing the solar plexus chakra
>
> DEITIES: Erzuli, Hecate
>
> PLANET: Venus
>
> ELEMENT: Fire
>
> SIGN: Aries

CARROT SEED (*Daucus carota*) Extracted by steam distillation from the dried seeds, this oil has a subtle earthy smell. It is an antiseptic and a disinfectant. Carrot seed oil is rejuvenating for the skin and helpful in cases of wrinkles, liver spots, psoriasis, eczema, sores, ulcers, boils, and carbuncles. It helps release toxins in the muscles and joints and benefits arthritis, gout, fluid retention, and rheumatism. It blends well with bergamot, juniper, lavender, citrus oils, cedarwood, and geranium.

> MAGICAL VIRTUES: Aligning the root, third
>   eye, and crown chakras; grounding
>
> PLANET: Mars, Mercury
>
> ELEMENT: Earth, fire
>
> SIGN: Sagittarius

CASSIA (*Cinnamomum cassia* syn. *C. aromaticum/Laurus cassia*) This brownish-yellow spicy oil is extracted from the leaves, bark, twigs, and stalks by steam distillation. Cassia oil helps fight viral infections such as coughs and colds, is warming and stimulates circulation. It benefits arthritis and rheumatism, and it supports lifting the mood. It blends well with caraway, coriander, frankincense, ginger, nutmeg, and rosemary.

Caution: May irritate the skin and mucus membranes. Avoid during pregnancy.

• • • • •

MAGICAL VIRTUES: Purification

PLANET: Sun

ELEMENT: Fire

SIGN: Leo

CEDARWOOD (*Juniperus virginiana*) This viscous, pale yellow oil is extracted by steam distillation from the wood chips and sawdust of the tree. It is antiseptic and a fungicide. Cedarwood has sedative properties and helps sooth nerves and anxiety. It is also useful for arthritis and rheumatism. It has an astringent action useful for skin problems such as acne and oily or itchy skin. Used in a vaporizer, it can help relieve respiratory congestion and catarrh. Cedarwood blends well with cypress, frankincense, juniper, lavender, and rose.

Caution: Use double diluted; may irritate the skin. Do not use for more than two weeks. Avoid during pregnancy.

MAGICAL VIRTUES: Purification, psychic powers, healing, luck,
   banishing, exorcism, wealth, protection, harmony, autumn equinox

DEITIES: Amun Ra, Cernunnos, Isis, Indra,
   Jupiter, Osiris, Pan, Poseidon, Wotan

PLANET: Mercury, Sun

ELEMENT: Air

CHAMOMILE, GERMAN (*Matricaria chamomilla* syn. *M. recutica*) This hay-scented, medium-thick oil is blue in colour and is extracted by steam distillation from the flower heads. Its uses are similar to those of Roman chamomile, except that it has greater anti-inflammatory properties owing to its higher levels of azulene. It has antibiotic, painkilling, and bactericidal actions, as well as sedative, mood-calming properties that soothe impatience and irritation, making it especially useful for premenstrual and menopausal mood swings. It's also helpful for the skin, healing and regenerating, calming inflammation in cases of eczema, psoriasis, and allergies. It blends well with geranium, lavender, bergamot, lemon, lavender, and ylang-ylang.

Caution: Avoid during pregnancy. It may cause dermatitis in sensitive individuals.

MAGICAL VIRTUES: Love, money-drawing, purification,
   protection, justice, meditation, Midsummer, anointing
   and aligning the heart and crown chakras

DEITIES: Cernunnos, Ra, sun gods

PLANET: Sun

ELEMENT: Water

SIGN: Leo

CHAMOMILE, ROMAN (*Anthemis nobilis* syn. *Chamaemelum nobile*) Extracted by steam distillation from the flower heads, Roman chamomile oil has a warm, sweet fragrance and is pale clear blue in colour, though it turns yellow with keeping. Like German chamomile, it is calming and helpful in relieving anxiety, headaches, migraines, insomnia, and other stress-related symptoms. It is wonderful for the skin and can be used for acne, allergies, burns, dermatitis, eczema, broken veins, dry skin, insect bites, rashes, and wounds. Use in the bath or with massage to relieve muscular aches and pains, arthritis, rheumatism, or painful periods and menopausal symptoms. Chamomile blends well with bergamot, clary sage, jasmine, lavender, geranium, and rose.

Caution: May cause dermatitis in some sensitive individuals. Avoid during pregnancy.

MAGICAL VIRTUES: Love, money-drawing, purification,
    protection, justice, meditation, Midsummer, anointing
    and aligning the heart and crown chakras

DEITIES: Cernunnos, Ra, sun gods

PLANET: Sun

ELEMENT: Water

SIGN: Leo

CINNAMON (*Cinnamomum zeylanicum* syn. *C. verum/Laurus cinnamomum*) This spicy essential oil has powerful antirheumatic properties and is also useful for period pains. It blends well with clove, frankincense, ginger, and lavender.

Caution: May cause skin irritation.

MAGICAL VIRTUES: Meditation, divination, protection,
    success, astral projection, healing, love, lust, passion, wealth,
    purification, anointing and balancing the solar plexus chakra

DEITIES: Aesculapius, Aphrodite, Helios, Ra, Venus

PLANET: Sun

ELEMENT: Fire

• • • • •

CITRONELLA (*Cymbopogon nardus* syn. *Andropogon nardus*) Extracted by the steam distillation of the grass, this oil has a lemony scent. It is antibacterial and is useful as an insect repellent, for oily skin, and for deodorising sweaty feet. It blends well with bergamot, orange, and lavender.

Caution: Avoid during pregnancy. May irritate sensitive skin.

MAGICAL VIRTUES: Anointing and balancing the solar plexus chakra

CLARY SAGE (*Salvia sclarea*) A pale yellow sweet-scented oil, clary sage oil is extracted by steam distillation from the flowering tops and leaves. Clary sage has a calming effect and is good for mild depression, nervous anxiety, insomnia, stress, and tension. It may be used by menopausal women for hot flushes and night sweats. It also helps calm acne and boils. Clary sage has the reputation of being an aphrodisiac. It blends well with lavender, geranium, lemon, and orange.

Caution: Avoid during pregnancy or if you have epilepsy.

MAGICAL VIRTUES: Clarity, divination, anointing
    and aligning the root and sacral chakras

PLANET: Mercury, Moon

ELEMENT: Air

CLOVE (*Eugenia caryophyllata* syn. *Syzygium aromaticum, Eugenia aromatica, E. caro-phyllus*) A thinnish, pale yellow oil with a spicy scent, clove oil is extracted from the leaves, stem, and buds. Clove is a pain-relieving oil, especially useful for toothaches, arthritis, and rheumatism. On the skin it can be used for acne, skin sores, leg ulcers, and bruises. It also may be used as an insect repellent and has the reputation of being an aphrodisiac. Clove oil blends well with cinnamon, lavender, ginger, and sandalwood.

Caution: Do not use more than two weeks. Use double diluted; may irritate the skin. Avoid completely during pregnancy.

MAGICAL VIRTUES: Love, lust, divination, banishing, purification, wealth,
    anointing and aligning the solar plexus, heart, and throat chakras

PLANET: Sun, Jupiter

ELEMENT: Fire

SIGN: Sagittarius

CORIANDER (*Coriandrum sativum*) Extracted from the crushed seeds by steam distillation, coriander oil has a warm, spicy scent and is a pale yellow colour. It is a natural deodorant and fungicide. It is good for nervous tension, rheumatism, arthritis pain, and muscle spasms. Coriander oil is said to be an aphrodisiac. It blends well with bergamot, lemon, and orange.

    Caution: Do not use more than two weeks.

    MAGICAL VIRTUES: Love, healing, lust, handfasting,
        anointing and balancing the solar plexus chakra

    DEITIES: Aphrodite, Venus

    PLANET: Mars

    ELEMENT: Fire

CUMIN (*Cuminum cyminum* syn. *C. odorum*) With a spicy scent, cumin oil is extracted by steam distillation from the ripe seed. It is bactericidal and antiseptic. Cumin oil is warming and helps relieve muscle pains and arthritis, as well as being good for nervous tension and headaches. It blends well with caraway and chamomile.

    Caution: Phototoxic—do not expose the skin to sun after use, as it may cause pigmentation. Avoid during pregnancy.

    MAGICAL VIRTUES: Releasing, banishing, purification,
        anointing and balancing the solar plexus chakra

CYPRESS (*Cupressus sempervirens*) With a fresh, woody scent, cypress is a thin, pale yellow oil extracted from the needles and twigs of the tree. It is an astringent, antiseptic, and deodorant. Cypress oil is especially useful for varicose veins and haemorrhoids, and it soothes muscular cramps, arthritis, and rheumatism. It blends well with lavender, juniper, pine, sandalwood, and rosemary.

    Caution: Best avoided during pregnancy.

    MAGICAL VIRTUES: Harmony, peace, releasing, consecration, anointing,
        blessing, anointing and aligning the sacral and throat chakras

    DEITIES: Aphrodite, Apollo, Artemis, Ashtoreth, Bhavani,
        Cupid, Cyparissus, Demeter, Diana, the Fates, Freya, the
        Furies, Hades, Hecate, Hera, Herakles, Isis, Jupiter, Mithras,
        Mut, Nephthys, Persephone, Pluto, Rhea, and Saturn

    PLANET: Saturn

    ELEMENT: Earth

· · · · ·

DILL (*Anethum graveolens*) A thin, pale oil with a sweet, earthy scent, dill is extracted from the seeds or whole herb. Use in massage or the bath for scanty periods, indigestion, colic, and nervous tension. Dill oil blends well with bergamot, caraway, and nutmeg.

> **Caution:** Avoid during pregnancy.
>
> MAGICAL VIRTUES: Money-drawing, protection, love, Beltane, anointing and aligning the solar plexus and throat chakras
>
> PLANET: Mercury
>
> ELEMENT: Air

ELEMI (*Canarium luzonicum* syn. *C. commune*) Elemi is a slightly citrus-scented, pale-coloured oil extracted from the gum by steam distillation. It is antiseptic. Elemi can be useful with heavy perspiration, cuts, wounds, and skin infections, and it helps rejuvenate mature skin. It blends well with frankincense, lavender, and myrrh.

> **Caution:** May be irritating to sensitive skin.

EUCALYPTUS (*Eucalyptus globulus*) Extracted from the leaves and twigs of the tree, eucalyptus oil is thin and colourless with a fresh, sharp scent. It is anti-inflammatory, antiseptic, antibacterial, and stimulating, useful for coughs, colds, hay fever, and sinus congestion, as well as sore muscles, rheumatism, arthritis, and neuralgia. It blends well with thyme, lavender, lemon, and pine.

> **Caution:** Do not use more than two weeks. Use double diluted; may irritate the skin. Not compatible with homeopathic treatments. Avoid if you have high blood pressure or epilepsy.
>
> MAGICAL VIRTUES: Purification, protection, healing, anointing and aligning the solar plexus and heart chakras
>
> PLANET: Mercury
>
> ELEMENT: Air

FENNEL, SWEET (*Foeniculum officinale* syn. *Anethum foeniculum*) Extracted by steam distillation from the seeds, fennel is a clear oil with an aniseed-like scent. It is an antiseptic. Fennel is good for digestive problems, fights obesity and cellulite, and is helpful for oily or dull skin, wrinkles, bruises, and rheumatism. It blends well with geranium, lavender, and sandalwood.

> **Caution:** Do not use for more than two weeks. Avoid during pregnancy and breastfeeding if you have epilepsy, oestrogen-linked cancers, or endometriosis.

MAGICAL VIRTUES: Protection, healing, purification, Midsummer,
   aligning the base, sacral, solar plexus, and heart chakras

DEITIES: Apollo, Dionysus, Prometheus

PLANET: Mercury

ELEMENT: Fire

FRANKINCENSE (*Boswellia carteri*) Extracted by steam distillation from the resin,
frankincense is a pale green-yellow oil with a woody, spicy scent. It is an antiseptic
and disinfectant. Frankincense is a calming and soothing oil, good for relieving the
pain of rheumatism and aching muscles. It has a balancing, rejuvenating action on
the skin, making it great for mature skin, sores, scars, cracked or inflamed skin, and
bed sores. It blends well with benzoin, sandalwood, myrrh, pine, and orange.

MAGICAL VIRTUES: Sun blends, purification, cleansing, releasing ego,
   protection, raising spiritual vibrations, consecration, anointing, spiritual love,
   blessing, balancing and aligning the heart, throat, third eye, and crown chakras

DEITIES: Adonis, Apollo, Bel, Demeter, Hades, Helios, Jehovah, Jesus,
   moon goddesses, Pluto, Ra, other sun gods, Venus, Vishnu, Vulcan, Yama

PLANET: Sun

ELEMENT: Fire

SIGN: Leo

GERANIUM (*Pelargonium odorantissimum*) The thin, almost colourless oil is extracted
by steam distillation from the leaves and stalks. Geranium is used for treating hormo-
nal imbalances such as menstrual and menopausal problems and premenstrual tension (PMT or PMS). It is also good at repelling head lice and mosquitos and for the
healing of wounds, acne, burns, cuts, dermatitis, eczema, haemorrhoids, cellulite, and
bruises. It blends well with bergamot, cedarwood, lavender, and rosemary.

Caution: May cause sensitivity in some people. Avoid during pregnancy.

MAGICAL VIRTUES: Releasing, cleansing, anointing,
   aligning the heart and throat chakras

DEITIES: Aphrodite, Athene (Athena), Isis, Menthu, Minerva, Shiva, Venus

PLANET: Venus

ELEMENT: Water

GINGER (*Zingiberaceae officinale*) A pale yellow, medium-thick oil with a warm, spicy scent, ginger oil is extracted by means of steam distillation from the plant's roots. Ginger is a stimulating, soothing, and warming oil used for digestive problems and nausea, including travel sickness, sea sickness, and hangovers. It is pain relieving and may be used for rheumatism and arthritis. It is said to be an aphrodisiac. Ginger blends well with bergamot, frankincense, neroli, sandalwood, and ylang-ylang.

Caution: Use double diluted; may irritate the skin. Phototoxic—do not expose the skin to sun after use, as it may cause pigmentation.

MAGICAL VIRTUES: Sexuality, love, courage, money-drawing,
love, success, anointing and balancing the root chakra

PLANET: Mars

ELEMENT: Fire

GRAPEFRUIT (*Citrus paradisi* syn. *Citrus racemosa* and C. *maxima* var. *racemosa*) Extracted from the peel of the fruit by cold compression, grapefruit oil is thin and pale yellow with a sharp, refreshing scent. Grapefruit is good for cellulite, obesity, oily skin, and acne, as well as being an uplifting oil that combats general and muscle fatigue, depression, jet lag, and hangovers. It blends well with bergamot, lavender, and frankincense.

MAGICAL VIRTUES: Cleansing, purification, balancing
and anointing the solar plexus chakra

HELICHRYSUM (*Helichrysum angustifolium* syn. *Helichrysum italicum*) A thin, pale yellow oil with a strong herby scent, helichrysum oil is extracted from the flowers by steam distillation. It is an antiseptic, good for circulatory problems, and eases the pain of rheumatism and arthritis, as well as being beneficial in cases of colds, flu, bronchitis, coughs, and asthma. On the skin it helps with the healing of scars, acne, dermatitis, stretch marks, boils, and abscesses. It blends well with bergamot, chamomile, lavender, and mandarin.

Caution: Should not be used on children under twelve years.

MAGICAL VIRTUES: Releasing old wounds and trauma, emotional
healing, anointing and balancing the solar plexus chakra

HYSSOP (*Hyssopus officinalis*) Extracted from the flowering tops by steam distillation, hyssop oil is a pale yellow-green oil with a sweet scent. Hyssop oil is used for menstrual problems including water retention around the time of monthly periods. It is also helpful for respiratory ailments such as bronchitis, asthma, colds, and flu. On the skin it helps heal wounds, bruises, eczema, and dermatitis. It blends well with clary sage, orange, tangerine, melissa (lemon balm), and rosemary.

Caution: Do not use more than two weeks. Avoid completely during pregnancy and if you have high blood pressure or epilepsy.

MAGICAL VIRTUES: Cleansing sacred space and tools, purification, balancing the sacral and solar plexus chakras, aligning the root, sacral, and solar plexus chakras with the heart chakra

DEITIES: Pluto, Zeus

PLANET: Jupiter

ELEMENT: Fire

SIGN: Cancer

JASMINE (*Jasminum gradiflora* or J. *officinale*) This has always been one of the most expensive oils owing to the number of flowers needed to extract an essential oil, but a therapeutic-grade oil is virtually impossible to obtain today as growers have changed their extraction methods and produce a less pure oil for fragrance. It is relaxing and mentally uplifting, helping ease depression and soothe the nerves. It is wonderful for the skin, toning and improving elasticity, reducing stretch marks and scars, and soothing irritated and dry skin. Jasmine oil is reputedly an aphrodisiac. It blends well with rose and sandalwood.

Caution: Avoid during pregnancy.

MAGICAL VIRTUES: Love, sexual attraction, prosperity, luck, happiness, meditation, spiritual love, prophetic dreams, astral projection, balancing and anointing the heart chakra

DEITIES: Artemis, Diana, Ganesha, mother goddess, Quan Yin, Vishnu, Zeus, moon goddesses

PLANET: Moon

ELEMENT: Water

JUNIPER (*Juniperus communis*) Extracted from the berries by steam distillation, juniper is a pale, thin oil with a woody scent. It is antiseptic. It cleanses the blood of toxins and is helpful in cases of fluid retention, cellulite, rheumatism, arthritis, and gout. It can be used for psoriasis and weeping eczema, and it calms anxiety, stress, and insomnia. Juniper blends well with cedarwood, cypress, lavender, bergamot, lime, and clary sage.

Caution: Do not use more than two weeks. Avoid if you are pregnant or have kidney problems.

MAGICAL VIRTUES: Visions, home protection, love, exorcism, healing

DEITIES: Gods and goddesses of justice, the Furies, Pan

PLANET: Mars, Sun

ELEMENT: Fire

SIGN: Aries

LAVANDIN (*Lavandula × intermedia* syn. *L. hybrida* and *L. hortensis*) This clear, light floral oil is extracted from the fresh flowering tops of the plant by steam distillation. Lavandin is relaxing and eases sore and stiff muscles and joints. It helps wounds heal faster and is useful for dermatitis. It blends well with bergamot, cinnamon, clary sage, pine, thyme, patchouli, and rosemary.

MAGICAL VIRTUES: Attraction, love, peace, harmony, joy, healing, sleep, purification, psychic awareness, prosperity, anointing and aligning the heart and crown chakras

DEITIES: Cernunnos, Circe, Hecate, Medea, Saturn

PLANET: Mercury

ELEMENT: Air

LAVENDER (*Lavandula angustifolia/Lavandula officinalis*) This thin, clear floral oil is extracted from the flowering tops of the plant by steam distillation. Lavender is soothing, calming, relaxing, and antiseptic. It can be used for migraines, headaches, nervous tension, depression, panic, hysteria, and insomnia. It is nourishing and balancing for the skin, good for acne, rosacea, eczema, dermatitis, boils, burns, sunburn, wounds, and psoriasis, and may be used to deter insects and on insect bites. It helps reduce high blood pressure, lymph congestion, cystitis, palpitations, period pains, cellulite, and fluid retention. Lavender blends well with cedarwood, geranium, pine, and rosemary.

MAGICAL VIRTUES: Attraction, love, peace, harmony, joy,
   healing, sleep, purification, psychic awareness, prosperity,
   anointing and aligning the heart and crown chakras

DEITIES: Cernunnos, Circe, Hecate, Medea, Saturn

PLANET: Mercury

ELEMENT: Air

LEMON (*Citrus limonum* syn. *Citrus limon*) A cold-pressed oil obtained from the fruit, lemon is a thin, pale greenish-yellow oil with a sharp, fresh smell. It is antiseptic and reduces acidity in the body. It may be used for rheumatism, arthritis, gout, cellulite, abscesses, boils, carbuncles, high blood pressure, headaches, and migraines. It is an uplifting oil, helpful in cases of depression and fatigue. It may be used to ease acne, oily skin and hair, cold sores, mouth ulcers, and insect bites. It blends well with lavender, eucalyptus, geranium, fennel, and juniper.

Caution: May irritate the skin. Phototoxic—do not expose the skin to sun after use, as it may cause pigmentation.

MAGICAL VIRTUES: Moon oils, purification, healing, love,
   aligning and anointing the throat and heart chakras

DEITIES: Moon deities

PLANET: Moon

ELEMENT: Water

LEMONGRASS (*Cymbopogon citratus* syn. *Andropogon citratus*/*A. schoenathus*) With a fresh, lemony scent, this amber-coloured oil is extracted from the leaves of the plant by steam distillation. Lemongrass is an uplifting, stimulating, and revitalising oil that is useful in cases of jet lag, headaches, nervous exhaustion, and stress-related conditions. It may be used for cellulite, muscle pains, oily skin, acne, athlete's foot and other fungal infections, and excessive perspiration. It acts as an insect repellent. Lemongrass blends well with basil, cedarwood, lavender, and tea tree.

Caution: Avoid in pregnancy; lemongrass oil is a possible skin irritant.

MAGICAL VIRTUES: Psychic awareness, purification,
   anointing and balancing the solar plexus chakra

PLANET: Mercury

ELEMENT: Air

SIGN: Gemini

LEMON VERBENA (*Lippia citriodora* syn. *Aloysia triphylla/A. citriodora/Lippia triphylla/Verbena triphylla*) This pale yellow, lemony-scented oil is extracted from the leaves by steam distillation. Lemon verbena oil is calming and uplifting, useful for depression, stress, and nervous conditions. It softens the skin and reduces puffiness. It blends well with lavender and palmarosa.

> **Caution:** May cause skin sensitization and is phototoxic.

> MAGICAL VIRTUES: Love, purification, sexual attraction,
>   Ostara, air blends, Venus planetary blends

> PLANET: Venus, Mercury

> ELEMENT: Air

LIME (*Citrus aurantifolia* syn. *Citrus medica* var. *acida/C. latifolia*) This pale yellow citrus oil is extracted by expression or by distillation from the fruit. Lime oil is uplifting and refreshing, lightening the mood and helping with depression. It is useful for reducing cellulite, boosting the immune system, for coughs, bronchitis, arthritis, rheumatism, obesity, cellulite, oily skin, acne, cold sores, and insect bites. It blends well with neroli, lavender, and clary sage.

> **Caution:** Phototoxic—do not expose the skin to sun after use, as it may cause pigmentation.

> MAGICAL VIRTUES: Purification, protection, love, joy, aligning
>   and anointing the solar plexus and heart chakras

> PLANET: Sun

> ELEMENT: Fire

MARJORAM (*Origanum marjorana/Origanum hortensis*) This pale yellow oil is extracted from the leaves and flowering tops of the plant by steam distillation. Marjoram is a warming, calming oil with pain-relieving properties. It is useful for asthma, anxiety, stress, tense and painful muscles, rheumatic pains, sprains, strains, swollen joints, headaches, migraines, insomnia, menstrual cramps, chilblains, and bruises. It is reputed to diminish sexual desire. It blends well with lavender, cedarwood, chamomile, and bergamot.

> **Caution:** Avoid during pregnancy.

> MAGICAL VIRTUES: Protection, joy, cleansing, anointing
>   and aligning the heart and solar plexus chakras

DEITIES: Aphrodite, Jupiter, Osiris, Thor, Venus

PLANET: Mercury

ELEMENT: Air

SIGN: Aries

MELISSA AKA LEMON BALM (*Melissa officinalis*) This thin, pale yellow oil has a lemony scent and is extracted from the flowering tops, leaves, and stems by steam distillation. Melissa oil is calming and uplifting. It helps with nervous conditions, depression, nervous palpitations, menstrual problems, cold sores, fungal infections, high blood pressure, nausea, headaches, migraines, baldness, and hair loss. It blends well with basil, frankincense, and lavender.

Caution: May cause skin irritation; use double diluted. Avoid during pregnancy.

MAGICAL VIRTUES: Success, joy, balancing and anointing the heart chakra

DEITIES: Moon goddesses, Artemis, Diana

PLANET: Moon

ELEMENT: Water

SIGN: Cancer

MYRRH (*Commiphora myrrha* syn. *Commiphora molmol/Balsamodendron myrrha*) This amber oil is extracted by steam distillation of the gum. It is effective against colds, catarrh, coughs, sore throats, bronchitis, haemorrhoids, boils, skin ulcers, bedsores, chapped and cracked skin, ringworm, wounds, eczema, and athlete's foot. It blends well with benzoin, clove, frankincense, lavender, and sandalwood.

Caution: Avoid during pregnancy.

MAGICAL VIRTUES: Purification, meditation, consecration, anointing, spiritual awareness, healing, peace, anointing and aligning the solar plexus and heart chakras

DEITIES: Adonis, Bhavani, Cybele, Demeter, Freya, Hathor, Hecate, Hera, Isis, Juno, Marian, Mut, Neptune, Nephthys, Poseidon, Ra, Rhea, Saturn

PLANET: Moon

ELEMENT: Water

NEROLI (*Citrus aurantium* var. *amara* syn. *Citrus vulgaris/C. Bigardia*) This thin, pale yellow, floral-scented oil is extracted by steam distillation from the blossoms of the bitter orange tree. It is antiseptic, disinfectant, deodorant, and sedative; it even has the reputation of being an aphrodisiac. It relaxes the mind and body, easing muscle spasms, palpitations, anxiety, depression, fear, shock, stress, vertigo, and insomnia. For the skin, it stimulates cell growth and is regenerative, reducing scarring, stretch marks, and broken capillaries, and leaving the skin soft and smooth. Neroli blends well with benzoin, jasmine, lavender, sandalwood, and ylang-ylang.

Caution: Use sparingly, as it is very relaxing.

MAGICAL VIRTUES: Love, sex, anointing and balancing the heart chakra

PLANET: Sun

ELEMENT: Fire

NIAOULI (*Melaleuca viridiflora* syn. *Melaleuca quinquenervia*) This sweet, fresh, pale yellow oil is extracted from the young leaves and twigs of the tree by steam distillation. It has pain-killing properties and is antiseptic and bactericidal, an insecticide and a stimulant. It is useful for treating bronchitis, catarrh, acne, boils, burns, ulcers, cuts, and cystitis. It is useful in the treatment of rheumatism and neuralgia. It blends well with fennel, juniper, lavender, lime, and pine.

NUTMEG (*Myristica fragrans* syn. *Myristica officinalis/M. oromata/Nux moschata*) This spicy oil is extracted by steam distillation from the seeds. It is both a sedative and a stimulant, anti-inflammatory, antiseptic, and bactericidal. It helps reduce inflammations, muscle aches and pains, rheumatism, arthritis, gout, and stimulates the heart and circulation. It blends well with cypress, clary sage, rosemary, and orange.

Caution: Do not use for more than two weeks. Avoid during pregnancy.

MAGICAL VIRTUES: Luck, prosperity, money-drawing,
	psychic awareness, divination

PLANET: Jupiter

ELEMENT: Air

ORANGE, SWEET (*Citrus sinensis* syn. *Citrus aurantium* var. *dulcis /C. aurantium* var. *sinensis*) This thin yellow oil with a fresh, tangy scent is extracted by cold compression from the peels of the fruit. It is useful in cases of colds, flu, eliminating toxins, stimulating the lymphatic system, water retention, obesity, nervous tension, and stress. It supports collagen formation in the skin and is great for mature skin, dermatitis, acne, and dry, irritated skin. It even has the reputation of being an aphrodisiac. Orange blends well with black pepper, cinnamon, cloves, ginger, and frankincense.

Caution: Phototoxic—do not expose the skin to sun after use, as it may cause pigmentation. Like other citrus oils, the shelf life is approximately six months.

MAGICAL VIRTUES: Love, luck, divination, healing, harmony,
money-drawing, prosperity, psychic awareness, anointing
and aligning the sacral and solar plexus chakras

PLANET: Sun

ELEMENT: Fire

SIGN: Leo, Sagittarius

PALMAROSA (*Cymbopogon martini* syn. *Cymbopogon martinii* var. *martinii*) This thin, pale yellow oil has a sweet floral scent and is extracted from the grass by steam distillation. It is antiseptic, antiviral, bactericidal, and hydrating. It is calming and uplifting for stress and nervous exhaustion and is good for aching feet and stiff, sore muscles. It is very moisturising for the skin and stimulates cell regeneration, so it is good for wrinkles, acne, dermatitis, minor skin infections, and preventing scarring. It blends well with geranium, bergamot, rosemary, and lime.

MAGICAL VIRTUES: Love, healing, anointing
and balancing the heart chakra

PLANET: Venus

ELEMENT: Water

PATCHOULI (*Pogostemon cablin* syn. *Pogostemon patchouli*) This thick, rich, sweet oil, yellow to dark brown in colour, is extracted from the young leaves of the plant, which are fermented prior to steam distillation. It is grounding and balancing, antiseptic, deodorant, antifungal, and sedative. It is helpful for depression, anxiety, cellulite, fungal and bacterial infections, insect bites, water retention, and wound healing. It promotes tissue regeneration, aiding cracked and dry skin, acne, eczema, sores, ulcers, and insect bites. It is said to be an aphrodisiac. Patchouli blends well with bergamot, clary sage, lavender, myrrh, and ylang-ylang.

MAGICAL VIRTUES: Money-drawing, prosperity, fertility, love, protection,
banishing, aligning and anointing the heart and crown chakras

PLANET: Venus

ELEMENT: Earth

PEPPERMINT (*Mentha piperita*) This thin, menthol-scented oil is clear to pale yellow in colour and extracted by steam distillation from the aerial parts of the plant just before flowering. It is antiviral, antibacterial, and antifungal, with pain-reducing properties. It is anti-inflammatory and cooling to the skin, reducing redness, irritation, itchiness, dermatitis, acne, ringworm, sunburn, and scabies. It stimulates the circulation. The menthol it contains helps clear the respiratory tract, easing sinus and chest congestion as well as being refreshing and stimulating for fatigue, depression, concentration, apathy, headache, migraine, nervous stress, vertigo, and nausea. Its pain-relieving actions help aching feet, rheumatism, neuralgia, muscular pains, and painful periods. Peppermint oil blends well with eucalyptus, lavender, marjoram, lemon, and rosemary.

Caution: Use double diluted; may irritate the skin. Avoid during pregnancy. Not compatible with homeopathic treatments. Should not be used on children under seven.

MAGICAL VIRTUES: Purification, cleansing, psychic dreaming,
exorcism, healing, money-drawing, anointing and aligning
the root, sacral, solar plexus, and throat chakras

PLANET: Mercury

ELEMENT: Air

PETITGRAIN (*Citrus aurantium* var. *amara* syn. *Citrus bigardia/Petitgrain bigarade*) This woody, floral, thin, pale yellow oil is extracted from the fresh leaves and small twigs by steam distillation. It is relaxing, calming rapid heartbeats, helping insomnia, nervous exhaustion, anger, and panic. It relaxes muscle spasms and soothes aches and pains. It is good for oily skin, acne, and excessive perspiration. Petitgrain blends well with bergamot, lavender, palmarosa, geranium, and rosewood.

MAGICAL VIRTUES: Personal protection, concentration,
meditation, anointing and aligning the root and heart chakras

PLANET: Sun

ELEMENT: Fire

PINE (*Pinus sylvestris*) This thin, fresh-forest-scented oil is pale yellow in colour and extracted by steam distillation from the tree's twigs, buds, and needles. It is anti-inflammatory, antibacterial, and antifungal. It elevates the mood, relieving mental and physical fatigue. It is useful for cystitis and urinary infections, arthritis, rheumatism, gout, sciatica, arthritis, cuts, sores, scabies, lice, excessive perspiration, muscular aches and pains, bronchitis, asthma, catarrh, coughs, colds, and flu. Pine blends well with cedarwood, eucalyptus, lavender, and rosemary.

Caution: Use double diluted; may irritate the skin. Avoid during pregnancy.

MAGICAL VIRTUES: Group consciousness, purification, healing, joy, fertility, cleansing, consecration, protection, money-drawing, exorcism, peace, Ostara, aligning the root, sacral, throat, and third eye chakras

DEITIES: Astarte, Attis, Dionysus, Cernunnos, Cybele, the Great Mother, Herne, Osiris, Pan, Pitys, Poseidon, Rhea, sun gods, Sylvanus, Venus

PLANET: Mars

ELEMENT: Earth

ROSE (*Rosa damascene*) This fresh, floral-scented oil, clear to pale yellow in colour, is extracted from the fresh flowers by steam distillation. One of its prime uses is in soothing depression, grief, anger, fear, post-natal depression, and nervous tension. It is good for female problems such as regulating female hormones, irregular menstruation, leucorrhoea, and menorrhagia. It helps with poor circulation and heart problems, heart palpitations and high blood pressure. It is marvellous for the skin, moisturizing and hydrating, and is especially good for dry, mature, and irritated skin, broken capillaries, redness, and eczema. It has the reputation of being an aphrodisiac. Rose blends well with jasmine, clove, and palmarosa.

Caution: Avoid during pregnancy.

MAGICAL VIRTUES: Unconditional love, peace, lust, beauty, healing, health, psychic awareness, anointing, aligning and expanding the heart and crown chakras

DEITIES: Adonis, Aphrodite, Bacchus, Blodeuwedd, Christ, Cupid, Demeter, Eros, Flora, Freya, Hathor, Hulda, Hymen, Isis, Nike, Venus, Vishnu

PLANET: Venus

ELEMENT: Water

ROSEMARY (*Rosmarinus officinalis*) This thin, clear oil has a clean herbal scent and is extracted from the fresh flowering tops of the plant by steam distillation. It is analgesic, antibacterial, antifungal, and anti-inflammatory. It is famous for improving the memory, mental clarity, and lifting mental tiredness. It can help stiff muscles, headaches, migraines, aches and pains, arthritis, rheumatism, fluid retention, bronchitis, Candida albicans, the removal of toxins, varicose veins, low blood pressure, poor circulation, catarrh, colds, flu, and sinusitis. It helps tighten sagging skin, eases skin congestion and puffiness, acne, dermatitis, and eczema. It benefits scalp disorders such as dandruff and alopecia, and encourages hair growth. Rosemary blends well with cedarwood, geranium, lavender, lemongrass, and peppermint.

Caution: Avoid during pregnancy or if you have high blood pressure or epilepsy.

MAGICAL VIRTUES: Cleansing, purification, exorcism, healing, anointing and balancing the heart chakra

DEITIES: Fairies

PLANET: Sun

ELEMENT: Fire

SIGN: Aries

ROSEWOOD (*Aniba rosaeodora* syn. *Aniba rosaeodora* var. *amazonica*) The spicy, floral oil is extracted from the wood chippings by steam distillation. It is useful for the treatment of headaches, colds, coughs, infections, nausea, and stress-related problems. It stimulates cell growth and the regeneration of tissues, making it good for mature, wrinkled, dull, dry, and oily skin. It has the reputation of being an aphrodisiac. Rosewood oil blends well with all citrus and floral oils.

MAGICAL VIRTUES: Emotional release; expands all the chakras in the body but specifically the heart chakra

SAGE (*Salvia officinalis*) This thin, herbal-scented oil is extracted from the dried leaves of the plant by steam distillation. It helps regulate the hormones and is most useful for menstrual and menopausal problems. It is also good for rheumatism, dermatitis, sores, ulcers, insect bites, stiff muscles, fibrositis, trembling, and palsy. Sage oil blends well with bergamot, lavender, lemon, and rosemary.

Caution: Avoid during pregnancy or if you have high blood pressure or epilepsy. Sage oil should be used sparingly and in double dilution, as it is toxic in large doses.

MAGICAL VIRTUES: Trance states, spiritual awareness, consecration,
purification, healing, protection, money-drawing, anointing
and aligning the root, sacral, and solar plexus chakras

DEITIES: Consus, Jupiter, Zeus

PLANET: Jupiter

ELEMENT: Air

SANDALWOOD (*Santalum album*) This woody, pale yellow oil is extracted from the chipped heartwood of the tree by steam distillation. Sandalwood has a calming and relaxing effect that reduces tension, depression, fear, stress, nervous exhaustion, insomnia, and anxiety. It is great for anti-aging skin care and dry skin, and it relieves itching, inflammation, and dry eczema. It is rumoured to be an aphrodisiac. Sandalwood blends well with lavender, myrrh, rose, vetiver, and ylang-ylang.

MAGICAL VIRTUES: Protection, healing, spirit attraction,
purification, healing, astral protection, anointing
and aligning the root and sacral chakras

DEITIES: Freya, Hanuman, Hathor, Hermes, Nike, Venus, Vishnu

PLANET: Moon

ELEMENT: Air

SPEARMINT (*Mentha spicata*) This minty, pale greenish-yellow oil is extracted by steam distilling the flowering tops of the herb. It stimulates the mind but calms nausea, hiccups, headaches, migraines, nervous strain, fatigue, stress, bronchitis, catarrh, and sinusitis. It can help relieve itchy skin, acne, dermatitis, and congested skin. Spearmint blends well with basil, eucalyptus, lavender, and rosemary.

Caution: Best avoided during pregnancy.

MAGICAL VIRTUES: Healing, mental activity, protection,
anointing and aligning the solar plexus and heart chakras

SPIKENARD (*Nardostachys jatamansi*) This medium-thick, mossy-scented oil is pale yellow in colour and extracted from the rhizome of the plant by steam distillation. It is useful in cases of tension, stress, migraine, nervous indigestion, and insomnia. It is rejuvenating for mature skin and soothing for skin inflammations and rashes. Spikenard blends well with lavender, patchouli, petitgrain, rose, and vetiver.

MAGICAL VIRTUES: Meditation, anointing and
aligning the solar plexus and heart chakras

TAGETES (*Tagetes minuta/Tagetes glandulifera*) This sweet, thick yellow oil is extracted from the leaves, stalks, and flowers of the plant. It is used for chest infections, coughs, catarrh, skin infections, calluses, bunions, and as an insect repellent. It is especially helpful when treating weeping wounds. Tagetes blends well with lavender, lemon, myrrh, and tangerine.

Caution: Use sparingly and double diluted. May cause a reaction on sensitive skin or photosensitivity. Avoid during pregnancy.

TARRAGON (*Artemisia dracunculus*) This herby oil is extracted from the leaves and flowering tops of the plant by steam distillation. It increases the circulation and helps in eliminating toxins, so is good for arthritis and rheumatism. It is beneficial in deodorant preparations, as it inhibits the growth of odour-forming microbes. It stimulates the appetite, eases menstrual pains, and helps to regulate periods. It blends particularly well with lavender, lime, and rosewood.

Caution: Use in moderation. Avoid use during pregnancy or on children.

MAGICAL VIRTUES: Change, grounding, anointing and
aligning the root, sacral, solar plexus, and heart chakras

DEITIES: Lilith

PLANET: Mars

ELEMENT: Fire

TEA TREE (*Melaleuca alternifolia*) This thin, pungent oil is extracted from the leaves and twigs of the tree by steam distillation. It fights bacterial, fungal, and viral infections and can be used for flu, cold sores, catarrh, coughs, vaginal thrush, cystitis, abscesses, acne, burns, oily skin, athlete's foot, warts, sunburn, and infected wounds. It can be added to antidandruff preparations. Tea tree blends well with clary sage, lavender, lemon, rosemary, and thyme.

MAGICAL VIRTUES: Purification, health, anointing
and balancing all the chakras

THYME (*Thymus vulgaris*) This sweet, herby, amber-coloured oil is extracted from the flowering tops and leaves of the plant by water or steam distillation. It helps remove toxins and stimulate the circulation, so is of benefit in treating arthritis, gout, and rheumatism. It is strongly antiseptic and useful for fighting colds, coughs, catarrh, cystitis, and urethritis. It eases muscular aches and pains, sprains, and sport injuries. As a diuretic, it may be of benefit for cellulite, obesity, and oedema. Thyme blends well with bergamot, lemon, lavender, rosemary, and pine.

Caution: Use double diluted, as it may irritate the skin. Avoid completely during pregnancy or if you have high blood pressure.

MAGICAL VIRTUES: Purification, protection, cleansing, healing,
psychic awareness, energy, strength, courage, anointing
and aligning the heart and solar plexus chakras

DEITIES: Ares, Mars; also associated with fairies

PLANET: Venus

ELEMENT: Water

SIGN: Aries

VETIVER (*Vetiveria zizanoides* syn. *Andropogon muricatus*) This earthy, amber-coloured oil is extracted from the roots by steam distillation. It calms and soothes the mind, easing hysteria, anger, irritability, mental and physical exhaustion, nervous complaints, and insomnia. It helps heal wounds and ease muscular, rheumatic, and arthritic pain. It nourishes dry and irritated skin, reduces wrinkles and stretch marks, and tightens slack skin. It has the reputation of being an aphrodisiac. Vetiver blends well with benzoin, grapefruit, lavender, and ylang-ylang.

MAGICAL VIRTUES: Money-drawing, protection,
anointing and balancing the heart chakra

PLANET: Venus

ELEMENT: Earth

YARROW (*Achillea millefolium*) This thin, sweet, spicy oil is extracted from the dried herb by steam distillation. It improves circulatory disorders such as varicose veins and haemorrhoids and may reduce high blood pressure. It may help irregular menstruation and menopausal problems. It can be used for inflamed wounds, rashes, cuts, eczema, scars, and burns. In hair preparations it stimulates hair growth. Yarrow blends well with angelica, cedarwood, and verbena.

Caution: Avoid during pregnancy. May irritate sensitive skin.

MAGICAL VIRTUES: Exorcism, banishing, protection,
    purification, psychic awareness, divination

DEITIES: Cernunnos, Herne, Pan

PLANET: Venus

ELEMENT: Water

YLANG-YLANG (*Cananga odorata* var. *genuina* syn. *Unona odorantissimum*) This sweet, exotic pale yellow oil is extracted from the freshly picked flowers by water or steam distillation. It is useful in cases of high blood pressure, rapid breathing and heartbeat, anxiety, tension, shock, fear, panic, insomnia, depression, and stress. It has a stimulating effect on the scalp, which promotes hair growth. It is reputed to be an aphrodisiac. Ylang-ylang blends well with bergamot, grapefruit, lavender, patchouli, and sandalwood.

Caution: Avoid if you have low blood pressure.

MAGICAL VIRTUES: Love, lust, peace, balancing
    and anointing the heart chakra

PLANET: Venus

ELEMENT: Water

Essential Oils By Symptom

ACNE: bergamot, camphor, cedarwood, chamomile (German or Roman), clary
sage, clove, everlasting, geranium, grapefruit, juniper, lavandin, lavender, lemon,
lemongrass, lime, mandarin, neroli, palmarosa, patchouli, petitgrain, rose, rosemary,
rosewood, sandalwood, tea tree, thyme

AGING SKIN: bergamot, chamomile, cypress, geranium, jasmine, juniper, lavender,
lemon, lemongrass, neroli, palmarosa, petitgrain, rose, rosemary, rosewood,
sandalwood, ylang-ylang

ANTIBACTERIAL: basil, bergamot, chamomile, cinnamon, cypress, eucalyptus,
everlasting, geranium, lavender, lemon, lime, palmarosa, patchouli, pine, rose,
sandalwood, tea tree, thyme

ANTIBIOTIC: garlic, tea tree

ANTIFUNGAL: basil, cedarwood, cypress, eucalyptus, garlic, lemon, lemongrass,
patchouli, peppermint, sandalwood, tea tree, thyme

ANTI-INFLAMMATORY: chamomile, citronella, eucalyptus, geranium, ginger,
lavender, patchouli, peppermint, rose, sandalwood, spearmint

ANTIMICROBIAL: myrrh, tagetes, thyme

ANTISEPTIC: basil, bergamot, black pepper, cajuput, camphor, cedarwood,
chamomile, cinnamon, clary sage, cloves, eucalyptus, fir, frankincense, grapefruit,
geranium, ginger, jasmine, juniper, lavender, lemon, lemongrass, lime, nutmeg,
orange, palmarosa, parsley, patchouli, peppermint, pine, rose, rosemary, rosewood,
sandalwood, tea tree, thyme, mandarin, neroli, petitgrain

ANTIVIRAL: cinnamon, eucalyptus, garlic, helichrysum, lavender, lime, palmarosa,
tarragon, tea tree, thyme

ANXIETY: benzoin, chamomile (Roman), clary sage, jasmine, lavender, neroli,
sandalwood

APHRODISIAC: cardamom, clary sage, clove, coriander, ginger, jasmine, neroli,
orange, patchouli, rose, rosewood, sandalwood, vetiver, ylang-ylang

ARTHRITIS: angelica, benzoin, birch, black pepper, cajeput, carrot seed, cedarwood, chamomile, clove, coriander, ginger, juniper, lemon, marjoram, peppermint, pine, sage, thyme, vetiver, yarrow

ASTHMA: cedarwood, cypress, eucalyptus, frankincense, lavender, Roman chamomile

ASTRINGENT: bay, benzoin, cedarwood, cypress, frankincense, geranium, hyssop, helichrysum, juniper, lemon, lime, myrrh, peppermint, rose, rosemary, sandalwood, yarrow

ATHLETE'S FOOT: clove, eucalyptus, lavender, lemon, lemongrass, marjoram, myrrh, patchouli, tea tree

BALDNESS: bay, birch, juniper, rosemary

BOILS: bergamot, chamomile, lavender, tea tree

BRUISES: calendula, chamomile, clove, fennel, geranium, hyssop, lavender, yarrow

BURNS: calendula, chamomile, lavender

CANDIDA: chamomile, eucalyptus, geranium, lavender, patchouli, rosemary, tea tree, thyme

CELLULITE: basil, cedarwood, cypress, fennel, grapefruit, juniper, lavender, lemon, lemongrass, mandarin, pine, rosemary

CELLULITIS: birch, cypress, fennel, grapefruit, lemon, rosemary

CHAPPED SKIN: benzoin, myrrh, patchouli, sandalwood

CHILBLAINS: black pepper, chamomile, lemon, lime, marjoram

CIRCULATION: cypress, geranium, ginger, juniper, lavender, lemon, neroli, peppermint, rose, rosemary, thyme

COLD SORES: bergamot, chamomile, eucalyptus, geranium, lavender, lemon, melissa (lemon balm), tea tree

CORNS: cinnamon, lemon, lime, tea tree

COUGHS: angelica, basil, bergamot, cajuput, cedarwood, garlic, ginger, hyssop, lavender, myrrh, oregano, peppermint, pine, sandalwood, thyme

CUTS: benzoin, chamomile, clove, eucalyptus, lavender, lemon, sage, tea tree, thyme

CYSTITIS: bergamot, chamomile, frankincense, juniper, lavender, pine, thyme, yarrow

DANDRUFF: bay, cedarwood, eucalyptus, lavender, lemon, rosemary, sage, tea tree

DECONGESTANT: cajuput, eucalyptus, garlic, lavender, niaouli, peppermint, pine

DERMATITIS: birch, carrot seed, cedarwood, chamomile, geranium, helichrysum, hyssop, juniper, lavender, peppermint, palmorosa, patchouli, rosemary, sage

DEODORANT: benzoin, bergamot, citronella, clary sage, coriander, cypress, geranium, lavender, lemon, lemongrass, myrrh, patchouli, peppermint, petitgrain, pine, rosewood, tea tree

DEPRESSION: benzoin, bergamot, carnation, chamomile, cinnamon, clary sage, cypress, eucalyptus, geranium, grapefruit, juniper, lavender, lemon, lemongrass, lime, melissa (lemon balm), neroli, orange, patchouli, peppermint, rose, rosemary, sandalwood, spearmint, tangerine, ylang-ylang

DIGESTIVE: black pepper, coriander, ginger, lemon, lemongrass, peppermint

DISINFECTANT: caraway, clove, juniper, lime, myrrh, pine

DRY SKIN: chamomile, frankincense, jasmine, lavender, neroli, palmarosa, patchouli, rose, rosewood, sandalwood, ylang-ylang

DULL SKIN: angelica, birch, fennel, grapefruit, lavender, lemon, rosemary, ylang-ylang

ECZEMA: bergamot, birch, calendula, carrot seed, chamomile, geranium, helichrysum, juniper, lavender, patchouli, rose, rosemary, sage, sandalwood, tea tree, thyme, yarrow

FATIGUE: black pepper, clary sage, frankincense, grapefruit, lemon, mandarin, ylang-ylang

FEVER: bergamot, black pepper, chamomile, eucalyptus, ginger, lemon, melissa (lemon balm)

GOUT: basil, benzoin, carrot seed, juniper, geranium, peppermint, rosemary

HAEMORRHOIDS: coriander, cypress, juniper, myrrh, yarrow

HANGOVER: cypress, grapefruit, juniper, pine, rosemary

HAYFEVER: eucalyptus, German chamomile, lavender, melissa (lemon balm)

HEADACHE: basil, eucalyptus, grapefruit, lavender, melissa (lemon balm), peppermint

HOT FLASHES: clary sage, chamomile, fennel, geranium, lavender, sage

HYPERTENSION: clary sage, lavender, melissa (lemon balm), marjoram, yarrow, ylang-ylang

HYPOTENSION: benzoin, birch, ginger, lavender, lemon, lemongrass, melissa (lemon balm), pine, rosemary, thyme

IMMUNE STIMULANT: cinnamon, geranium, lavender, lemon, rose, rosemary, tea tree

INDIGESTION: angelica, aniseed, basil, bergamot, black pepper, carrot seed, cinnamon, cloves, ginger, hyssop, juniper, lemon, lemongrass, melissa (lemon balm), nutmeg, orange, oregano, parsley, peppermint, pimento, rosemary, spearmint, thyme

INFECTION: black pepper, cinnamon, juniper, lavender, lemon, lemongrass, myrrh, pine, rosemary

INFLUENZA: bay, black pepper, cinnamon, cloves, cypress, ginger, lemon, peppermint

INSECT BITES: basil, bergamot, cajeput, calendula, chamomile, eucalyptus, lavender, lemon, melissa (lemon balm), sage, tea tree, thyme

INSECT REPELLENT: basil, bergamot, cedarwood, citronella, eucalyptus, lavender, lemongrass, melissa (lemon balm), peppermint, rosemary

INSOMNIA: lavender, clary sage, neroli, petitgrain, Roman chamomile, sandalwood

IRRITABILITY: benzoin, clary sage, geranium, lavender, neroli, Roman chamomile, sandalwood

IRRITATED SKIN: angelica, benzoin, calendula, cedarwood, clary sage, helichrysum, hyssop, jasmine, lavender, myrrh, patchouli, rose

JET LAG: basil, geranium, grapefruit, peppermint, rosemary

MEASLES: bergamot, eucalyptus, geranium, German chamomile, lavender, tea tree

MEMORY PROBLEMS: basil, rosemary

MENOPAUSE: clary sage, cypress, geranium, jasmine, lavender, Roman chamomile, sandalwood

MENSTRUAL PROBLEMS: clary sage, geranium, lavender, marjoram, Roman chamomile

MIGRAINE: lavender, peppermint, Roman chamomile, rosemary

MUSCLE CRAMPS: allspice, black pepper, coriander, cypress, grapefruit, jasmine, lavandin, lavender, marjoram, pine, rosemary, thyme, vetiver

MUSCLE PAIN: basil, bay, black pepper, clary sage, marjoram, peppermint, Roman chamomile, rosemary

MUSCLE STIFFNESS: allspice, black pepper, coriander, cypress, grapefruit, jasmine, lavandin, lavender, marjoram, pine, rosemary, thyme, vetiver

NAUSEA: clove, ginger, melissa (lemon balm), peppermint

NEURALGIA: bay, benzoin, black pepper, cajuput, chamomile, clary sage, cloves, geranium, lemon, peppermint

NORMAL/COMBINATION SKIN: bergamot, cedarwood, chamomile, clary sage, geranium, jasmine, lavender, mandarin, neroli, orange, palmarosa, patchouli, petitgrain, rose, rosemary, sandalwood, ylang-ylang

OILY SKIN: basil, bay, bergamot, cajeput, camphor, carrot seed, cedarwood, citronella, clary sage, cypress, fennel, geranium, grapefruit, juniper, lavender, lemon, lemongrass, lime, mandarin, petitgrain, rosemary, rosewood, sandalwood, tea tree, thyme

OVERINDULGENCE: grapefruit, juniper, lemon, peppermint

OVER-WORK: clary sage, lavender, neroli

PALPITATIONS: orange, rose, ylang-ylang

PERSPIRATION: citronella, cypress, lemongrass, pine, sage

PMS/PMT: bergamot, cedarwood, citronella, clary sage, cypress, fennel, geranium, grapefruit, jasmine, juniper, lavender, lemon, neroli, orange, pine, Roman chamomile rose, rosemary, sandalwood

PSORIASIS: angelica, bergamot, birch, chamomile, lavender

RASH: calendula, carrot seed, chamomile, lavender, sandalwood, tea tree, yarrow

REFRESHING: cypress, eucalyptus, grapefruit, juniper, lemon, lime, mandarin, orange, peppermint, rosemary, tangerine, ylang-ylang

RELAXING: benzoin, carnation, clary sage, geranium, jasmine, lavender, lemongrass, neroli, patchouli, sandalwood, ylang-ylang

RESPIRATORY PROBLEMS: basil, benzoin, cedarwood, eucalyptus, peppermint, rosemary, sandalwood

RHEUMATISM: black pepper, cajuput, cedarwood, chamomile, clove, coriander, cypress, eucalyptus, fennel, frankincense, ginger, hyssop, juniper, lavender, lemon, niaouli, oregano, pine, rosemary, thyme, yarrow

RINGWORM: geranium, lavender, marjoram, myrrh, patchouli, peppermint, tea tree

SCABIES: bergamot, cinnamon leaf, lavender, lemongrass, peppermint, pine, rosemary, thyme

SCAR TISSUE: helichrysum, jasmine, neroli, petitgrain, sandalwood

SCIATICA: allspice, chamomile, citronella, eucalyptus, lavender, marjoram, peppermint, pine, rosemary

SEASICKNESS: ginger

SEDATIVE: benzoin, bergamot, cedarwood, clary sage, cypress, frankincense, jasmine, lavender, mandarin, melissa (lemon balm), neroli, petitgrain, rose, sandalwood, ylang-ylang

SHOCK: basil, lavender

SINUSITIS: basil, eucalyptus, lavender, peppermint, pine, rosemary, tea tree

SPOTS: bergamot, cajeput, camphor, eucalyptus, helichrysum, lavender, lemon, lime, mandarin, sage, tea tree, thyme

SPRAINS: black pepper, chamomile, clove, eucalyptus, ginger, lavender, marjoram, pine, rosemary

STRESS: angelica, basil, cedarwood, chamomile, cypress, geranium, jasmine, lavender, lemon, mandarin, neroli, orange, palmarosa, patchouli, petitgrain, rose, tangerine, tarragon, ylang-ylang

STRETCH MARKS: chamomile, frankincense, lavender, mandarin, patchouli, rosemary, rosewood, yarrow

SUNBURN: eucalyptus, lavender, Roman chamomile

SWEATY FEET: cypress, clary sage, geranium, peppermint

SWELLING: chamomile, cinnamon, cypress, eucalyptus, fennel, geranium, grapefruit, juniper, lavender, lemon, peppermint, petitgrain, rose, rosemary, ylang-ylang

THRUSH: bergamot, geranium, myrrh, tea tree

TICKS: marjoram

TOOTHACHE: cajuput, cinnamon, cloves, nutmeg, peppermint, pimento

VARICOSE VEINS: cypress, geranium, lemon, lime, yarrow

VERRUCAE: tea tree

VERTIGO: lavender, melissa (lemon balm), peppermint

WARTS: cinnamon leaf, lemon, lime, tea tree

WATER RETENTION: bay, benzoin, black pepper, carrot seed, cedarwood, cypress, eucalyptus, hyssop, juniper, lavender, lemon, lemongrass, parsley, pine, rose, rosemary, sandalwood

WINDBURN: lavender, chamomile (Roman)

WRINKLES: carrot seed, fennel, frankincense, geranium, jasmine, lavender, mandarin, myrrh, palmorosa, patchouli, rose, rosewood, sandalwood, ylang-ylang

WOUNDS: bergamot, cajuput, calendula, chamomile, clary sage, clove, cypress, eucalyptus, frankincense, geranium, helichrysum, hyssop, juniper, lavender, tea tree

Magical Oils

Essential oils are sometimes called the soul or life blood of a plant, and these concentrated essences are powerful magical tools, drawing on all the magical qualities and vibrations of a particular herb in a concentrated form. You will need to purchase good quality oils from reputable suppliers. You can't make real essential oils at home since it is a lengthy, complicated, and expensive process that requires vast quantities of raw materials, but you can make macerated and infused oils from home-grown or wild plants to use in magic (see pages 269–270).

One very important thing must be said first, though, which is that you *cannot* use synthetic perfumes for magical work any more than you can use them for aromatherapy, and for the same reason. When we use an herb or essential oil for magic, we are using the inherent powers of that plant. Over the course of millennia, medical and magical herbalists have determined the qualities of plants—which herbs heal which conditions, which cleanse negative energies, which create feelings of peace and harmony, and so on—and magic using herbs or oils draws on these qualities. Synthetic perfumes are chemical blends made to imitate the perfume of a flower; fake lavender oil will not have the same effect as real lavender oil. You probably won't know what's in the synthetic oil, but it is not magically inert—what's in it will have its own energy and vibration, and that may have the opposite effect to the working you intend; you should never introduce an unknown quantity into a magical operation. Furthermore, most synthetic fragrance oils contain petroleum solvents, which produce carcinogens when burned.

When you create a magical oil, you make it for specific purposes, blending it with intent and choosing the ingredients very carefully to achieve a magical task. It can be used in a number of ways:

- To anoint a candle for use in candle magic. For example, you could anoint a green candle with money-drawing oil, focusing your intent into the candle as you do, and burn it to release the magic. This blends the energies of the oil with the magical symbolism of the candle's colour and the energy of the flame itself.

- You can evaporate oils in place of incense, using a purpose-made oil evaporator or in a dish of hot water placed on a radiator.

- To consecrate and empower magical tools or robes.

- To consecrate and empower amulets, talismans, charms, and crystals.

- Use as an anointing oil for the body during ritual.

- In the bath add two teaspoons of blended magical oil to the bath after it has run. Treat it as a ritual, not a wash. A purification bath, for example, is a prerequisite to any ritual, and you could use a purification oil or you might use an appropriate oil, such as Beltane oil, to help you attune to the ceremony to come.

- Like an amulet, a magical oil can create a focus for a specific magical intention. Wear it as a perfume or carry a handkerchief infused with it and you will be drawing on that energy all day, however subconsciously. If you need extra courage to face a difficult situation, for example, you might wear a courage oil.

- Use a protection oil to magically seal the doors and windows of your home, to prevent negativity entering or to protect you from magical attacks.

- Use a peace oil or harmony oil to calm the atmosphere in the house after an argument.

- Use a clearing oil to cleanse negativity from a home or ritual space.

- Put a drop of money-drawing oil in your purse or on the till of your shop.

BLENDING A MAGICAL OIL

The following recipes are blends, made with a carrier oil with drops of pure essential oils added. Remember that the carrier oil has its own magical qualities, so choose it with care. I simply put the carrier oil in a dark glass 20 millilitre bottle, add the requisite number of drops of the various essential oils, and gently swirl it to blend them, concentrating on the intent or purpose of the oil as I carry out each step. The bottle should then be capped and labelled. The shelf life of the oil can be extended by adding 20 drops of vitamin E oil. I keep reading that they last six months, but I opened an anointing oil I made fifteen years ago yesterday, and its scent was as strong and true as the day I made it; it depends which oils are used and how it is stored.

The time and season you blend the oil will affect its magical qualities, since they will become an intrinsic part of the blend. A really effective full moon oil, for example, can only be made under the influence of a full moon, and don't even think about making a Beltane oil at Samhain! For more on this topic, please see page 423.

CHARGING A MAGICAL OIL

Magical oils are already imbued with the power of the plants and the intent you put into their blending, but before you use them you can charge (magically empower) them, which reinforces their purpose. Taking your wand or your forefinger, tap the bottle and say, "Let the Lord and Lady witness that I charge this oil that it may (state purpose)."

MAGICAL OIL RECIPES

The following recipes are based on using 20 millilitres of carrier oil plus 20 drops of vitamin E oil to act as a preservative, then adding the advocated number of drops of essential oil. Follow the recipes below or use the tables of correspondences and substitutions at the back of this book.

DEITY OILS	
AMUN RA	FRANKINCENSE 5, CINNAMON 5, ROSE 8, MYRRH 4
APOLLO	CINNAMON 9, MYRRH 4, FRANKINCENSE 2
ARADIA	FRANKINCENSE 5, SANDALWOOD 5, MYRRH 4, LEMON 3, ROSE 20
ARTEMIS	JASMINE 20, VERBENA 4
ASTARTE	SANDALWOOD 4, ROSE 15, ORANGE 5, JASMINE 15
ATHENE	GERANIUM 6, MYRRH 4
BRAN	FRANKINCENSE 5, PINE 5, ROSEWOOD 5

DEITY OILS	
CERNUNNOS	SANDALWOOD 8, PATCHOULI 5, LAVENDER 5, OAKMOSS 5
DEMETER	MYRRH 9, VETIVER 6, OAKMOSS 3
EARTH MOTHER	PINE 9, PATCHOULI 9, ROSE 20
FREYA	CYPRESS 7, ROSE 15, SANDALWOOD 5
HATHOR	ROSE 15, SANDALWOOD 15, BENZOIN 5
HECATE	CYPRESS 10, SANDALWOOD 4, PATCHOULI 6
HERNE	VETIVER 10, PINE 6, JUNIPER 3
HORNED GOD	PATCHOULI 8, PINE 6, CEDAR 4, JUNIPER 4
HORUS	MARJORAM 5, BERGAMOT 10, SANDALWOOD 10
ISIS	ROSE 10, CYPRESS 8, MYRRH 4, GERANIUM 4, CEDAR 5
KALI	JASMINE 12, ROSE 12, SANDALWOOD 6

DEITY OILS

LORD AND LADY	ROSE 10, CINNAMON 4, MYRRH 3, FRANKINCENSE 3
MERLIN	JUNIPER 5, CEDAR 7, ROSEWOOD 4
PAN	PATCHOULI 3, PINE 5, CEDAR 5, JUNIPER 1
SUN GODDESS	CINNAMON 6, LEMON VERBENA 6, YLANG-YLANG 6
TRIPLE GODDESS	JASMINE 10, PATCHOULI 4, ROSE 20

ELEMENTAL OILS

AIR	LAVENDER 8, MARJORAM 8, LEMONGRASS 4
EARTH	PATCHOULI 5, PINE 3, VETIVER 4
FIRE	ORANGE 12, FRANKINCENSE 4, SANDALWOOD 4
WATER	LEMON 10, SANDALWOOD 6, PALMAROSA 6, YLANG-YLANG 4, JASMINE 2

PLANETARY OILS

EARTH	CYPRESS 9, PATCHOULI 9, OAKMOSS 3
JUPITER	CINNAMON 3, CLOVE 1, YLANG-YLANG 5
MARS	CINNAMON 8, CLOVE 8, BLACK PEPPER 2
MERCURY	CLOVE 4, LAVENDER 5, LEMONGRASS 5
MOON	FRANKINCENSE 10, LEMON 3, LEMON BALM 3
NEPTUNE	LEMON 6, JASMINE 7, ROSE 8
PLUTO	EUCALYPTUS 4, PATCHOULI 4, PINE 10
SATURN	CYPRESS 5, PATCHOULI 6, CLOVE 1
SUN	ORANGE 10, CINNAMON 5
VENUS	THYME 7, CEDAR 9, BENZOIN 4

PSYCHIC WORK

ASTRAL PROJECTION	SANDALWOOD 3, BAY 7, LEMONGRASS 7, THYME 7
CLAIRVOYANCE	LEMON 5, FRANKINCENSE 5, SANDALWOOD 5
CLEARING	FRANKINCENSE 5, MYRRH 6, SANDALWOOD 4, ROSEMARY 5
DIVINATION	LEMONGRASS 5, LEMON 5, THYME 5, CLOVE 4
MEDITATION	SANDALWOOD 4, ROSE 20
PROTECTION #1	FRANKINCENSE 6, MYRRH 2, SANDALWOOD 2, ROSEMARY 2, DILL 1
PROTECTION #2	ROSEMARY 3, GERANIUM 4, CYPRESS 4
PSYCHIC	SANDALWOOD 3, ORANGE 6, CLOVE 1
RUNE READING	BAY 6, THYME 6
SCRYING	VALERIAN 5, BAY 2, ANISE 2, CLARY SAGE 3
SPIRIT DEPART	MYRRH 10, RUE 2, MINT 5
SPIRIT GUIDE	LEMONGRASS 7, DILL 4

TO GET THE SIGHT	CINNAMON 3, JUNIPER 3, SANDALWOOD 3, PATCHOULI 2
VISION	FRANKINCENSE 5, THYME 10, LEMONGRASS 2

RITUAL OILS

ALTAR CONSECRATION	FRANKINCENSE 5, MYRRH 5, CINNAMON 10
ANOINTING	MYRRH 4, CINNAMON 4
BABYLONIAN	JUNIPER 10, CEDAR 10, CYPRESS 10
CIRCLE	ROSEMARY 5, LAVENDER 4, MYRRH 4
CONSECRATION	CLOVE 4, LEMONGRASS 8, THYME 8
EGYPTIAN	CEDAR 5, MYRRH 2, JUNIPER 2, FRANKINCENSE 3, CINNAMON 2
ESBAT	SANDALWOOD 10, ROSE 15, MYRRH 3, THYME 2, FRANKINCENSE 5
FULL MOON	SANDALWOOD 10, FRANKINCENSE 4, ROSE 10

RITUAL OILS

HANDFASTING	ROSE 10, ORANGE 4, CINNAMON 2
HEX BREAKER	ROSEMARY 10, FRANKINCENSE 3, BAY 10, JUNIPER 10
INITIATION	FRANKINCENSE 4, SANDALWOOD 4, ROSEMARY 4
KYPHI	JUNIPER 6, FRANKINCENSE 4, CINNAMON 5, CEDAR 6, MYRRH 5, PATCHOULI 4, CYPRESS 6, CAMPHOR 6, SANDALWOOD 4
MEDICINE WHEEL	SAGE 8, PINE 8
PURIFICATION	ROSEMARY 10, LAVENDER 10
SABBAT	FRANKINCENSE 4, MYRRH 4, FENNEL 1, THYME 2, CHAMOMILE 4, ROSE 8
TEMPLE	ROSEMARY 3, FRANKINCENSE 3, THYME 4
UNIVERSAL	FRANKINCENSE 6, MYRRH 6, SANDALWOOD 6, ROSEMARY 6

SABBAT OILS

BELTANE	FRANKINCENSE 3, CALENDULA 10, ROSE 20
MIDSUMMER	CHAMOMILE 5, LAVENDER 10, ROSE 10, VERBENA 10, ORANGE 10, FRANKINCENSE 3
AUTUMN EQUINOX	JUNIPER 12, MYRRH 5, ROSE 10
IMBOLC	BENZOIN 3, MYRRH 10, BASIL 4, CINNAMON 2
LUGHNASA	PINE 6, PATCHOULI 5, SANDALWOOD 10, CEDAR 6, FRANKINCENSE 2
OSTARA	FRANKINCENSE 5, VIOLET 10, ORANGE 6, ROSE 10
SAMHAIN	CYPRESS 5, LEMONGRASS 5, PATCHOULI 5
YULE	FRANKINCENSE 8, ORANGE 5, BAY 1, CINNAMON 3, CLOVE 2

SPELLS

ATTRACT MEN	JASMINE 6, ROSE 3, YLANG-YLANG 2, LAVENDER 3
ATTRACT WOMEN	CEDAR 6, PATCHOULI 4, CINNAMON 7
BUSINESS	BENZOIN 10, CINNAMON 5, BASIL 5
COME TO ME	JASMINE 8, GERANIUM 1, SANDALWOOD 4, ROSE 5
COMPELLING	VERBENA 4, JASMINE 7, ROSE 7, MYRRH 4, LAVENDER 6,
COURAGE	FRANKINCENSE 5, THYME 5
ENERGY	ORANGE 16, LIME 6, CARDAMOM 3
FAST MONEY	PATCHOULI 14, CEDARWOOD 10, VETIVER 8, GINGER 4
HEALING	ROSEMARY 10, JUNIPER 10
INTERVIEW	YLANG-YLANG 8, LAVENDER 6, ROSE 2
LOVE	BERGAMOT 5, LAVENDER 5, CLOVE 1, CINNAMON 1

SPELLS	
LOVE # 2	BERGAMOT 1, LAVENDER 1, CLOVE 1, ORANGE 8, GERANIUM 10
LOVE-DRAWING	ROSE 15 LAVENDER 5
LUCK-CHANGING	CINNAMON 9, PINE 7, VERBENA 7
MONEY-DRAWING #1	PATCHOULI 14, CEDAR 10, VETIVER 8, GINGER 4
MONEY-DRAWING #2	PATCHOULI 5, OAKMOSS 5, PINE 8
PEACE	YLANG-YLANG 6, LAVENDER 6, CHAMOMILE 4, ROSE 2
PERSONAL BLESSING	CINNAMON 3, LAVENDER 3, VETIVER 5
POWER DRAWING	SANDALWOOD 4, ORANGE 8, PINE 7
SUCCESS	VERBENA 7, SANDALWOOD 7, VETIVER 7
VENUS LOVE OIL	VERBENA 2, LEMON 5, ORANGE 5
WEALTH	CINNAMON 8, PATCHOULI 8, BASIL 2

ZODIAC OILS	
AQUARIUS	CYPRESS 10, CEDAR 10
ARIES	BERGAMOT 8, ALLSPICE 3, LIME 2
CANCER	ROSE 20, LEMON 4, SANDALWOOD 20
CAPRICORN	PATCHOULI 4, CYPRESS 4, CINNAMON 2, CEDARWOOD 4, VETIVER 4
GEMINI	LAVENDER 5, LEMONGRASS 4, JUNIPER 3
LEO	JUNIPER 10, ORANGE 10, CINNAMON 5
LIBRA	THYME 2, SANDALWOOD 10, ROSE 10
PISCES	JASMINE 20, LEMON 9, LIME 1
SAGITTARIUS	YLANG-YLANG 15, ORANGE 4
SCORPIO	MYRRH 8, SANDALWOOD 10, BASIL 1, GINGER 1
TAURUS	SANDALWOOD 10, PATCHOULI 3, THYME 2, BENZOIN 5
VIRGO	JUNIPER 5, CYPRESS 10, LEMONGRASS 10, LAVENDER 10, VERBENA 5

COLOURING MAGICAL OILS

Personally, I never colour my magical oils, but some people like to do so to add a further magical resonance. In the occult and in healing, colours are also seen as having a certain vibration, or wavelength. For example, red is a low light vibration, activating the root chakra, producing feelings of strength, passion, etc. At the other end of the scale, violet is a high vibration colour that activates the third eye chakra, producing feelings of inspiration, dream activity, and spirituality. Oils may be coloured with candle wax dyes. See appendix 1 for suitable colours.

USING COLOURED OILS TO BALANCE THE CHAKRAS

RED: Red is a stimulating colour that can be applied to the root chakra to activate it and stimulate the flow of the physical life force, improving vitality. Use ginger, black pepper, cardamom, patchouli, or cinnamon oil.

ORANGE: Orange has a tonic effect and is applied to the spleen chakra to activate it and to stimulate emotional health and well-being. Use clove, fennel, mandarin, marjoram, melissa (lemon balm), neroli, or orange oil.

YELLOW: Yellow stimulates the solar plexus chakra and the mental faculties. Use bergamot, lavender, aniseed, lemongrass, eucalyptus, melissa (lemon balm), or rosemary oils.

GREEN: Green has a calming effect. It is used to stimulate the heart chakra and the emotions and to awaken compassion. Use rose, jasmine, caraway, or lavender oil.

BLUE: Blue is a calming colour and is used to stimulate the throat chakra and awaken intuition. Use benzoin, calendula, lavender, aniseed, or bergamot oil.

VIOLET: Violet is a healing colour that works on both the physical and spiritual levels. It is used to stimulate the third eye chakra and awaken deeper levels of consciousness. Use aniseed, cedar, chamomile, clary sage, juniper, lemongrass, or neroli oil.

WHITE: White is a cleansing and purifying colour. It is used to balance the crown chakra. Use frankincense, myrrh, sage, clary sage, or sandalwood oil.

MAGICAL BATH SALTS

Take a cup of cooking salt, colour with a few drops of food colouring (optional), add 16 drops in total of the required oils (you can use the previous recipes for magical oils), and blend with the back of a spoon. The colour should be added before the oil and blended until it is smooth throughout.

Store immediately in an airtight container. Add a handful to your ritual bath for cleansing the body and aura and to help you attune to the matter at hand. You can vary the oils used to your taste using the tables of correspondences and substitutions at the back of this book.

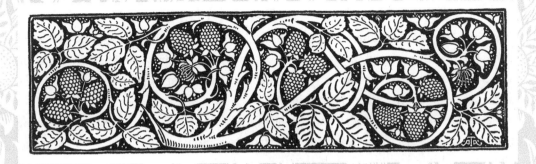

CHAPTER 12

Magical Herbalism

The worldview of the Pagan is different from the normally accepted one of western materialistic society. For the Pagan, everything possesses spirit: a living force within it. People talk about "using" herbs for magic, but this is to misunderstand the relationship. True magical herbalism is not a case of following a kind of cookbook, a pinch of this and a pinch of that; it is many years of intimate study with the plants themselves as the teachers.

When working with plant allies, the spirit of the plant is more important than any "active ingredient." Each plant is a living teacher and must be approached as an individual, which may (or may not) become your ally. It is a knowledge that cannot be bought and that cannot be learned from books, only by doing.

Gathering Ritual Herbs

If you want to work with herbs the hearth witch way, then you must begin by getting to know the plants that grow in your local area—those vegetation spirits that live with you along your local hedgerow, meadow, park, road, or garden. Get yourself a good field guide so that you can identify plants in your locality.

Few western magicians today understand or work with the Old Knowledge concerning plants. So-called "magical herbals" give instructions on how to collect a plant by drawing a circle around it and telling it a little rhyme before hacking it about and leaving it a coin or pinch of tobacco in recompense for its trauma. What good these are to it remains a mystery. Some books will tell you that you must ask a tree or plant for its favours—walk round it three times and ask if you can have a bit. How many people know when they have got an answer? Is the plant even listening? You might as well buy some herbs off the shelf in the supermarket or pick up a dead twig from the forest floor.

Spend time with the plants, noting where they live—in sun or shade, on chalky soil or sandy soil, and so on—their growth habits, when they flower, and when they set their seeds. Note the shape of the leaves, their texture and colour; their taste, if edible. In this way you will begin to learn from the plants themselves. Each plant must be approached as an individual spirit, a vital life force approached with love and respect. You must learn to speak its language by listening with an open heart and using the inner senses, as well as the everyday senses of taste, smell, and touch. Don't expect to learn everything at once, as it will likely be over several seasons that the plant reveals its nature to you. The plant itself is always the teacher.

Sometimes a plant or tree will call to you, and you should listen and trust your inner wisdom. Accept any insight that is given to you, no matter what the circumstances. No two oak trees have the same personality, and no two yarrows have the same qualities. Some plants will give willingly, some must be courted, some hunted with stealth. Some will never give you anything, no matter how persistent you are.

Each plant must be correctly approached and harvested in perfect condition; its life force is the essence of its power. This force is harnessed by taking the plant internally, fresh or as an infusion; by employing it in an incense or bathing herb, by using it as a magical potion, or by using it in a spell or ritual. If the herb is approached with love and trust, its force will harmonise with the witch and share its secrets. If the plant is taken with the wrong motives or if it is mistreated or misused, it may cause discomfort, mislead, or seek to gain control of the witch. If an enemy is made of the plant spirit, it can destroy.

Finally, remember that all herbs are infused with the energy of the moon. As the moon waxes and wanes, pulling with her the tides of the sea, she influences all that is living. As the moon waxes, the energy flows upwards into the leaves and stalks of the plant; as it wanes, the virtue travels to the roots. Plants to be harvested for their roots should be gathered at the waning moon, and plants required for their flowers, leaves, and fruits should be gathered at the waxing moon.

Identifying Herbs

Plant names can be a bit confusing. For example, "marigold" is applied to *Calendula officinalis*, a useful medicinal herb, and *Tagetes*, an annual flower used as a bedding plant, which is poisonous. Then again, many plants have local and folk names, but there are a dozen different species called bachelor's buttons, and you don't want to get the wrong one for your purposes.

The only way to be sure is to refer to the official botanical name, usually in Latin or Greek. This normally has two parts, the first referring to the genus the plant belongs to, and the second referring to the specific species and usually descriptive, so that *Quercus rubra* translates as "oak red," with *quercus* meaning "oak" and *rubra* meaning "red." The second part of the name can tell you a lot about the plant: *officinalis*, for example, means that it was a medicinal herb listed in the official pharmacopeia, while *azurea* means "blue," *chinensis* means "from China," *vulgaris* means "common," *sylvestris* means "of the woods," *sativa* means "cultivated," and *stellata* means "starry." Using botanical names isn't entirely foolproof, as they are sometimes changed as the plants are reclassified and may appear differently in older books. Throughout this work I've tried to give both old and new botanical names.

On Correspondences

The subject of magical correspondences is a complex one created from a variety of sources. To begin with, we have the traditional uses for herbs, both magical and medicinal, which come down to us in the accounts and survivals of folklore; some herbs were thought to attract fairies, others to dispel disease and negativity, some were hung up as a protective measure, and so on. We also have the assignations given to herbs by various religions and different plants used in the worship of specific gods or associated with them in mythology. Where I have assigned gods and goddesses to herbs it is because those plants were connected with those particular deities either in their mythology or worship. I have seen books and websites that arbitrarily assign gods to herbs, while others ascribe them based on their planetary rulers, but this is incorrect. Why would a plant from China or the New World be sacred to a Greek god when those plants were unknown in ancient Greece, for example? Treat such assignations with caution.

When you look up the correspondences of a plant, you may read that such-and-such an herb is ruled by the sun or Mercury and so on. Most of this lore is from mediaeval astrologers, who believed that all herbs and plants came under the rulership of the planets, as follows:

- Sun: The sun is dynamic and expansive. Herbs ruled by the sun turn towards the sun or have yellow flowers, such as marigold, St. John's wort, and dandelion.

- Mars: Mars is the planet of war, so Mars plants symbolise a warlike spirit and generally have thorns or stings, such as thistles and nettles.

- Saturn: Saturn is the planet of aging, limitation, and death, so Saturn plants are slow growing or long living and woody, thrive in the shade, and have deep roots, or they are poisonous, foul smelling, or considered evil, such as hemlock and henbane.

- Mercury: Mercury is the planet of communication, so Mercury plants include fast-growing weeds, creepers, and winding plants or plants with hairy, fuzzy, or finely divided leaves. They may be aromatic.

- Venus: Venus is the planet of love and beauty, so Venus plants overwhelm the senses with sweet scents and lovely flowers, red fruits, or soft, furry leaves.

- Moon: The moon governs the tides, and moon plants often grow near water or have a high water content or juicy leaves. They may have white flowers or moon-shaped leaves or seed pods.

- Jupiter: Jupiter is the bringer of abundance, so Jupiter plants are usually big and bold and often edible.

For at least a couple of thousand years and right up to the seventeenth century and beyond, it was usual for physicians to take astrological influences into account when formulating treatments for their patients, based on which planet had caused the disease or which part of the body was afflicted:

- Sun: heart, spine, general vitality

- Moon: stomach, digestive system

- Mercury: brain, five senses, hands

- Venus: throat, kidneys, ovaries

- Mars: muscles, head

- Jupiter: liver, thighs, feet, growth

- Saturn: skin, hair, teeth, bones

This means that if you had a heart problem, you would treat it with herbs of the sun; if you had a bone problem, you would treat it with herbs of Saturn. The astrologer-herbalist tradition was recorded most comprehensively in *The Compleat Herbal* (1653) by Nicholas Culpeper.

Naturally, ritual magicians also worked to the same astrological principles:

- Sun: dynamic, male, expansive energy; the sun rules over prosperity and general protection

- Moon: subtle, feminine, and inward-looking energy; the moon rules the instinct, emotions, and psychic abilities

- Mercury: rules the mind, intellect, and communication

- Venus: feminine, creative, harmonious, and loving energy

- Mars: male, assertive, spontaneous, and daring energy

- Jupiter: benign, expansive, and optimistic energy

- Saturn: Saturn's energy is to do with limitation, change, the crystallisation of efforts, and with endings

The more recently discovered planets have also been assigned traits:

- Uranus: inspirational, inventive, and intuitive

- Neptune: passive, visionary, and dreamy

- Pluto: sexual energy

The old astrologer-herbalists of Europe assigned planets and elements to each known herb according to its characteristics and virtues. This means that New World and oriental plants generally do not have such attributions, though modern magical herbalists are attempting to rectify this: some with more skill and understanding than others, it has to be said, so be wary when you come across them.

· · · · ·

The Elements

In modern Pagan magic we also work with the four elements of earth, air, fire, and water. The four elements as the basic building blocks of creation were first defined by Empedocles, a fifth-century BCE philosopher from Sicily who was an initiate of several mystery traditions. His *Tetrasomia*, or "Doctrine of the Four Elements," influenced Western philosophy and magic in the succeeding millennia. He didn't actually call these four principles elements (*stoikheia*), but roots (*rhizai*), since he was a magical herbalist. For him, the elements were not just physical forms but manifested spiritual essences or even god energies; they were the fourfold roots of everything that had existed in fixed quantities since the beginning of the universe, not as isolated things but as parts of the whole.

AIR: The powers of air are concerned with the intellect, the powers of the mind, knowledge (as opposed to wisdom), logic, inspiration, information, teaching, memory, thought, and communication. Like the other elements, the powers of air can be constructive or destructive. Air magic is usually concerned with the intellectual or the spiritual, and in ritual air is symbolised through the use of perfume or incense. Air plants tend to be freshly fragrant, such as bergamot, lavender, lemon grass, mint, and pine.

EARTH: The powers of earth are concerned with what is manifest—the material, the fixed, the solid, the practical—and with what is rooted. Earth magic is concerned with manifestation, business, health, practicality, wealth, stability, grounding and centring, fertility and agriculture. Earth plants tend to be nourishing or earthy-smelling, such as cypress and patchouli.

FIRE: Fire is the most mysterious of all the elements. It seems almost supernatural in comparison to earth, air, or water, which are states of matter while fire is energy. Fire magic is concerned with creativity, life energy, and zeal. Fire gives us vitality, igniting action, animation, and movement. It sparks courage and acts of bravery. It heats passion and enthusiasm. Fire is the power of inner sight and creative vision, directing it and controlling it to make it manifest in the world. Fire plants tend to have fiery sap or to taste hot, like ginger, or have warm perfumes, like carnation, clove, and cinnamon.

WATER: Water is a liquid, like the blood that flows through our veins. It is associated with the emotions, feelings, and the subconscious, and water magic is usually concerned with divination and scrying. Water plants are juicy and fleshy or grow near water, such as iris, lemon, and jasmine.

· · · · ·

The Magical Virtues of Plants

ACACIA (*Acacia senegal*): Relaxation, regeneration, spring, meditation, protection. Sacred to Adonis, Apollo, Astarte, Christ, Diana, Ishtar, Jehovah, Osiris, Ra, Vishnu. Ruled by the sun and the element of air. See Arabic Gum.

ACONITE (*Aconitum napellus*): Death, black magic, gods and goddesses of death and the underworld. Ruled by the planet of Saturn and the element of water. **Note:** poisonous.

ACORN (*Quercus spp.*): Growth, luck, money, protection.

AFRICAN VIOLET (*Saintpaulia spp.*): Home protection, spirituality. Ruled by the planet Venus and the element of water.

AGAPANTHUS (*Agapanthus* spp.): Aphrodisiac, fertility, love. Ruled by the planet Mars.

AGRIMONY (*Agrimonia eupatoria*): Emotional healing, protection, psychic, smudge, counter-magic. Ruled by the planet Jupiter, the element of air, and the star sign Cancer.

ALDER (*Alnus glutinosa*): Ostara, divination, scrying. Ruled by the planet Venus and the elements of fire, water, and earth. Sacred to Apollo, Arawn, Arthur, Bran, Branwen, Circe, Cronos, fairies, Guinevere, Gwern, Herakles, Marsyas, Orpheus, Phoroneus, and Rinda.

ALECOST (*Crysanthemum balsamita* syn. *Tanacetum balsamita*): Women's rituals and rites of mother goddesses. Ruled by the moon and the element of air.

ALEXANDERS (*Smyrnium olusatrum*): Male magic and the god principle. Ruled by Jupiter and the element of fire. Sacred to Zeus.

ALFALFA (*Medicago sativa*): Grounding, money, prosperity, protection. Ruled by the planet Venus and the element of earth.

ALKANET (*Anchusa officinalis*): Purification, prosperity.

ALLSPICE (*Pimenta dioica*): Energy, healing, luck, money, virility. Ruled by the planet Mars and the element of fire.

ALMOND (*Prunus dulcis*, syn. *Prunus amygdalus/Amygdalus communis/Amygdalus dulcis*): Ostara, regeneration, divination, fertility, love, luck, money. Ruled by the planets Mercury and the sun, the element of air, and the star sign of Gemini. Sacred to Amacas, Attis, Car, Carmenta, the Caryatids, Cybele, Demophoon, Freya, Metis, Nana, Phyllis, and Zeus.

ALOE VERA (*Aloe barbadensis, Aloe indica, Aloe perfoliata, Aloe vulgaris*): Healing, love, home protection, divination, spiritual development. Ruled by the moon and the element of water. Sacred to Aeacus, Amun Ra, Artemis, Chandra, Indra, moon goddesses, Rhadamanthus, Venus, Vulcan, and Yama.

ALOES, WOOD (*Aquilaria malaccensis*): Love and spirituality. Ruled by the planet Saturn, the elements of earth and water, and the star signs Capricorn and Cancer.

ALYSSUM (*Alyssum* spp.): Balance, calm, peace, protection. Ruled by the planet Mercury and the element of air.

AMARANTH (*Amaranthus* spp.): Death, funerals, healing, immortality, protection. Sacred to Artemis and Demeter. It is ruled by the planet Saturn, the element of fire, and the star signs Capricorn and Aquarius.

ANEMONE (*Anemone* spp.): Ostara, healing, hope, renewal. Sacred to Adonis, Aphrodite, and Tammuz. Ruled by the planet Mars, the element of fire, and the star signs Aries and Scorpio.

ANGELICA (*Angelica archangelica* syn. *Angelica officinalis*): Beltane, Midsummer, south, healing, protection, cleansing, exorcism, purification, banishing, blessing, clairvoyance, visions, warding, peace. Ruled by the sun, the element of fire, and the sign of Leo. Sacred to sun gods and Venus.

ANISE (*Pimpinella anisum*): Clairvoyance, banishing, divination, exorcism, protection. Ruled by the planet Mercury, the element of air, and the sign of Gemini. Sacred to Apollo, Hermes, and Mercury.

APPLE (*Malus* spp.): Fertility, lust, love, marriage, immortality, fidelity, harvest, initiation, wisdom. Ruled by the sun and Venus, the element of water, and the sign of Taurus. Sacred to Aphrodite, Apollo, Bel, Ceridwen, Demeter, Diana, Eve, Flora, Godiva, Herakles, Hesperides, Iduna, Inanna, Kore, Lugh, Mêliae, Morgana, Nehallenia, Olwen, Persephone, Pomona, sun gods, Titaea, Venus, and Zeus.

APRICOT (*Prunus armeniaca*): Love. Ruled by the planet Venus, the element of water, and the star signs Taurus and Libra.

ARABIC GUM (*Acacia senegal*): Purification, attracting positive energy. Ruled by the sun, the element of air, and the star sign of Leo. Sacred to Apollo, Helios, and Sol. See Acacia.

ARBUTUS (*Arbutus* spp.): Protection, exorcism. Ruled by the planet Mars, the element of fire, and the star signs Aries and Scorpio.

ARNICA (*Arnica montana*): Fertility, protection. Ruled by the sun and the element of fire. Sacred to Apollo, Freya, Helios, and Ra.

ASAFOETIDA (*Ferula foetida*): Exorcism, purification, prophetic dreams, fertility. Ruled by Saturn and Mars, the element of fire, and the star signs Aries and Scorpio. Sacred to Athene, Priapus, and Saturn.

ASH (*Fraxinus* spp.): The world tree, astral travel, all rites of passage, healing, protection, initiation, autumn equinox, Midsummer, Ostara, and Yule. Sacred to Ares, Athene, Cernunnos, Fates, Furies, Gwydion, Herne, Jupiter, Llyr, Mars, Minerva, Neptune, Norns, Odin, Poseidon, Thor, Uranus, Woden, Wyrd, Ymir, and Zeus. Ruled by the sun, the elements of water and fire, and the star sign Leo.

ASPARAGUS (*Asparagus officinalis*): Fertility, lust, potency. Ruled by the planets Mars and Jupiter, the element of fire, and the signs Gemini and Virgo. Sacred to Hermes, Mercury, and Zeus.

ASPEN (*Populus tremula*): Protection on all levels, communication with spirit, resurrection, the world tree, underworld journeys, Samhain, and Yule. Ruled by the sun and the element of fire. Sacred to Apollo, death goddesses, Hercules, Jupiter, Mut, Nun, Valkyries, and the White Goddess.

ASPHODEL (*Asphodelus albus*): Fertility, peace, love. Ruled by the planets Saturn and Venus, the element of water, and the signs Tauris, Libra, Capricorn, and Aquarius. Sacred to Aphrodite, Hades, Hecate, Persephone, Pluto, Saturn, and Venus. **Note:** poisonous.

ASTRAGALUS (*Astragalus* spp.): Life-force enhancing, healing.

ASTER (*Aster* spp.): Calming, astral projection, love. Ruled by the planet Venus, the element of water, and the star signs Taurus and Libra. Sacred to Aphrodite and Venus.

AUBERGINE AKA EGGPLANT (*Solanum melongena*): Prosperity, wealth. Ruled by the planet Jupiter.

AVENS (*Guem urbanum*): Exorcism, purification. Ruled by the planet Jupiter, the element of fire, and the star signs Sagittarius and Pisces. Sacred to Jupiter, Thor, and Zeus.

AVOCADO (*Persea americana*): Happiness, wealth, longevity, love, lust.

AZALEA (*Rhododendron* spp.): Attraction. **Note:** poisonous.

BALM OF GILEAD (*Commiphora gileadensis*): Love, attracting spirits, protection, psychic healing. Ruled by the planets Jupiter and Venus, the element of water, and the star signs Taurus and Libra. Sacred to Aphrodite and Venus.

BAMBOO (*Bambuseae* spp.): Protection, luck, hex breaking, banishing.

BANANA (*Musa* spp.): Passion, fertility, potency, prosperity.

BASIL (*Ocimum basilicum*): Healing, revitalising, love, initiation, business, fidelity, happiness, harmony, home, money. Ruled by the planet Mars, the element of fire, and the sign of Scorpio. Sacred to Erzulie, Krishna, Lakshmi, and Vishnu.

BARLEY (*Hordeum vulgare*): Fertility, initiation, harvest, Lughnasa, autumn equinox. Sacred to Ceres and Demeter.

BAY (*Laurus nobilis*): Prophecy, divination, healing, consecrating tarot cards, protection, banishing negativity, cleansing, spiritual purification, prophetic dreams, sealing. Ruled by the sun, the element of fire, and the star sign Leo. Sacred to Adonis, Aesculapius, Apollo, Ares, Ceres, Ceridwen, Cupid, Daphne, Eros, Faunus, gods of healing, Mars, Ra, sun and dawn gods and goddesses, and Vishnu.

BAYBERRY (*Myrica cerifera*): Money, prosperity, luck, blessings, Yule. Ruled by the planets Jupiter and Mercury and the element of earth.

BEAN (*Fabaceae/Leguminosae* spp.): Death, spirits of the dead, funerals, banishing negativity and evil. Ruled by the planet Mercury and the element of air. Sacred to Blodeuwedd, Cardea, Carnea, and Demeter.

BEECH (*Fagus sylvatica*): Ruled by the planets Mars and Saturn. Sacred to Artemis, Diana, Jupiter, Odin, Thor, and Zeus. Used to consecrate magical books or while studying magical scripts and alphabets.

BELLADONNA (*Atropa belladonna*): Trance, visions, divination, death and the underworld, underworld deities, Samhain. Ruled by the planet Saturn and the element of water. Sacred to Atropos, Bellona, Circe, Dionysus, and Hecate. **Note:** deadly poisonous.

BENZOIN (*Styrax benzoin*): Cleansing, purifying, spiritual development, astral projection, meditation, balance, equinoxes. Ruled by the sun, the element of fire, and the signs Leo and Aquarius. Sacred to Aphrodite, Ares, Freya, Hathor, Khephera, Mut, Nike, Typhon, and Venus.

BERGAMOT, MONARDA (*Monarda didyma*): Protection, meditation. Ruled by the planet Mercury, the element of air, and the star signs Gemini and Virgo.

BERGAMOT, CITRUS (*Citrus bergamia*): Money and success. Ruled by the planet Mercury, the element of air, and the signs Gemini and Virgo.

BETONY (*Betonica officinalis*): Healing, dispelling negativity, protection. Ruled by the sign of Aries, the element of fire, and the planet Jupiter. Sacred to gods of medicine and healing, such as Aesculapius and Chiron, and stag-horned gods, such as Herne and Cernunnos.

BILBERRY (*Vaccinium myrtillus*): Counter-magic, protection, luck, money. Ruled by the planet Jupiter, the elements fire and water, and the signs Sagittarius and Pisces.

BINDWEED (*Convolvulus* spp.): Binding. Ruled by Saturn and the element of water.

BIRCH (*Betula alba*): The passage of the sun, new beginnings, birth, purification, protection, warding, Beltane, Midsummer, growth, healing, fertility, love, otherworld travel, vision, divination. Ruled by the planet Venus and the element of water. Sacred to Brigantia, Brighid, Earth Mother, Kupala, Kupalo, the Rusalki, and Thor.

BIRTHWORT (*Aristolochia longa*): Afterbirth, sacred to goddesses of childbirth. Ruled by the planet Venus and the element of water. Sacred to Artemis and Diana.

BISTORT (*Polygonum bistorta*): Cleansing, banishing, exorcism, fertility, Ostara. Ruled by the planet Saturn and the element of earth. Sacred to Apollo, Bel, Brighid, Cernunnos, Helios, Kneph, and Pythios.

BLACKBERRY (*Rubus fructicosus*): Autumn equinox, harvest, abundance, death, consecrating the cup or cauldron. Ruled by the planet Venus, the element of water, and the sign of Aries. Sacred to Brigantia, Brighid, fairies, and harvest goddesses.

BLACKTHORN (*Prunus spinosa*): Samhain, death aspects of the Goddess, particularly Ceridwen. Ruled by the element of earth and the planet Saturn.

BLADDERWRACK (*Fucus vesiculosis*): Sea magic, money, protection. Ruled by the moon, the element of water, and the star sign Cancer. Sacred to moon goddesses.

BLOODROOT (*Sanguinaria candensis*): Harmony, marriage, love, protection, purification. **Note:** poisonous.

BLUEBELL (*Hyacinthoides non-scripta/Endymion non-scriptus/Scilla non-scriptus*): Constancy, fairy contact, joy, love, death, funerals, Beltane. Ruled by the moon or Saturn, the element of air, and the signs Libra and Cancer. Sacred to Diana, Endymion, fairies, and Pan.

BORAGE (*Borago officinalis*): Rouses from lethargy, excites activity, courage, Lughnasa, psychic awareness, meditation, inner journeys. Ruled by the planet Jupiter and the zodiac sign of Leo. Sacred to Llew and Lugh.

BROOM (*Genista* sp.): Coming of summer, cleansing and purification, sweeps away negativity, Beltane. Ruled by the planet Mars. Sacred to Blodeuwedd.

BRYONY (*Bryonia alba*): Poppets, money-drawing, underworld journeys, protection. Ruled by the planet Mars and the element of earth.

BUCHU (*Agathosma betulina*): Psychic powers, prophetic dreams, esbats. Ruled by the moon, the element of water, and the star sign Cancer. Sacred to moon goddesses.

BUCKTHORN (*Rhamnus* spp.): Protection, exorcism, justice.

BUCKWHEAT (*Fagopyrum esculentum*): Protection from negativity, poverty, and evil; money attraction and wealth; autumn equinox. Ruled by the planet Venus and the element of earth. Sacred to harvest gods and goddesses.

BUGLEWEED (*Lycopus virginicus*): Love and protection. Ruled by the planet Venus, the elements of earth and air, and the signs Taurus and Libra.

BURDOCK (*Arctium lappa*: greater dock and *Arctium minus*: lesser dock): Protection against magic, healing. Ruled by the planet Venus and the element of water. Sacred to Blodeuwedd.

CALAMUS AKA SWEET FLAG (*Acorus calamus/Calamus aromaticus*): Compelling, luck, healing, money, protection.

CALENDULA (*Calendula officinalis*): Consecration, constancy, love, protection. Ruled by the sun, the element of fire, and the sign Leo. Sacred to sun gods.

CAMELLIA (*Camellia* spp.): Love.

CAMPHOR (*Cinnamonum camphora*): Chastity, health, cleansing, divination, prophetic dreams. Ruled by the moon and the element of water. Sacred to Artemis and Chandra.

CARAWAY (*Carum carvi*): Protection, cycle of the year, faithfulness, cleansing. Ruled by the sun and Mercury and the element of air.

CARDAMOM (*Elettaria cardamomum*): Love, passion, lust. Ruled by the planet Venus and the element of water. Sacred to Erzulie, Hecate, and Medea.

CARNATION (*Dianthus* spp.): Celebrations, handfasting, protection, luck, south, Midsummer. Ruled by the sun and the element of fire. Sacred to Jupiter and Zeus.

CAROB (*Ceratonia siliqua*): Health, wealth. Ruled by the planet Jupiter, the element of fire, and the sign Sagittarius. Sacred to Jupiter and Zeus.

CARROT (*Daucus carota*): Fertility. Ruled by the planet Mercury, the element of fire, and the signs Gemini and Virgo.

CATNIP (*Nepeta cataria*): Trances, shapeshifting work. Ruled by the planet Venus and the element of water. Sacred to Bast and Sekhmet.

CEDAR (*Cedrus* spp.): True cedars belong to the genus *Cedrus* and are associated with eternity and preservation from decay and corruption, the continuation of the soul, and longevity. Ruled by Mercury and the sun and the element of fire. Sacred to Amun Ra, Cernunnos, Indra, Isis, Jupiter, Osiris, Pan, Poseidon, and Wotan.

CELANDINE, GREATER (*Chelidonium majus*): Protection, happiness, Ostara, Beltane. Ruled by the sun and the element of fire. Sacred to sun gods.

CELANDINE, LESSER (*Ranunculus ficaria*): Visions, cleansing crystal balls and scrying tools, Ostara. Ruled by the sun and the element of fire. Sacred to Artemis, Diana, Hecate, and sun gods.

CENTAURY (*Centaurium erythraea* syn. *Eurythraea centaurium*): Trance states, the craft of herbalism, communication with plant spirits. Ruled by the sun and the element of fire. Sacred to Chiron, the patron of herbalists.

CHAMOMILE (*Anthemis nobilis* syn. *Chamaemelum nobile*: Roman chamomile and *Matricaria chamomilla* syn. *M. recutita* and *Chamomilla recutita*: German chamomile): Regeneration, healing, protection, peace, money, luck, Midsummer. Ruled by the sun, the element of water, and the sign of Leo. Sacred to Cernunnos, Ra, and sun gods.

CHERRY (*Prunus avium*): Happiness, love, and divination.

CHERVIL (*Anthriscus cerefolium*): Mental activity, clarity, Samhain, initiation, connection to the higher self. Ruled by the planet Jupiter and the elements of air and water. Sacred to the goddess Ceridwen.

CHESTNUT, HORSE (*Aesculus hippocastanum*): Abundance, conception, fertility, justice, success. Ruled by the planet Jupiter and the element of fire. Sacred to Zeus.

CHICKWEED (*Stellaria media*): Fertility, love, Imbolc. Ruled by the planet Venus and the element of earth. Sacred to Brigantia.

CHICORY (*Cichorium intybus*): Removal of obstacles, invisibility, Lughnasa, autumn equinox. Ruled by Jupiter and the element of air. Sacred to harvest gods and goddesses.

CHILI PEPPER (*Capsicum* spp.): Fidelity, love, counter-magic. Ruled by the planet Mars, the element of fire, and the signs Aries and Scorpio.

CHINA BERRY (*Melia azedarach*): Luck and change.

CHRYSANTHEMUM (*Chrysanthemum* spp.): Ancestors, funerals, home, strength, protection, cheerfulness. Ruled by the sun and the element of fire.

CINNAMON (*Cinnamonum zeylanicum* syn. *Cinnamonum lauraceae*): Purification, raises magical vibration, peace, healing, blessing, lust, money, healing. Ruled by the sun and fire. Sacred to Aesculapius, Aphrodite, Helios, Ra, and Venus.

CINQUEFOIL (*Potentilla* spp.): Protection, purification. Ruled by the planet Jupiter and the element of fire. Sacred to Mother Earth.

CLARY SAGE (*Salvia sclarea*): Visions, getting the sight, opening the third eye. Ruled by Mercury and the moon and the element of air.

CLEAVERS (*Gallium aparine*): Renewal, Ostara, purification. Ruled by the moon and the element of water.

CLOVE (*Carophyllus aromaticus* syn. *Syzygium aromaticum*): Aphrodisiac, lust, money, prosperity. Ruled by the planet Jupiter and the element of fire.

CLOVER (*Trifolium* spp.): Visionary herb, Beltane, faithfulness. Ruled by the planet Mercury and all four elements. Sacred to Aphrodite, Freya, Hathor, and Venus.

COCONUT (*Cocos nucifera*): Luck, purification, protection, chastity.

COHOSH, BLACK (*Actaea racemosa*): Banishing, courage, love, protection, potency.

COHOSH, BLUE (*Caulophyllum thalictroides*): Protection, healing, purification, women's magic.

COLTSFOOT (*Tussilago farfara*): Ostara, Beltane, divination, love, money, healing, tranquillity. Ruled by the planet Venus and the element of water.

COLUMBINE (*Aquilegia vulgaris*): Healing, childbirth, gifts of the spirit, courage, love, spiritual warrior, second-degree initiation, otherworld journeys. Ruled by the planet Venus and the element of water.

COMFREY (*Symphylum officinale*): Cleansing, divination, luck, healing, love, safety whilst travelling, protection. Ruled by the planet Saturn, the element of air, and the star sign of Capricorn. Sacred to Hecate.

COPAL (*Protium copal*): Love and purification.

CORIANDER (*Coriandrum sativum*): Healing, eternal life, aphrodisiac, love, protection, peace. Ruled by the planet Mars and the element of fire. Sacred to Aphrodite and Venus.

CORN (i.e., all grain crops): Abundance, harvest, autumn equinox, Lughnasa. Ruled by the sun and the element of fire. Sacred to gods and goddesses of the harvest, such as Ceres and Demeter.

CORNFLOWER (*Centaurea cyanus*): Opens the third eye chakra, clairvoyance, autumn equinox, Lughnasa. Ruled by the planet Saturn and the element of water. Sacred to Chiron (the patron deity of herbalism), Flora, and gods and goddesses of the harvest.

COSTMARY: see Alecost

CROCUS (*Crocus* spp.): Friendship, love, peace, Imbolc, Ostara. Ruled by the planets Mercury and Venus and the element of water. Sacred to Aphrodite, Cupid, Eros, Persephone, and Venus.

CUCKOO PINT (*Arum maculatum*): Beltane, sacred marriage. Ruled by the planet Mars and the element of fire. Sacred to the Lord and Lady. **Note:** poisonous.

CUCUMBER (*Cucumis sativus*): Chastity, healing, fertility, astral travel. Ruled by the moon and the element of water.

CYCLAMEN (*Cyclamen* spp.): Banishing, fertility, protection, happiness, lust. Ruled by the planet Mars and the element of water. Sacred to Hecate.

CYPRESS (*Cupressus* spp.): Fire worship, the sun, death, mourning, funerals, the incorruptible nature of the spirit, Yule, calming. Ruled by the planet Saturn and the element of earth. Sacred to Aesculapius, Ahuramazda, Aphrodite, Apollo, Artemis, Ashtoreth, Athene, Bhavani, Calypso, Cronos, Cupid, Cyparissos, Daphne, Demeter, Diana, Fates, Freya, Furies, Gaia, Hades, Hebe, Hecate, Hera, Herakles, Isis, Jupiter, maiden goddesses, Mithras, Mut, Nephthys, Persephone, Pluto, Rhea, Saturn, Sylvanus, and Zarathustra.

DAFFODIL (*Narcissus pseudonarcissus*): Love, luck, fertility, death. Ruled by the planet Mars.

DAISY, ENGLISH (*Bellis perennis*): Purity, innocence, faithful love, attracting true love, Beltane, Midsummer. Ruled by the planet Venus, the element of water, and the sign of Cancer. Sacred to Alcestis, Aphrodite, Apollo, Artemis, Belenos, Belidis, Christ, Dryads, Freya, Saule, sun gods and goddesses, Thor, and Venus.

DAMIANA (*Turnera diffusa* syn. *Turnera aphrodisiaca*): Love, lust, aphrodisiac, tantric magic, Great Rite, visions. Ruled by the planet Pluto, the element of water, and the sign Scorpio. Sacred to Artemis, Diana, Ganesha, Vishnu, and Zeus.

DANDELION (*Taraxacum officinale*): Sun emblem, energy, vitality, divination, Beltane. Sacred to Brighid, Green George, and Hecate. Ruled by the planet Jupiter, the element of air, and the sign Sagittarius.

DATE PALM (*Phoenix dactylifera*): Regeneration, fertility, rebirth. Sacred to Amun, Demeter, Inanna, Isis, Lat, Leto, Nephthys, and Nike.

DATURA (*Datura stramonium*): Sleep, protection, astral projection and hex breaking. **Note:** poisonous.

DEADLY NIGHTSHADE: see Belladonna

DEVIL'S CLAW (*Harpagophytum procumbens*): Banishing, exorcism. Ruled by the planet Mars and the element of fire.

DILL (*Anethum graveolens*): Protection against witchcraft, clears the mind, protection, cleansing sacred space, Midsummer, Beltane. Ruled by the planet Mercury and the element of fire or air.

DITTANY OF CRETE (*Origanum dictamnus*): Death and the afterlife, childbirth, astral projection. Ruled by the planet Venus. Sacred to the goddess Lucine and Zeus.

DOCK (*Rumex crispus*): Healing, money, fertility, divination, warrior magic. Ruled by the planet Jupiter and the element of air.

DOGWOOD (*Cornus sanguinea*): Protection and safety for home and children, protection against witchcraft, divination. Sacred to Ares and Mars.

DRAGON'S BLOOD (*Dracaena draco*): Eternal life, love, faithfulness, potency, astral projection, add to incenses to increase their potency, consecration. Ruled by the planet Mars and the element of fire. Sacred to Ares, Athene, Horus, Isis, Menthu, Minerva, and Shiva.

ECHINACEA (*Echinacea* spp.): Healing, prosperity, protection. Ruled by the planet Mars.

ELECAMPANE (*Inula helenium*): Love, protection against magic, psychic powers, Midsummer, connection with nature spirits, luck. Ruled by the planet Mercury, the element of air, and the signs Virgo and Gemini.

ELDER (*Sambucus nigra*): The dried blossom makes a good fixative for herbal incenses. It can be particularly added to Beltane and Midsummer incense, and is sacred to dryads, fairies, and Venus. The leaves should be gathered on Midsummer morning to add to healing incense. The bark and berries may be collected in the early autumn for crone aspects of the Goddess, including Holda, Hulda, the Elder Mother, and Hel. Ruled by the planet Venus and the element of air.

ELM (*Ulmus* spp.): Prophetic dreams, fairy contact. Ruled by the planet Saturn and the element of earth. Sacred to elves, Hoenin, Lodr, Odin, and Orpheus.

ENCHANTER'S NIGHTSHADE (*Circaea lutetiana*): Attraction, drawing, enchantment, shapeshifting. Ruled by the planet Saturn. Sacred to Circe.

EUCALYPTUS (*Eucalyptus globulus*): Healing, dispelling negativity. Ruled by the planet Mercury and the element of air.

EVENING PRIMROSE (*Oenothera biennis*): Beauty, success, friendship. Ruled by the moon. Sacred to Diana.

EYEBRIGHT (*Euphrasia officinalis*): Clarity, joy, inspiration. Ruled by the sun, the element of air, and the star sign Leo.

FENNEL (*Foeniculum vulgare*): Courage, Lughnasa, Midsummer, purification, protection. Ruled by the planet Mercury and the element of fire. Sacred to Apollo, Dionysus, and Prometheus.

FENUGREEK (*Trigonella foenum-graecum*): Lughnasa, music, poetry, healing. Ruled by the planet Mercury and the element of air. Sacred to Apollo.

FEVERFEW (*Tanacetum parthenium* syn. *Chrysanthemum parthenium*): Protection, Midsummer, meditation, healing. Ruled by the planet Venus and the element of water.

FERN, MALE (*Dryopeteris felix-mas*): Used for home protection, divination, fairy contact, and Midsummer. Ruled by the planet Mars and the element of air. Sacred to dawn and sun gods and goddesses, the Great Goddess, Hades, Kupala, Kupalo, Pluto, and sky gods of thunder and lightning (especially at Midsummer).

FIG (*Ficus carica*): Love, fertility. Ruled by the planet Jupiter, the element of fire, and the sign Sagittarius. Sacred to Bacchus, Dionysus, Isis, Juno, and Pan.

FIR, SILVER (*Abies alba*): Yule, childbirth, women's rites. Ruled by the moon, the element of earth, and the sign Sagittarius. Sacred to Adonis, Artemis, Attis, Bacchus, centaurs, Cybele, Dionysus, Druantia, mother goddesses, Neptune, Osiris, Poseidon, and Vesta.

FLAX (*Linum usitatissimum*): Web of life, wyrd, Midsummer. Ruled by the planet Mercury and the element of fire. Sacred to Arachne, Arianrhod, Athene, Brighid, Fates, Frigg, Hulda, Inanna, Isis, Meith, Minerva, Neith, and the Norns.

FORGET-ME-NOT (*Myosotis sylvatica*): Love, memory, the underworld, shamanic initiation, spring, remembrance, the dead. Ruled by the planet Venus and the element of water. Sacred to Persephone.

FOXGLOVE (*Digitalis* spp.): Protection, fairy contact, third-degree initiation. Ruled by the planet Venus and the element of water. Sacred to fairies.

FRANGIPANI (*Plumaria* spp.): Love, attraction.

FRANKINCENSE (*Boswellia thurifera*): Cleanses, purifies, consecrates, raises vibrations, drives away negativity, anointing, blessing. It is ruled by the sun, the element of fire, and the zodiac sign Leo. Sacred to Adonis, Aphrodite, Apollo, Bel, Demeter, Hades, Helios, Jehovah, Jesus, moon goddesses, Pluto, Ra, sun gods, Venus, Vishnu, Vulcan, and Yama.

FUMITORY (*Fumaria officinalis*): Earth spirit connection, Samhain, spirit attraction, protection, consecration, aura cleansing, exorcism. Ruled by the planet Saturn and the element of earth.

GALANGAL (*Kaempferia galanga*): Visions, energy. Ruled by the planet Mars and the element of fire.

GARDENIA (*Gardenia* spp.): Protection, attraction.

GARLIC (*Allium sativum*): Banishing, exorcism, protection. Ruled by the planet Mars, the element of fire, and the star sign Aries. Sacred to Circe, Cybele, and Hecate.

GERANIUM (*Pelargonium* spp.): Hex breaking, love, protection, healing, prosperity. Ruled by the planet Venus and the element of water. Sacred to Aphrodite, Athene, Isis, Menthu, Minerva, Shiva, and Venus.

GINGER (*Zingiber officinale*): Energy, passion, lust. Ruled by the planet Mars and the element of fire. Sacred to Aries and Mars.

GOLDENROD (*Solidago* spp.): Divination, love, luck, money, and prosperity. Ruled by the planet Venus and the element of air.

GORSE (*Ulex eurpaeus*): Brings hope and positivity, ruled by the sun and the element of fire. Sacred to Jupiter, Onniona, spring goddesses, sun gods, and Thor.

GRAPE: see Vine

GROUND IVY (*Glechoma hederacea* syn. *Nepeta glechoma*): Ostara, discovering the source of negative magic. Ruled by the planet Venus. Sacred to spring goddesses.

HAWTHORN (*Crataegus monogyna*): Beltane, fairy contact, Great Rite, death, fertility. Ruled by the planet Mars. Sacred to Ares, Artemis, Blodeuwedd, Cardea, Creiddylad, Eris, Flora, Hymen, Olwen, and Thor.

HAZEL (*Corylus avellana*): Autumn equinox, wisdom, inspiration, making and consecrating wands, dowsing, protection. Ruled by the planet Mercury and the element of air. Sacred to Aengus, Artemis, Boann, Chandra, Connla, Diana, Fionn, Hecate, Lleu, Lugh, Mac Coll, Manannan, Mercury, Ogma, Taliesin, and Thor.

HEATHER (*Calluna vulgaris*): Third-degree initiation, shamanic initiation, Midsummer, fairy contact, protection, luck, money. Ruled by the planet Venus, the star sign Gemini, and the element of water. Sacred to Aphrodite Erycina, Attis, Butes, Cybele, Isis, Osiris, summer goddesses, Uroica, and Venus.

HELIOTROPE (*Heliotropium arborescens*): Protection, wealth, devotion, prophetic dreams, banishing. Ruled by the sun and the element of fire. Sacred to Apollo, Clytie, and Helios. **Note:** poisonous.

HELLEBORE (*Helleborus niger*): Astral projection, exorcism, banishing. Sacred to Athene and Hecate. Ruled by the planet Saturn and the element of water. **Note:** poisonous.

HEMLOCK (*Conium maculatum*): Astral travel, Samhain. Ruled by the planet Saturn and the element of water. Sacred to Hecate. **Note:** poisonous.

HEMP (*Cannabis sativa*): Trance states, otherworld travel. Ruled by the planet Saturn and the element of water. Sacred to Bacchus, Pan, Priapus, and Vesta.

HEMP AGRIMONY (*Eupatoria cannabinum*): Healing, love, bonding a magical group. Ruled by the planet Jupiter.

HENBANE (*Hyoscyamus niger*): Death, underworld, prophetic trance, clairvoyance, ancestor contact, visions. It is ruled by the planets Saturn and Jupiter and the element of water. Sacred to Bil, Ceridwen, crone goddesses, Demeter in her death aspect of Phorcis the Sow, Freya, Rinda, thunder and sky gods, and Verdani. **Note:** poisonous.

HIBISCUS (*Hibiscus* spp.): Love, lust, divination.

HOLLY (*Ilex aquifolium*): Protection against negativity, counter-magic, Yule, warrior magic. The berries symbolise the sun, light, fire, and warmth. Ruled by the planets Saturn and Mars and the element of fire. Sacred to crone aspects of the Goddess, such as the Cailleach Bheur and the Morrigu, and to sky and thunder gods, such as Lleu, Lugh, Mars, Saturn, Tannus, Taran, and Thor.

HOLLYHOCK (*Althea rosea* syn. *Alcea rosea*): Healing, success, money, protection, meditation. Ruled by the planet Venus and the element of earth. Sacred to plant devas.

HONEYSUCKLE (*Lonicera* spp.): Beltane, Midsummer, harvest, Samhain, divination, dreams, love. Ruled by the planets Jupiter and Mars, the sign of Cancer, and the element of earth. Sacred to Ceridwen, fairies, and Pan.

HOP (*Humulus lupulus*): Lughnasa, underworld travel, wolf totems. Ruled by the planet Mars and the element of air. Sacred to Brighid and Leto.

HOREHOUND (*Marrubium vulgare*): Intuition, exorcism, temple and aura cleansing. Ruled by the planet Mercury and the element of air. Sacred to Horus, Isis, and Osiris.

HOUSELEEK (*Sempervivum tectorum*): Protection, aphrodisiac, love. Ruled by the planet Jupiter and the element of air. Sacred to Jupiter and Zeus.

HYACINTH (*Hyacinthus orientalis*): Love, happiness, protection.

HYSSOP (*Hyssopus officinalis*): Purification, dispelling negativity, smudging, protection, cleansing. Ruled by the planet Jupiter, the element of fire, and the zodiac sign of Cancer. Sacred to Pluto and Zeus.

INDIGO (*Indigofera tinctoria*): Bindings, endings. Ruled by the planet Saturn and the element of water. Sacred to the Dark Mother.

IRIS (*Iris* spp.): Orris (iris) root may be added as a fixative to incense and used for spiritual protection and to connect with the Higher Self. Ruled by the planets Venus and the moon and the element of water. Sacred to Aphrodite, Demeter, Hera, Iris, Isis, Juno, Osiris, Persephone, and Venus, and used to placate the Furies.

IVY (*Hedera helix*): Changing consciousness, prophecy, vision, rebirth, regeneration, initiation, Yule. Ruled by the planet Saturn and the element of water. Sacred to Ariadne, Arianrhod, Bacchus, Bran, Ceridwen, Cissia, Cronos, Dionysus, Gorgopa, Hymen, Isis, Kundalini, Lakshmi, Mars, Osiris, Persephone, Psyche, Rhea, Saturn, White Goddess, and Zeus.

JASMINE (*Jasminum officinalis*): Meditation, psychic dreams, aphrodisiac, love, sex, boosting a depleted aura and giving it protection. Ruled by the moon and the element of water. Sacred to Artemis, Diana, Ganesha, maternal aspects of the Goddess, Quan Yin, Virgin Mary, Vishnu, and Zeus.

JOJOBA (*Simmondsia chinensis*): Beauty, healing. Ruled by the planet Jupiter and the element of water.

JUNIPER (*Juniperis communis*): Truth, justice, healing, Yule, Samhain, driving out the old year. Ruled by the planets Mars, the sun, and Saturn, the element of fire, and the zodiac sign of Aries. Sacred to the Furies and Pan.

LARKSPUR (*Delphinium Consolida*): Joy, protection. Ruled by the planet Venus and the element of water.

LAVENDER (*Lavendula* spp.): Purification, healing, cleansing, meditation, peace, harmony, Midsummer. Ruled by the planet Mercury and the element of air. Sacred to Cernunnos, Circe, Hecate, Medea, Saturn, and serpent goddesses.

LEMON BALM AKA MELISSA (*Melissa officinalis*): Healing, particularly emotional problems. Ruled by the moon, the element of water, and the zodiac sign of Cancer. Sacred to Artemis, Diana, and other moon goddesses.

LEMON (*Citrus × lemon*): Cleansing, love, protection. Ruled by the moon and the element of water.

LEMONGRASS (*Cymbopogon citratus*): Psychic powers, lust.

LEMON VERBENA (*Aloysia citrodora*): Love, attraction, preventing bad dreams, Ostara, peace, joy. Ruled by the planets Venus and Mercury, the signs Gemini and Virgo, and the element of air.

LILAC (*Syringa vulgaris*): Exorcism, protection.

LILY (*Lilium* spp.): New moon, Imbolc. Ruled by the moon and the element of water. Sacred to Adonis, Astarte, Athene, Attis, Ceres, Isis, Jupiter, Kundalini, Lakshmi, maiden goddesses, moon goddesses, Osiris, Psyche, Sophia, and Venus.

LIME (*Citrus acida*): Healing, love, protection. Ruled by the element of fire.

LINDEN (*Tilia* spp.): Divination, healing, restoration, working with magical scripts and alphabets. Ruled by the planet Jupiter. Sacred to Chiron, earth deities, Philyra, and Saule.

MAGNOLIA (*Magnolia* spp.): Attraction, fidelity, love, marriage. Ruled by the planet Venus, the element of water, and the signs Libra and Taurus.

MANDRAKE, TRUE (*Mandragora officinarum*): Protection, poppets, prosperity, fertility, love. Ruled by the planet Mercury and the element of fire. Sacred to Circe, Diana, Hathor, Hecate, and Saturn. **Note:** poisonous.

MANDRAKE, AMERICAN (*Podophyllum peltatum*): Death, protection, guarding secrets, fertility, virility. **Note:** poisonous.

MANDRAKE, ENGLISH: see Bryony

MAPLE (*Acer* spp.): Travel protection, abundance, divination. Ruled by the planet Jupiter and the elements of air and earth.

MARIGOLD: see Calendula

MARJORAM (*Origanum majorana*): Protection, repels negativity, happiness, love, weddings, handfastings, healing, unblocking the heart chakra. Ruled by the planet Mercury, the element of air, and the zodiac sign of Aries. Sacred to Aphrodite, Hera, Jupiter, Osiris, Thor, and Venus.

MARSHMALLOW (*Althaea officinalis*): Love attraction, aphrodisiac, banishing, exorcism, protection, otherworld travel, handfasting, tantric magic, the Great Rite, Lughnasa. It is ruled by the planet Venus and the moon, the element of water, and the star signs Cancer and Gemini.

MEADOWSWEET (*Filipendula ulmaria* syn. *Spiraea ulmaria*): Beltane, Midsummer, love, marriage, handfasting, fertility, plenty. Ruled by the planets Venus and Jupiter, the element of water, and the zodiac sign of Gemini. Sacred to Aine, Blodeuwedd, Gwena, and Venus.

MIMOSA (*Mimosa pudica*): Prophetic dreams, joy, love, healing, protection. Ruled by the planet Saturn and the element of water.

MISTLETOE (*Viscum album*): Protection, healing, divination, prophetic dreams, Midsummer, Yule, fertility, rebirth. Ruled by the planets of the sun and Jupiter and the element of air. Sacred to Apollo, Balder, Cerridwen, Freya, Frigga, Odin, and Venus.

MONKSHOOD: see Aconite

MOTHERWORT (*Leonurus cardiaca*): Astral travel, counter-magic, healing, women's magic.

MUGWORT (*Artemisia vulgaris*): Travel protection, protection, women's rituals, Imbolc, Ostara, Midsummer, Lughnasa, croning rituals, clairvoyance, prophetic dreams. Ruled by the moon and the planet Mercury, the element of water, and the signs of Taurus and Libra. Sacred to Artemis, Chandra, Diana, and Hecate.

MULBERRY (*Morus nigra*): Child protection, wisdom. Ruled by the planet Mercury and the element of air. It is sacred to goddesses of wisdom, spinning, and weaving. Use to invoke Asherah, Athene, Chih, Ma Ku, Minerva, Sien-tsan, Singarmati, and Ts'an Nü.

MULLEIN (*Verbascum thapsus*): Protection, courage, attraction, Samhain, ancestor contact. The powdered root is known as "graveyard dust." Ruled by the planet Saturn and the element of water. Sacred to Circe, crone goddesses, and Jupiter.

MYRRH (*Commiphora myrrha*): Love, fertility, death, regeneration, rebirth, Ostara, Samhain, autumn equinox, funerals, memorials, weddings, handfastings, spiritual awareness. Ruled by the moon, the planets Jupiter and Saturn, and the element of water. Sacred to Adonis, Aphrodite, Bhavani, Cybele, Demeter, Dionysus, Freya, Hathor, Hecate, Hera, Isis, Juno, Marian, Mut, Nephthys, Neptune, Pamphile, Persephone, Poseidon, Ra, Rhea, Saturn, Tammuz, and Yahweh.

MYRTLE (*Myrtus communis*): Prophecy, love, fertility, marriage, death, regeneration. Ruled by the planets Venus and the moon and the element of water. Sacred to Aphrodite, Artemis, Ashtoreth, Astarte, Freya, the Graces, Hathor, Hera, Marian, Myrrha, Thetis, and Venus.

NARCISSUS (*Narcissus* sp.): Beginnings, hope, peace, fertility, love, death, renewal. Ruled by the planet Venus and the element of water.

NETTLE, STINGING (*Urtica dioica*): Healing, protection, dispelling negativity, underworld journeys, and rites of birth, initiation, and death. Ruled by the planet Mars and the element of fire. Sacred to Agni, Blodeuwedd, Cernunnos, Hades, Horus, Jupiter, Osiris, Pcuvus (earth fairies), Pluto, thunder gods, Thor, Vishnu, Vulcan, and Yama.

NICOTIANA (*Nicotiana* spp.): Cleansing, purification.

NUTMEG (*Myristica fragrans*): Counter-magic, luck, justice, money, virility, Yule. Ruled by the planet Jupiter, the element of air, and the sign of Pisces.

OAK (*Quercus robur*): Doorway to knowledge, Beltane, Midsummer, Lughnasa, Yule, fertility, strength, stability. Ruled by the planet Jupiter and the element of fire. Sacred to Ares, Arianrhod, Artemis, Athene, Balder, Blodeuwedd, Brighid, Ceirddylad, Ceridwen, Cernunnos, Circe, Cybele, Dagda, Dianus, Donar, Dryads, Erato, Erinnyes, Hades, Hecate, Herakles, Herne, Horus, Indra, Janicot, Janus, Jehovah, Jupiter, Llyr, Mars, Nephthys, Odin, Pan, Pluto, Rhea, Taran, Taranis, Thor, Ukko, Vishnu, and Zeus.

OLIVE (*Olea europaea*): New beginnings, peace, continuity, the expulsion of evil and negativity, consecration, purification, blessing. Ruled by the sun and the element of fire. Sacred to Amun Ra, Apollo, Artemis, Athene, Auxesia Hera, Damia, Demeter, Ganymede, Hercules, Hermes, Indra, Isis, Juno, Jupiter, Nut, Poseidon, sun gods, and Zeus.

ORANGE (*Citrus × sinensis*): Love, energy, joy. Ruled by the sun and the element of fire.

OREGANO (*Origanum vulgare*): Healing, joy, luck, protection. Ruled by the planet Venus and the element of air.

ORRIS: see Iris

PARSLEY (*Petroselinum crispum* syn. *P. satirum*): The underworld, ancestral knowledge, the dead, autumn equinox, Samhain. Ruled by the planet Mercury and the element of air. Sacred to Aphrodite, Archemorus, death gods and goddesses, Persephone, and Venus.

PASSIONFLOWER (*Passiflora incarnata*): Tranquillity, trance.

PATCHOULI (*Pogostemon patchouli*): Aphrodisiac, sexual attraction. Ruled by the planet Venus and the element of earth.

PEAR (*Pyrus communis*): Love, marriage, fertility. Ruled by the planet Venus and the element of water. Sacred to Hera and Juno.

PENNYROYAL (*Mentha pulegium*): Counter-magic, aura cleansing, protection, healing. Ruled by the planets Mars and Venus and the element of earth.

PEONY (*Paeonia* spp.): Healing, protection against evil spirits and nightmares. Ruled by the sun or the moon and the element of fire. Sacred to Aesculapius, Apollo, Leto, and Paeon.

PERIWINKLE (*Vinca minor*): Binding, death, funerals, afterlife, love, passion, protection against evil spirits, attract money, home protection, goddess rituals, Imbolc. Ruled by the planet Venus and the element of water. Sacred to mother goddesses.

PEPPERMINT (*Mentha × piperita*): Clarity, cleansing. Ruled by the planet Venus, the element of air, and the star signs Virgo and Aquarius. Sacred to Hades and Minthe.

PHLOX (*Phlox* spp.): Love, healing, weddings and handfastings, bonding, harmony.

PLANTAIN, GREATER (*Plantago major*): Strength, healing, protection. Ruled by the planet Venus and the element of earth. Sacred to Odin.

PINE (*Pinus sylvestris*): Purification, cleansing, dispelling negativity, spring equinox, fertility, regeneration, new beginnings. Ruled by the planet Mars and the elements of earth and air. Sacred to Astarte, Attis, Cernunnos, Cybele, Dionysus, the Great Mother, Herne, Osiris, Pan, Pitys, Poseidon, Rhea, sun gods, Sylvanus, and Venus.

POKEWEED (*Phytolacca american*): Exorcism, protection from negativity, counter-magic. Ruled by the planet Uranus.

POPLAR (*Populus alba*): Dispelling disease, protection, endurance, connection with the higher self. Ruled by the sun and Saturn and the element of fire. Sacred to Apollo, Calypso, death goddesses, Dryope, Heliades, Helios, Hespera, Jupiter, Mut, Nun, Persephone, Phaeton, sun gods, and Valkyries.

POPPY, FIELD (*Papaver rhoeas*): Fertility, harvest, luck, money, love, autumn equinox, Lughnasa, abundance, death. Ruled by the moon and water. Sacred to Agni, Ceres, Demeter, Hades, harvest goddesses, Hypnos, Jupiter, mother goddesses, Nyx, Persephone, Pluto, Proserpine, Somnus, Vulcan, and Yama.

POPPY, OPIUM (*Papaver somniferum*): Sleep, visions, rites of the Mother Goddess. Ruled by the moon and the element of water. Sacred to Anubis, Bhavani, Demeter, Freya, Hecate, Hera, Hypnos, Isis, Mut, Neptune, Nepthys, Rhea, Saturn, Somnos, and Thanatos.

PRIMROSE (*Primula vulgaris*): Song and poetry, bardic initiation, purification, protection, attracting love, Ostara, Beltane. Ruled by the planet Venus and the element of earth. Sacred to Blodeuwedd, fairies, Freya, and goddesses of the spring and love.

PURSLANE (*Portulaca oleracea*): Protection against witchcraft, evil spirits, the evil eye, and nightmares; brings harmony in the home. Ruled by the moon and the element of water.

REED (*Phragmites communis*): Rebirth, voice of the spirits, royalty and sun gods, Midsummer. Sacred to Attis, Cybele, fairies, Faunus, Hermes, Horus, Inanna, Isis, Lugh, Osiris, Pan, Ra, Taliesin, and Unkulunkulu. Ruled by the sun and the element of fire.

RICE (*Oryza sativa*): Blessing, money, prosperity, fertility, protection, wealth. Ruled by the sun and the element of earth.

ROSE (*Rosa* spp.): Rebirth, resurrection, funerals, memorials, initiations, luck, love, passion, sexuality, sensuality, seduction, marriage, Great Rite, handfasting, Beltane. The white rose represents purity, perfection, innocence, virginity, and the Maiden Goddess, while the red is earthly passion, fertility, and the Mother Goddess. Red roses are ruled by Jupiter, damask roses by the planet Venus, and white roses by the moon. All fall under the element of water. Sacred to Adonis, Aphrodite, Artemis, Aurora, Bacchus, Blodeuwedd, Christ, Cupid, Demeter, Dionysus, Eros, Flora, Freya, Hathor, Horus, Hulda, Hymen, Inanna, Ishtar, Isis, Kubaba, the Mothers, Nike, Ninsianna, Saule, Venus, Virgin Mary, and Vishnu.

ROSEMARY (*Rosmarinus officinalis*): Mind and the memory, concentration, meditation, healing, love, marriage, births, funerals, memorial services, protection, dispelling negativity and evil, attracting fairies, spells designed to retain youth. Ruled by the sun, the element of fire, and the zodiac sign of Aries.

ROWAN (*Sorbus aucuparia* syn. *Pyrus aucuparia*): Witchcraft, protection, divination, the dead, invoking spirits and familiars, visions, Samhain, banishing undesirable entities, Imbolc, awen. Ruled by the moon and the element of water. Sacred to Akka, Brigantia, Brighid, Cuchulain, Maa-Emoinen, Rauni, and Thor.

RUE (*Ruta graveolens*): Anaphrodisiac, inner vision, clairvoyance, banishes negative energies, exorcism, purification. It is ruled by the sun, the element of fire, and the sign of Leo. Sacred to Aradia, Diana, Hermes, Horus, Mars, Menthu, Mercury, and Odysseus.

SAFFRON (*Crocus sativus*): Love, marriage, handfasting, lifts the spirits, divination, aphrodisiac, beginnings, dawn, strength, wealth. Though given to the sun by the astrologer-herbalists for its golden stamens and dye, the ancients thought saffron was sacred to moon goddesses. It is ruled by the sun, the element of fire, and the sign of Leo. Sacred to the deities Amun Ra, Ashtoreth, Eos, Indra, Jupiter, and Zeus.

SAGE (*Salvia officinalis*): Wisdom, prophetic dreams, warding off the evil eye, purification, cleansing, aura cleansing, immortality. Ruled by the planet Jupiter and the element of air. Sacred to Consus, Jupiter, and Zeus.

SANDALWOOD (*Santalum* spp.): Peace, meditation, scrying, divination and trance work. Ruled by the moon and the element of air. Sacred to Hanuman, Hathor, Hermes, Nike, Venus, and Vishnu.

SASSAFRAS (*Sassafras* spp.): Money attraction, healing. Ruled by the planet Jupiter and the element of fire.

SKULLCAP (*Scutellaria lateriflora*): Protection, meditation, peace, trance work. Ruled by the planet Saturn and the element of water.

SMALLAGE (*Apium graveolens*): Funerals, lust, victory, psychic powers, underworld journeys, autumn equinox, Samhain. Ruled by the planet Mercury and the element of fire. Sacred to Zeus.

SNEEZEWORT (*Achillea ptarmica*): Warrior magic, Lughnasa, invoking fire elementals, Ostara, Midsummer, grounding and head clearing after trance work. Ruled by the planet Mars and the element of fire.

SNOWDROP (*Galanthus nivalis*): Imbolc, purity, cleansing. Ruled by the moon and water. Sacred to Adonis, Attis, Brigantia, Brighid, Ceres, Isis, and the Virgin Mary.

SOAPWORT (*Saponaria officinalis*): Cleansing, purification. Ruled by the planet Venus and the element of earth.

SOLOMON'S SEAL (*Polygonatum multiflorum*): Banishing negativity and evil spirits, brings about change. Ruled by the planet Saturn and the element of water.

SORREL (*Rumex acetosa*): Love. Ruled by the planet Venus and the element of earth. Sacred to Aphrodite and Venus.

SOUTHERNWOOD (*Artemisia abrotanum*): Attraction, love-drawing, sex, lust, changing bad luck, curse breaking, men's rituals, Lughnasa. Ruled by the planet Mercury and the element of air.

ST. JOHN'S WORT (*Hypericum perforatum*): Counter-magic, protection, clearing, Midsummer, repels negativity, purification, and exorcism. It is ruled by the sun, the element of fire, and the sign of Leo. Sacred to sun gods, particularly Baldur.

STRAWBERRY (*Fragaria vesca*): Blessing, love, Midsummer, fertility. Ruled by the planet Venus and the elements of earth or water. Sacred to fairies, Freya, love goddesses, and mother goddesses.

SUNFLOWER (*Helianthus annus*): Sun rituals, Midsummer, happiness, blessings, fertility, strength, courage, action, self-image, consecrating healing stones and gems. Ruled by the sun, the element of fire, and the star sign Leo. Sacred to Apollo, Demeter, Helios, and Venus.

SWEET CICELY (*Myrrhis oderata*): Midsummer, Beltane, joy, happiness. Ruled by the planet Jupiter and the element of air. Sacred to summer goddesses.

SWEET PEA (*Lathyrus odoratus*): Attracts loyalty and affection. Ruled by the element of air and the planet Venus.

TANGERINE (*Citrus tangerina*): Energy, strength, power. Ruled by the sun and the element of fire.

TANSY (*Tanacetum vulgare* syn. *Chrysanthemum vulgare*): Death and immortality, funerals, cleansing, Ostara. Ruled by the planet Venus, the element of earth, and the star sign Gemini. Sacred to Ganymede.

TARRAGON (*Artemisia dracunculus*): Underworld journeys, warrior magic, vision quests. Ruled by the planet Mars and the element of fire. Sacred to Lilith.

THISTLE (all): Endurance, Samhain. Ruled by the planet Mars, the element of fire, and the star sign Aries. Sacred to Bacchus, Pan, Priapus, Thor, and Vesta.

THYME (*Thymus vulgaris*): Warrior path, courage, strength, purification, protection (especially from nightmares), remembrance of the dead, healing, love attraction. Ruled by the planet Venus, the element of water, and the star sign Aries. Sacred to Ares, fairies, and Mars.

TOADFLAX (*Linaria vulgaris*): Protection, hex breaking. Ruled by the planet Mars and the element of fire.

TOMATO (*Solanum lycopersicum*): Love, protection.

UNICORN PLANT (*Proboscidea althaeifolia*): Retrieving lost objects, binding, protection.

VALERIAN (*Valeriana officinalis*): Healing, love, soothing quarrels, protection from lightning, working with cat familiars. The powdered root is one of the roots called "graveyard dust." Ruled by the planet Mercury, the element of water, and the star sign Virgo.

VANILLA (*Vanilla planifolia*): Happiness, good fortune.

VERBENA: see Vervain or Lemon Verbena

VERVAIN (*Verbena officinalis*): First-degree initiation, bardic initiation, Midsummer, Samhain, cleansing, purifying, poetry and song, clairvoyance, divination, protection from negativity and evil magic, home protection, purification, love. Ruled by the planets Venus and Mercury, the element of water, and the star sign Gemini. Sacred to Aphrodite, Aradia, Ceridwen, Diana, Horus, Isis, Jupiter, Mars, Ra, Thor, Venus, and Zeus.

VINE (*Vitis vinafera*): Everlasting life, divine intoxication, entheogen, negating the ego, Lughnasa, autumn equinox. Ruled by the sun and the element of fire. Sacred to Adonis, Apollo, Bacchus, Dionysus, Flora, Inanna, Ishtar, Liber Pater, Orpheus, Osiris, and Ra.

VIOLET (*Viola odorata*): Fertility, love, faithfulness, luck, death, otherworld journeys, peace, Midsummer. Ruled by the planet Venus and the element of water. Sacred to Aphrodite, goddesses of love, Io, Orpheus, and Venus.

WALNUT (*Juglans regia*): Fertility, anointing, wishes. Ruled by the sun and the element of fire. Sacred to Adonis, Apollo, and Jupiter.

WATER LILY (*Nymphaeaceae* spp.): Rebirth of the sun from the underworld, Yule, funerals, anaphrodisiac, moon rituals. Ruled by the planets Neptune and the moon, the element of water, and the star sign Cancer.

WILLOW (*Salix* spp.): Water, the underworld, poetry, death, witches, the moon, birth, the feminine, intuition, inspiration. Sacred to Artemis, Anatha, Belili, Belin, Belinos, Brigantia, Brighid, Cailleach, Callisto, Calypso, Ceres, Circe, Europa, Hecate, Hera, Hermes, Isis, Kundalini, Lakshmi, Mercury, moon goddesses, Muses, Neith, O-Ryu, Osiris, Persephone, Poseidon, Psyche, the Rusalki, and Zeus.

WISTERIA (*Wisteria* spp.): Good fortune, prosperity.

WOAD (*Isatis tinctoria*): Healing, warrior magic. Ruled by the planet Saturn and the element of water. Sacred to warrior gods.

WOLFSBANE: see Aconite

WOODRUFF (*Galium oderatum* syn. *Asperula oderata*): Victory, reward, prosperity, Beltane, a fixative for perfumes and incense. Ruled by the planet Mars and the element of fire. Sacred to summer goddesses.

WORMWOOD (*Artemisia absinthium*): Divination, scrying, women's rites, Imbolc, banishing negativity. Ruled by the planet Mars and the element of air. Sacred to Aesculapius, Artemis, Castor, Diana, Horus, Iris, Isis, maiden goddesses, Menthu, and Pollux.

YARROW (*Achillea millefolium*): Male principle, Midsummer, healing, divination, clairvoyance, aura cleansing, protection. Ruled by the planet Venus and the element of water. Sacred to Cernunnos, Herne, and Pan.

YEW (*Taxus baccata*): Death, regeneration from death, Yule. Ruled by Saturn and the element of water. Sacred to Athene, Banbha, Deidre, Hecate, Naoise, Saturn, and underworld goddesses.

Using Herbs for Magic

There are hundreds of ways you can bring your hearth witch's herb craft into your magical work. We've already covered making ritual wine and food, but you can also use herbs in talismans, amulets, charms, spells, teas, potions, incense, and oils just to start with. Always remember that you are working with the virtues inherent in the plant to achieve the result you want, whether that is to evoke the energy of a particular deity or season or for protection, cleansing, purification, abundance, or banishing.

. . . .

KITCHEN PROTECTION CHARM

To keep your home and family safe and happy, take a sprig of each of the following herbs:

SAGE FOR WISDOM

ROSEMARY FOR REMEMBRANCE

LEMON BALM FOR JOY

ST. JOHN'S WORT FOR PROTECTION

LAVENDER FOR PEACE

Tie the herbs with a red thread, making sure that some herbs are tied one way and some the other so that you are left with a bunch with herbs sticking out both sides instead of one end herbs, the other stalks. As you tie them, visualise creating protection and happiness for your home and family as you say:

I tie this sage for wisdom, to know what is truly important

I tie this rosemary for remembrance, so that I might never forget it

I tie this lemon balm for joy, that I might celebrate it

I tie this St. John's wort to protect it

And I tie this lavender to keep it in peace and harmony

Herbal Talismans

This is one of the simplest forms of magic using herbs. Herbal talismans are fabric pouches filled with dried herbs. You can either buy a pouch (wedding favour bags work well) or, better still, make one yourself. It doesn't have to be a work of art; it is the intent that is important.

You will need an oblong piece of cloth, big enough to take all the ingredients when folded in half and sewn up. Choose a sturdy fabric; the right colour adds extra strength to the magic (see appendix 1). Take the cloth and fold it in half, right sides together. Sew up three sides, reinforcing your intent with each stitch (you can chant it as you sew), and then turn it right-side out. Put the ingredients into the pouch one by one, stating your desire each time. (If you don't have the exact herbs listed, you can make substitutions using the tables of correspondences in appendix 3.) Sew it shut and then either carry it with you, put it in the appropriate room of your house, or sleep with it under your pillow, according to its purpose.

FERTILITY TALISMAN

GREEN CLOTH

3 ALMONDS

3 GRAINS OF BARLEY

3 VIOLET FLOWERS

2 WALNUT HALVES

3 ACORNS

3 SUNFLOWER SEEDS

3 GRAINS OF RICE

3 RED ROSE PETALS

Assemble at the full moon. Place it under your pillow or under the bed.

FRIENDSHIP TALISMAN

PINK CLOTH

1 CROCUS BULB

3 PRIMROSE FLOWERS

3 CARDAMOM PODS

1 CLOVER STEM

3 CORIANDER SEEDS

1 PIECE DRIED ORANGE PEEL

To attract new friendships, assemble at the waxing moon.

LOVE-DRAWING TALISMAN

PINK CLOTH

DRIED PEEL OF 1 APPLE

7 DRIED BASIL LEAVES

HALF A CINNAMON STICK

3 CLOVES

7 DRIED RED ROSE PETALS

1 VANILLA POD

Make at the waxing moon and carry close to your heart.

. . . .

Money-Drawing Talisman

GREEN CLOTH

3 ALMONDS

1 NUTMEG

A PINCH OF CINNAMON POWDER

3 CLOVES

A FEW PINE NEEDLES

3 SAGE LEAVES

Assemble at the waxing moon and place in your purse or your business's cash register.

. . . .

"Peace in the Home" Talisman

BLUE CLOTH

PIECE OF ANGELICA ROOT

2 TEASPOONS DRIED CHAMOMILE FLOWERS

2 TEASPOONS DRIED LAVENDER FLOWERS

2 TEASPOONS DRIED LEMON VERBENA

3 OLIVE LEAVES

1 TEASPOON SANDALWOOD BARK OR POWDER

SMALL ROSE QUARTZ CRYSTAL

Assemble at the full moon and place in the kitchen or sitting room.

Home Protection Talisman

WHITE CLOTH

1 ACORN

PIECE OF ANGELICA ROOT

3 BAY LEAVES

A PINCH OF DRIED CALENDULA PETALS

3 HOLLY LEAVES

9 ROWAN BERRIES

A PINCH OF DRIED VERVAIN

Assemble at the full moon and place in your porch, kitchen, or the highest part of the house.

Prophetic Dream Pillow

PURPLE CLOTH

9 BAY LEAVES, POWDERED

2 TABLESPOONS POWDERED MUGWORT

2 TABLESPOONS POWDERED SAGE

Prepare at the full moon and sleep with it beneath your pillow.

Potions

Potion is a generic term for herbal preparations made in a ritual way. They are made according to the same methods as infusions and decoctions made for healing, but they are brewed with magical intent at the correct moon phase and season and perhaps with appropriate words and symbolic actions.

You may also come across the word *philtre*, which is the specific name for a love potion, used to make one person fall in love with another. Picture the victim of unrequited love stealing away to the village wise woman or cunning man and purchasing, under cover of night, a concoction to feed to his or her unsuspecting would-be lover. Often philtres were made from wine infused with poisonous herbs such as mandrake root and bryony. Sometimes they had human urine or ground-up animal organs in them. Modern witches eschew such arts, believing it to be very wrong to manipulate the will of another. Instead, it is permissible to ask for love to come to you and let the universe decide who it shall be.

SOLAR AND LUNAR INFUSIONS

Sometimes potions are given extra magical energy by being placed in sunlight or moonlight for two or three days or nights, according to their purpose. You can either brew the herbs in the usual way and then place them outside or make a cold infusion by placing your herbs in a jar, covering them with water, and leaving them under the sun or moon for three days or nights.

Solar infusions are generally used for spells and rituals of energy, strength, growth, joy, happiness, and courage, but this will be affected by the time of year that they are made. One made at Midsummer will embody all of the qualities listed above, but one made at or around Lughnasa will carry them in a lesser degree. One made at Samhain will incorporate the energies of winter, death, and bane, so bear the season in mind.

Lunar infusions can be made according to the moon's phases. At the waxing moon you can make potions to be used in spells and rituals to make things grow, to attract things that are to come towards you. At the waning moon make potions for banishing, cleansing, and clearing. The full moon is the most powerful time for potions of divination and love.

USING POTIONS

Potions can be used in a number of ways:

- Take as a tea to absorb the herb's energy. Using one herb at a time is a good way to get to know them.

- Infuse the herbs in wine for the ritual cup.

- Use a consecration potion to consecrate magical objects.

- Use a purification potion to cleanse the temple or working area.

- Use a purification potion in the bath for a pre-ritual cleansing.

- Use a banishing potion as a wash to cleanse a place of negative energies.

- Use a protection potion to wash around the doors and windows of your house, or bathe in it.

PROTECTION POTION

1 PINT BOILING WATER

½ TEASPOON ANGELICA

½ TEASPOON CHAMOMILE

½ TEASPOON DILL

½ TEASPOON HYSSOP

½ TEASPOON LAVENDER

½ TEASPOON ROSEMARY

½ TEASPOON ROWAN BERRIES, CRUSHED

½ TEASPOON ST. JOHN'S WORT

½ TEASPOON VERVAIN

Pour the water over the herbs and infuse, covered, for 20 minutes. Strain and use to wipe around the doors and windows of your house or any other areas you feel need protecting. Make at the full moon. Do not take internally.

. . . .
LOVE POTION

1 BOTTLE RED WINE

3 CARDAMOM PODS

½ CINNAMON STICK

2 CLOVES

RED ROSE PETALS

Place all ingredients except the rose petals in a pan. Warm gently but do not boil for 15 minutes. Strain into cups and sprinkle the rose petals on top. Drink with your love (with their permission) at the full moon.

. . . .
PURIFICATION POTION

1 PINT BOILING WATER

1 TEASPOON HYSSOP

3 SAGE LEAVES

7 BASIL LEAVES

3 BAY LEAVES

1 TEASPOON ROSEMARY

Pour the water over the herbs and infuse, covered, for 20 minutes. Strain and use to wash the temple or working area, magical tools, sprinkle around the ritual space using a sprig of fresh hyssop or rosemary, or use in the pre-ritual bath. Do not take internally.

. . . .
DIVINATION TEA

½ PINT BOILING WATER

½ TEASPOON CALENDULA PETALS

¼ TEASPOON GROUND CINNAMON

½ TEASPOON CLARY SAGE

Pour the boiling water over the herbs and infuse, covered, for 10 minutes. Strain and drink before performing acts of divination.

. . . . .

AURA-CLEANSING POTION

1 PINT BOILING WATER

1 TEASPOON ANGELICA LEAVES

1 TEASPOON JASMINE FLOWERS

1 TEASPOON ROSEMARY LEAVES

3 SAGE LEAVES

Pour the water over the herbs and infuse, covered, for 20 minutes. Strain and use to sprinkle around the aura, using a sprig of rosemary, or use in the bath. Do not take internally.

CONSECRATION POTION

1 PINT BOILING WATER

3 BAY LEAVES

7 GRAINS OF FRANKINCENSE

1 TEASPOON HYSSOP

1 TEASPOON MINT LEAVES

Pour the water over the herbs and infuse, covered, for 20 minutes. Strain and use to consecrate magical tools or robes, or to anoint participants in a ritual. If possible, make at the full moon. Do not take internally.

BANISHING POTION

1 PINT BOILING WATER

1 TEASPOON BIRCH BARK

1 CLOVE GARLIC, CRUSHED

1 TEASPOON JUNIPER BERRIES, CRUSHED

1 TEASPOON RUE

1 TEASPOON ST. JOHN'S WORT

Pour the water over the herbs and infuse, covered, for 20 minutes. Strain and use to sprinkle around the area you need to banish negative energies or spirits from, using a sprig of fresh hyssop or rosemary. Make at the waning moon. Do not take internally.

Herbal Inks

I like to use herbal inks for magical work, as they are entirely natural and biodegradable. The herbs can be collected in a ritual way, at the right time and season, and add their own power to the spell or amulet. The ink can be made with intent. Homemade inks often are not very permanent, but using an appropriate herb and colour adds great power to an act of magic.

Modern ink is mostly made from petroleum products, but originally inks were made from plants or household items, such as soot, honey, and egg white. Black herbal inks can be made from plants that contain dark pigments and tannin; these include alder, dogwood, blackthorn, and oak galls. Red ink can be made from field poppies, brown ink from onion skins, and a blue ink from elderberries.

BASIC METHOD

The herb used (husks or galls need to be crushed first) should be just covered with boiling water. This should be allowed to infuse overnight and then strained. Add alcohol (10 percent of the total volume should be alcohol) and bottle.

. . . .

BEETROOT INK (RED)

9 OUNCES FRESH BEETROOT

35 FLUID OUNCES WATER

2 TEASPOONS WHITE VINEGAR OR VODKA

Chop and grind the beetroots. Add the water and boil until the liquid is reduced by half. Filter through muslin twice, add the vinegar, and bottle. Store away from sunlight.

. . . .

TURMERIC (*CURCUMA LONGA*) INK (YELLOW)

1 OUNCE TURMERIC POWDER

20 FLUID OUNCES WATER

1 TEASPOON WHITE VINEGAR OR VODKA

Add the turmeric and water to a pan and boil until the liquid has reduced by a half and a good colour has been obtained. Filter twice through muslin and add the vinegar. Store in an airtight glass bottle in a cool place away from sunlight.

. . . . .

INVISIBLE INK

If you write on paper with lemon juice, the words will be invisible but magically appear if the paper is warmed slightly.

BLACKBERRY INK (PURPLE)

9 OUNCES FRESH BLACKBERRIES

35 FLUID OUNCES WATER

2 TEASPOONS WHITE VINEGAR OR VODKA

Mash the blackberries. Add the water and boil until the liquid is reduced by half. Filter through muslin twice, add the vinegar, and bottle. Store away from sunlight.

Ritual Fumigation

SMUDGING

If you feel that your home has accumulated negative energy, or if there is a bad atmosphere lingering after an argument, you can take several measures to cleanse it. (It is a good idea to do this on a regular basis, in any case.) One of the simplest ways of cleansing your home of negative energy is to use a smudge stick or carry a dish of white sage burning on charcoal as you walk from room to room. You can also use rosemary or frankincense. See chapter 13 for more cleansing incenses.

BANISHING

If you need a more heavy-duty cleansing, you can use this method. In each room of your house place a dish with a peeled clove of garlic ringed with salt. These will absorb negative energies. Leave them for an hour. Take the dishes of garlic and salt outside and burn the contents completely.

Open all the windows and doors. Carry a dish of banishing incense (see chapter 13) around the house, starting at the top and working your way down. In each room allow the smoke to go in each corner, and say:

> *In the name of the God and Goddess,*
>
> *I command all evil and negativity to be gone.*
>
> *This do I will. So mote it be!*

Close the doors and windows. Using a protection oil, dip in your finger and draw it round the edges of all the doors and windows, saying:

> *In the name of the God and Goddess,*
>
> *I seal this place so that no evil may enter.*
>
> *This do I will. So mote it be!*

Light a white candle on your altar or hearth. Say:

> *Lord and Lady, grant me your protection*
>
> *as I give you my thanks and my service.*
>
> *So mote it be.*

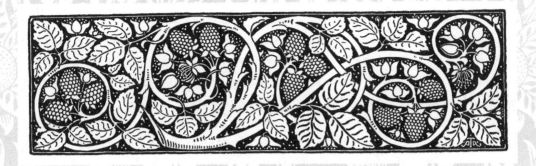

CHAPTER 13

Incense

The magical use of incense needs a chapter of its own. Incense—perfumes burned to release fragrant smoke—has been used all over the world, from ancient times till the present day. Rising smoke has always been associated with prayers rising to the gods, whether from the domestic hearth, the Pagan altar, the Druids' needfire, or the Catholic Church's incense burner.

In ancient Egyptian temples priests formulated and used aromatics like cedarwood, frankincense, myrrh, juniper, and caraway in their rites. One legendary blend was Kyphi, made from sixteen different essences, which would be breathed in by the priests and pharaohs during meditation. The Roman historian Plutarch wrote of it that "the smell of this perfume penetrates your body by the nose. It makes you feel well and relaxed, the mind floats and you find yourself in a dreamy state of happiness, as if listening to beautiful music."[41]

---

41 Quoted from Daniele Ryman, *The Aromatherapy Handbook: The Secret Healing Power of Essential Oils* (C. W. Daniel, 1989).

Everyone knows that during rituals witches and magicians use incenses—powerful perfumes that somehow help the magic. Ask many of these witches and magicians why they use incenses or how they work and they may struggle to explain. Ask them why they use the ingredients they do or how those ingredients are decided and they might mumble about following some recipes or charts of correspondences.

In this book I want to show you how to make magical incenses, how to choose suitable ingredients, and how to use those incenses, but first of all I want you to be clear about why you are going through all the trouble. Incenses work on several levels:

1. First is the effect incense has on the mood of the magician. Any aromatherapist will tell you that perfumes affect the emotions. They may be stimulating or calming, soothing or invigorating, and raise or depress the spirits. Magicians through the ages have developed this into a precise art.

2. A perfume may have certain associations for the person who experiences it. There is a famous story of the philosopher Proust who smelled the baking of madeleine cakes and it powerfully brought back to him all the experiences and emotions of his childhood. If you associate certain perfumes with a ritual setting, it can induce the mood required and concentrate the mind on the task in hand. If you condition yourself to associate different perfumes with different rituals or deities, this will act as a subconscious shortcut.

3. Lastly, on a more profound level, is the effect of the perfume's *vibration*. When something vibrates at a certain frequency, any object near it will begin to vibrate with the same frequency: a principle used in both healing and magic. Each plant, like every crystal or stone, has a particular vibration. When we use plants for incense making, we really mean using the combined vibrational force of the chosen plants rather than their medicinal qualities or even their perfumes. When we use an incense, it is for the purpose of changing the vibration of the atmosphere to the level needed for a specific magical operation, not because it has a "nice smell."

Types of Incense

There are many types of incense available in shops, from the joss sticks and cones you can buy in supermarkets to the loose incense obtained from occult shops, which is burned on charcoal or thrown straight onto the ritual bonfire.

However, there are several reasons why it is better to make your own incenses for magical purposes. Commercial joss and cones are made with a compound base and often synthetic mineral–derived oils that have no magical value. Some commercially prepared loose incenses are just designed to look attractive and smell nice, even if you buy them from an occult shop. A careful examination of the contents will often reveal inexplicable ingredients, besides which, they are made in bulk at any old time. Make your own and you will be sure that they contain the correct ingredients and are blended in the proper manner at the right magically empowering time.

The Ingredients

Every plant has its own magical vibration, which is utilised in incenses. When it comes to blending incenses, plants can be used in many forms. Traditional Craft incenses are composed largely of flowers and herbs (leaves and stems), but incenses that contain resins, essential oils, and aesthetically pleasing shapes such as star anise have become popular in recent years. Any herbs, flowers, berries, or barks used should be dried.

Let's look at some types of plant matter you might include in an incense:

RESINS

Resins such as frankincense, myrrh, copal, benzoin, acacia, and pine improve the burning quality, the perfume, and the keeping quality of an incense. Resins should be crushed into small pieces but not powdered.

ESSENTIAL OILS

For a real boost to the strength of an incense's perfume, add a few drops of essential oil. Please note that any oil you add to an incense must be 100 percent non-diluted essential oil. Synthetic and mineral oils smell foul when they are burning, often reminiscent of burning plastic or rubber tyres, and have absolutely no magical value—or at least none we can predict, since we do not know what is in them.

WOODS AND BARKS

Wood improves the bulk and burning quality of an incense. Some, such as cedar or sandalwood, are also highly fragrant. Woods are usually added in the form of shavings or bark chips if you are collecting your own. These need to be quite small if you want them to blend in well with the other ingredients. If you really must buy them rather than collecting them yourself, they can often be bought powdered. Do remember that anything you collect yourself is always going to be much more powerful, and sawdust picked up from the floor is not going to be very magical. Woods and barks that might be added include willow, cinnamon, oak, apple, pine, cedar, ash, alder, and birch.

ROOTS

In some plants, such as mandrake, briony, dragon's blood, and galangal, the power of the plant is concentrated in the root. Small chips of dried root may be added to incense, or occasionally roots are available in powdered form. Orris root powder will fix the perfume of an incense (i.e., make it last longer) and improve its shelf life; it is a particularly valuable addition if you are not including any resins to fix the incense.

POWDERED SPICES

Spices like ginger, cinnamon, cardamom, etc., are readily available in powdered form. These are easily added to an incense, but be careful: a little goes a long way.

DRIED BERRIES

Dried berries make a useful addition to incenses, adding bulk, perfume, and sometimes acting as a binding ingredient. The most commonly used berries include juniper, rowan, hawthorn, and elder, but dried berries of any type can be used (though take care that they do not have toxic fumes, like yew). They are crushed in a mortar with a pestle before they are added to the incense. This releases the oils and the perfume within them.

DRIED HERBS

Dried herbs usually consist of the stems and leaves of a plant in a shredded or crumbled form. These might include familiar culinary herbs such as basil, sage, rosemary, and thyme, or more exotic herbs. They are freely available from herbal suppliers and occult shops, but growing or collecting your own is best.

DRIED FLOWERS

Dried flowers add colour and attractiveness to the look of an incense, and also perfume and texture. Some flowers keep their colour and perfume better than others in the drying process. Commonly used petals and flowers include rose, sunflower, marigold, jasmine, honeysuckle, and clover.

SEEDS AND PODS

Seeds and pods, such as poppy, cardamom, cloves, and star anise, make an interesting visual addition to an incense.

Tools Needed

You will need few specialist tools for making incense, but it is worthwhile investing in the following:

PESTLE AND MORTAR

These are readily available in kitchen shops and are relatively inexpensive. They should be made from stone or marble or be ceramic but not metal, which will taint the ingredients as well as earth any magical charge that you put into the incenses. If you only intend to make a small amount of incense at any one time, just enough for a single ritual or working, then you will not need a large mortar. If you intend to make large batches for the whole coven, you may need something bigger. Keep this just for incense making; do not also use it for food.

SPOONS AND MEASURING CUPS

These should be made from silver, copper, horn, or plastic. Again, this is so you do not earth any magic in the incenses when they have been charged.

JARS

Glass jars with screw-on lids are best for keeping your incenses. I save and wash out all of my jam jars. Store the finished products in a cool, dark place. Don't forget to label the jars!

Blending Loose Incense

Loose incense is probably the easiest type of incense to make and the most useful kind for magical ritual. The recipes in this chapter are all for loose incense.

First of all, assemble your ingredients, your pestle and mortar, your mixing spoons, and your jars and labels ready for the finished product.

All the measurements in this chapter are by volume, not weight. I use a spoon to measure out small quantities when I am making a single jar of incense, but I use a cup for large quantities and big batches. Therefore, when the recipe says 3 parts frankincense, ½ part thyme, and 1 part myrrh, this means three spoons of frankincense, half a spoon of thyme, and 1 spoon of myrrh.

When using resins and essential oils, these should be combined together first, stirring lightly with the pestle and left to go a little sticky before you add any woods, barks, and crushed berries. Next add any herbs and powders and lastly any flowers.

Charging the Incense

As you blend the incense, concentrate on the purpose for which the incense will be used and "project" this into the blend. If you like, you can make a whole ritual of the event, picking and drying your own herbs, then laying out the tools and ingredients on the altar, lighting a candle, and asking the God and Goddess for help:

> *God and Goddess, deign to bless this incense that I would consecrate in your names.*
>
> *Let it obtain the necessary virtues for acts of love and beauty in your honour.*
>
> *Let blessing be.*

Burning Incenses

To use your incenses, take a self-igniting charcoal block (available from occult and church suppliers) and apply a match to it. It will begin to spark across its surface and eventually glow red. Place it on a flame-proof dish with a mat underneath (it will get very hot). When the charcoal block is glowing, sprinkle a pinch of the incense on top—a little goes a long way. Alternatively, if you are celebrating outdoors and have a bonfire, you can throw much larger quantities of incense directly onto the flames. I have also sprinkled it on the hot plate of my woodburners, and this smoulders away quite nicely, though it would really mess up a gas or electric hob!

When a packet of charcoal blocks has been opened, they will quickly start to absorb moisture from the air. This makes them difficult to ignite. Pop them in the oven for ten minutes on a low heat to dry them out, and they will light easily.

Times for Blending

To make extra-powerful ritual incenses, they should be blended at the proper time and season. Witches and Pagans pay attention to the phases of the moon and work their magic by its tides.[42] I will make incense for a sabbat during the tide of that sabbat or use one I made on that sabbat the previous year. For other incenses, I usually blend them according to the phases of the moon.

WAXING MOON

The waxing moon is a good time for starting new projects, new relationships, and for planting flowers and vegetables. It is a time for beginnings, things that will grow to fullness in the future. Use this time to prepare incenses for protection, changing your luck, consecration, initiation, and for honouring the Maiden Goddess.

FULL MOON

The full moon is a good time for positive magic—healing, blessing, and so on. You will feel the benefit when working on creative projects and celebrating the fertile, positive, productive forces in the world and in yourself. Use this time to prepare incenses for love, fertility, blessing, creativity, healing, the full moon esbat, and for honouring the Mother Goddess.

WANING MOON

The waning moon is a time for letting go of bad habits and negative thinking. It is a time of winding down, relinquishing old relationships and situations. It is the time to perform purifications, exorcisms, and cleansing magic. Use this time to make incenses for purification, banishing, exorcism, cleansing, and for honouring the Crone Goddess.

THE DARK MOON

During the three days of the dark moon, the moon regenerates itself and begins life anew, just as all life generates in the darkness of the womb or seeds in the dark earth, growing to maturity in the light. The days of the dark moon are good for deep inner journeys and

---

42   A sabbat is not just a fixed moment but a tide of change during which the shifting energies can be felt for a few days on each side. Making your incense during this period will incorporate these energies into the blend.

meditations. The goddess of death and the underworld rules the dark moon. Use this time to make incenses for scrying, clairvoyance, divination, meditation, underworld travel, shapeshifting, and shamanic work.

PLANETARY RULERSHIPS

You might also wish to make your incenses according to the rulerships of the planets. It is an involved subject and there is not space to discuss it here, but basically each day is ruled by a planet, which in turn influences certain purposes:

SUNDAY (SUN) rules employers, friendship, healing, and work.

MONDAY (MOON) rules agriculture, psychic ability, the home, and medicine.

TUESDAY (MARS) rules conflict, competition, debates, courage, and lust.

WEDNESDAY (MERCURY) rules study, teaching, divination, and communications.

THURSDAY (JUPITER) rules material things, money, property, and luck.

FRIDAY (VENUS) rules love, art, music, incense, and perfume making.

SATURDAY (SATURN) rules the elderly, death, reincarnation, wills, destruction, and endings.

Collecting Ingredients for Incense

The most powerful incenses are made from ingredients you mindfully and ritually collect yourself. I'm writing this at the beginning of May, and as I look around I can see that it's time to gather hawthorn blossoms, horse chestnut candles, yellow dandelion heads, flowering rosemary and sage, marigold petals, and raspberry leaves. If you gather your own ingredients, you will be certain that they have been gathered in a reverent, magically empowered manner. When you come to blend the incense and later to burn it, you will remember the atmosphere of the meadow, riverbank, or garden where you picked the herbs, as well as the day and the season and the enchanted feelings you had at the time.

Make sure the herbs you collect are not growing near a busy road, as they will be polluted. Do not use iron or steel to cut them, as it earths their life force, and don't let them touch the ground after they've been picked, as this has the same effect. You should ask permission of the plant first and state why you want its gifts. If you don't think you've had a reply or are not sure, leave it alone. Only take a little of any one plant; don't strip it bare so that it will die. Place the plant matter in a clean paper, plastic, or fabric bag.

Nature will provide you with all the ingredients you need for your incense making. It is not necessary to use resins and oils if you do not wish to do so. What nature provides is seasonal, and gathering ingredients for incense can be a magical lesson in itself, attuning you to the turning of the seasons and teaching you about herb craft. Gather produce on a dry day, as any damp can have a tendency to turn to mildew. All herbs should be dried before using in an incense.

BUYING INGREDIENTS FOR INCENSE

If you want to buy your ingredients (and you will have to buy non-native plant products such as frankincense if you want to use them), go to a reputable herbal supplier. These will have a regular turnover of stock, and you are not going to finish up with some dusty old herbs that are years old. It is much, much cheaper to buy in bulk, say a kilo at a time. You can share out extra quantities among your friends. Some occult shops charge well over the odds for herbs, so it pays to shop around. Try Asian and ethnic shops for spices.

CHOOSING SUITABLE HERBS FOR INCENSE

Every herb has been attributed to a planet, zodiac sign, element, and god or goddess. This work has been done over thousands of years by observation, experiments, intuition, and inspiration. Over the centuries the work of witches, magicians, and herbalists has given us the knowledge to work with our materials. An incense may be one single herb or a blend of many. Each ingredient should be chosen for its attributes and correspondences. Never use synthetic ingredients, as they will not have the effect you intend; also, they are not magically inert and may have the opposite effect.

Incense Recipes

For all recipes, blend together and burn on charcoal.

APHRODITE

½ PART CYPRESS NEEDLES

A FEW DROPS OF CYPRESS OIL

3 PARTS BENZOIN

½ PART ROSE PETALS

1 PART APPLE WOOD

¼ PART CINNAMON STICKS

¼ PART DAISY FLOWERS

A FEW DROPS OF GERANIUM OIL

¼ PART VIOLET FLOWERS

APOLLO

½ PART BAY LAUREL LEAVES

½ PART PEONY FLOWERS

2 PARTS ASPEN WOOD

2 PARTS FRANKINCENSE

½ PART CYPRESS NEEDLES

½ PART FENNEL SEEDS

2 PARTS ACACIA

A FEW DROPS OF BAY OIL

INCENSE

ATHENE

2 PARTS APPLE WOOD

½ PART OLIVE LEAVES

A FEW DROPS OF GERANIUM OIL

1 PART ASH WOOD

½ PART CYPRESS NEEDLES

A FEW DROPS OF CYPRESS OIL

A PINCH OF DRAGON'S BLOOD

4 PARTS BENZOIN

½ PART MULBERRY LEAVES

BAST

1 PART CATNIP

½ PART VALERIAN ROOT POWDER

2 PARTS MYRRH

A FEW DROPS OF MYRRH OIL

BELINOS

2 PARTS WILLOW BARK

½ PART DAISY FLOWERS

½ PART CELANDINE FLOWERS

2 PARTS FRANKINCENSE (OPTIONAL)

BLODEUWEDD

1 PART BROOM FLOWERS

1 PART BEAN FLOWERS

1 PART HORSE CHESTNUT FLOWERS

1 PART OAK FLOWERS

1 PART MEADOWSWEET FLOWERS

1 PART FLOWERING NETTLE

1 PART PRIMROSE FLOWERS

1 PART HAWTHORN FLOWERS

1 PART FLOWERING BURDOCK

1 PART BLACKTHORN FLOWERS

1 PART CORN COCKLE FLOWERS

BRIGHID

½ PART DRIED ROWAN BERRIES

½ PART BLACKBERRY WOOD

1 PART BIRCH BARK

1 PART WILLOW WOOD

½ PART BISTORT ROOT

1 PART OAK WOOD

½ PART SNOWDROP FLOWERS

½ PART FLAX LEAVES AND FLOWERS

. . . .
CAILLEACH

2 PARTS ASPEN WOOD OR BARK

½ PART BLACKBERRY LEAVES OR WOOD

½ PART CRUSHED ELDERBERRIES

5 PARTS MYRRH

½ PART PARSLEY

1 PART WILLOW BARK

. . . .
CERIDWEN

½ PART BAY LAUREL LEAVES

½ PART WHEAT GRAINS

½ PART IVY LEAVES

3 PARTS OAK WOOD

½ PART VERVAIN HERB

½ PART CHERVIL HERB

1 PART HONEYSUCKLE BLOSSOMS

½ PART MISTLETOE

½ PART APPLE BLOSSOMS

1 PART BLACKTHORN WOOD

INCENSE

Cernunnos

½ PART BETONY HERB

1 PART PINE RESIN

A FEW DROPS OF PINE OIL

2 PARTS OAK WOOD

½ PART CHAMOMILE FLOWERS

½ PART YARROW HERB

1 PART LAVENDER FLOWERS

1 PART CEDAR WOOD

1 PART ASH WOOD

½ PART BISTORT ROOT

½ PART NETTLE LEAVES

Demeter

½ PART KERNELS OF WHEAT OR BARLEY

1 PART ROSE PETALS

2 PARTS FRANKINCENSE

2 PARTS MYRRH

½ PART PENNYROYAL HERB

½ PART BEAN FLOWERS

½ PART RED POPPY PETALS

½ PART CYPRESS NEEDLES

A FEW DROPS OF CYPRESS OIL

A FEW DROPS OF ROSE OIL (OPTIONAL)

EARTH MOTHER

1 PART PINE RESIN

1 PART MANDRAKE ROOT

1 PART ROSE PETALS

½ PART PATCHOULI LEAVES

A FEW DROPS OF PATCHOULI OIL

FREYA

½ PART PRIMROSE FLOWERS

½ PART COWSLIP FLOWERS

½ PART CYPRESS NEEDLES

1 PART MISTLETOE TWIGS AND LEAVES

½ PART ROSE PETALS

½ PART DAISY PETALS

½ PART STRAWBERRY LEAVES

½ PART MYRTLE

½ PART RED CLOVER FLOWERS

5 PARTS MYRRH

2 PARTS BENZOIN

3 PARTS RED SANDALWOOD

A FEW DROPS OF SANDALWOOD OIL

A FEW DROPS OF ROSE OIL (OPTIONAL)

INCENSE

HECATE

½ PART CRUSHED GARLIC

½ PART MANDRAKE ROOT

2 PARTS WILLOW BARK

1 PART LAVENDER

4 PARTS MYRRH

A FEW DROPS OF MYRRH OIL

A FEW DROPS OF CYPRESS OIL

½ PART MUGWORT

ODIN

2 PARTS ASH WOOD

½ PART MISTLETOE

1 PART OAK WOOD

½ PART STORAX

1 PART ELM WOOD

½ PART AMARANTH (OPTIONAL)

PERSEPHONE

1 PART CYPRESS NEEDLES

A FEW DROPS OF CYPRESS OIL

½ PART DRIED POMEGRANATE RIND

4 PARTS WILLOW WOOD

¼ PART DITTANY OF CRETE

¼ PART PARSLEY

¼ PART IVY LEAVES

½ PART RED POPPY SEEDS

½ PART RED POPPY PETALS

¼ PART FORGET-ME-NOT FLOWERS AND LEAVES

Earth (Element)

2 PARTS PINE WOOD

A FEW DROPS OF PATCHOULI OIL

½ PART BISTORT ROOT

½ PART HONEYSUCKLE

½ PART PINE RESIN

½ PART CYPRESS NEEDLES

½ PART SAGE

Air (Element)

2 PARTS ACACIA

2 PARTS BENZOIN

A FEW DROPS OF LAVENDER OIL

1 PART LAVENDER FLOWERS

A FEW DROPS OF LEMON VERBENA OIL

1 PART CEDAR WOOD

½ PART MINT

Fire (Element)

1 PART ASH WOOD

¼ PART BAY LEAVES

½ PART CLOVES

1 PART COPAL

1 PART ORANGE PEEL

A FEW DROPS OF ORANGE OIL

¼ PART CORIANDER POWDER

A PINCH OF DRAGON'S BLOOD

2 PARTS FRANKINCENSE

1 PART GALANGAL ROOT

INCENSE

2 PARTS RED SANDALWOOD

¼ PART GINGER POWDER

3 PARTS CRUSHED JUNIPER BERRIES

½ PART MARIGOLD PETALS

½ PART ROSEMARY

. . . .

WATER (ELEMENT)

3 PARTS MYRRH

1 PART BENZOIN

2 PARTS WHITE SANDALWOOD

½ PART LEMON BALM (MELISSA)

A FEW DROPS OF LEMON BALM (MELISSA) OIL

½ PART CHAMOMILE FLOWERS

½ PART COMFREY LEAVES

½ PART EUCALYPTUS LEAVES

. . .

SUN

2 PARTS ACACIA RESIN

3 PARTS FRANKINCENSE

½ PART ORANGE PEEL

1 PART MYRRH

2 PARTS RED SANDALWOOD

½ PART ROSEMARY

¼ PART CINNAMON BARK

1 PART BENZOIN

A FEW DROPS OF CEDAR OIL

. . . . . .

SAMHAIN

4 PARTS MYRRH

A FEW DROPS OF MYRRH OIL

1 PART CRUSHED ROWAN BERRIES

1 PART ASPEN WOOD

1 PART ELDER WOOD

1 PART MULLEIN FLOWERS

½ PART IVY LEAVES

1 PART CRUSHED JUNIPER BERRIES

A FEW DROPS OF JUNIPER OIL

. . .

YULE

3 PARTS FRANKINCENSE

A FEW DROPS OF ORANGE OIL

A FEW DROPS OF JUNIPER OIL

1 PART CRUSHED JUNIPER BERRIES

½ PART MISTLETOE

. . . . .

IMBOLC

1 PART BENZOIN

3 PARTS MYRRH

½ PART BASIL LEAVES

A FEW DROPS OF BENZOIN OIL

1 PART CELANDINE FLOWERS

. . . . .

INCENSE

· · · · ·
OSTARA

3 PARTS FRANKINCENSE

1 PART BENZOIN

A PINCH OF DRAGON'S BLOOD

A PINCH OF NUTMEG

½ PART VIOLET FLOWERS

½ PART ORANGE PEEL

1 PART RED ROSE PETALS

· · · · ·
BELTANE

4 PARTS FRANKINCENSE

½ PART SORREL

1 PART HAWTHORN FLOWERS

½ PART PRIMROSE FLOWERS

½ PART APPLE BLOSSOMS

1 PART OAK BARK

· · · · · · · ·
MIDSUMMER

3 PARTS RED SANDALWOOD

½ PART MUGWORT

½ PART CHAMOMILE FLOWERS

½ PART ROSE PETALS

½ PART LAVENDER FLOWERS

INCENSE

Lughnasa

1 PART OAK BARK

½ PART PINE RESIN

A FEW DROPS OF PATCHOULI OIL

½ PART ASH LEAVES

2 PARTS SANDALWOOD

½ PART WORMWOOD

1 PART CEDAR WOOD

A FEW DROPS OF CEDAR OIL

3 PARTS FRANKINCENSE

Autumn Equinox

2 PARTS BENZOIN

2 PARTS MYRRH

1 PART HAZEL WOOD

½ PART CORN

½ PART RED POPPY FLOWERS

½ PART CORNFLOWER

½ PART IVY

Consecration

½ PART MACE

½ PART STORAX

1 PART BENZOIN

½ PART CLOVES

A FEW DROPS OF LEMONGRASS OIL

¼ PART THYME

INCENSE

WAXING MOON

1 PART WHITE ROSE PETALS

¼ PART CAMPHOR

½ PART LILY FLOWERS

½ PART CINQUEFOIL

¼ PART MUGWORT

½ PART DAISY FLOWERS

Blend during the waxing moon for workings connected with starting new projects, new relationships, and for beginnings—things that will grow to fullness in the future.

FULL MOON

3 PARTS WHITE SANDALWOOD

½ PART ORRIS ROOT POWDER

½ PART THYME

½ PART POPPY SEEDS

1 PART WHITE ROSE PETALS

1 PART BENZOIN

2 PARTS MYRRH

2 PARTS FRANKINCENSE

½ PART GARDENIA FLOWERS

Blend during the full moon for workings connected with positive magic—healing, blessing, and so on.

WANING MOON

½ PART GARLIC LEAVES

3 PARTS MYRRH

Blend during the waning moon and use for workings connected with letting go, winding down, relinquishing old relationships and situations, purifications, and cleansing magic.

DARK MOON

½ PART PARSLEY

2 PARTS WILLOW BARK

3 PARTS MYRRH

½ PART FORGET-ME-NOT FLOWERS

Blend during the three days of the dark moon and use for workings of deep inner journeys and meditations.

AURA CLEANSING

4 PARTS FRANKINCENSE

1 PART SAGE

½ PART ROSEMARY

½ PART JASMINE FLOWERS

A FEW DROPS OF ROSEMARY OIL

MEDITATION

4 PARTS ACACIA RESIN

2 PARTS SANDALWOOD

1 PART ROSE PETALS

A FEW DROPS OF ROSE OIL (OPTIONAL)

DIVINATION

2 PARTS WHITE SANDALWOOD

1 PART ACACIA

½ PART CALENDULA (MARIGOLD) PETALS

1 PART HAZEL WOOD

½ PART BAY

½ PART CLARY SAGE

A PINCH OF NUTMEG

. . . .

Cleansing

2 PARTS FRANKINCENSE

2 PARTS MYRRH

2 PARTS RED SANDALWOOD

1 PART ROSEMARY

A FEW DROPS OF ROSEMARY OIL

¼ PART DRAGON'S BLOOD

. . . .

Purification

3 PARTS FRANKINCENSE

¼ PART CINNAMON

1 PART ROSEMARY

1 PART LAVENDER FLOWERS

½ PART LEMON PEEL

A FEW DROPS OF ROSEMARY OIL

. . . .

Protection

½ PART BAY

½ PART AVENS

½ PART MUGWORT

½ PART YARROW

½ PART ROSEMARY

½ PART ST. JOHN'S WORT

½ PART ANGELICA ROOT

½ PART BASIL

2 PARTS CRUSHED JUNIPER BERRIES

A FEW DROPS OF JUNIPER OIL

3 PARTS FRANKINCENSE

2 PARTS MYRRH

INCENSE

· · · · · · ·
Banishing

3 PARTS MYRRH

1 PART RUE

½ PART MINT

A FEW DROPS OF MINT OIL

1 PART PEONY FLOWERS

· · ·
Love

3 PARTS FRANKINCENSE

½ PART HONEYSUCKLE FLOWERS

½ PART MUSK CRYSTALS

½ PART LILAC FLOWERS

A FEW DROPS OF LEMON VERBENA OIL

½ PART ORANGE PEEL

½ PART LEMON PEEL

Blend at the full moon and use in rituals and spells to attract love.

· · · · ·
Healing

½ PART BAY LEAVES

½ PART CHAMOMILE FLOWERS

½ PART LEMON BALM (MELISSA) LEAVES

A PINCH OF POWDERED CINNAMON

1 PART CRUSHED JUNIPER BERRIES

1 PART LAVENDER FLOWERS

A FEW DROPS OF LAVENDER OIL

¼ PART SAGE LEAVES

1 PART ROSEMARY LEAVES

A FEW DROPS OF ROSEMARY OIL

Blend at the full moon and use during candle magic and spells and rituals for healing.

. . . .

Peace

3 PARTS FRANKINCENSE

A FEW DROPS OF YLANG-YLANG OIL

A FEW DROPS OF LAVENDER OIL

1 PART LAVENDER FLOWERS

1 PART CHAMOMILE FLOWERS

1 PART ROSE PETALS

Blend at the waxing or full moon.

. . . .

Abundance

½ PART CINNAMON BARK

A FEW DROPS OF CINNAMON OIL

¼ PART NUTMEG POWDER

½ PART CRUSHED CLOVES

¼ PART MACE

½ PART SHREDDED GALANGAL ROOT

¼ PART BASIL LEAVES

A FEW DROPS OF BASIL OIL

½ PART CHAMOMILE FLOWERS

Blend at the waxing moon.

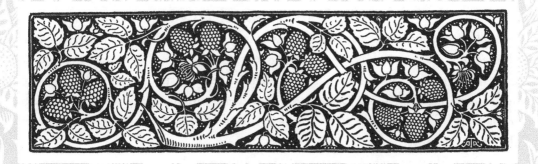

CHAPTER 14

Vegetable Dyes

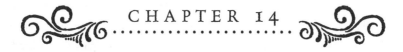

If you've ever tried to wash blackberry stains out of a white shirt, you will realise that plants can provide some pretty powerful dyes. People have been using plants to colour fabric and yarn for thousands of years. The oldest recorded example is the use of indigo in the Indus Valley four and a half thousand years ago. The ancient Egyptians are known to have used madder and safflower to colour fabric, while in early Ireland dyeing was considered to be a somewhat magical process and was strictly a women's craft, with a taboo on dyeing fabric in the presence of men. Dye craft was developed into a fine art by the great mediaeval guilds of dyers in Europe, and their recipes were closely guarded secrets. However, the first synthetic dye was invented in 1864 by a British chemist called William Perkins; by the end of the century most fabric was synthetically dyed, and much of the ancient knowledge was lost.

Why Use Natural Dyes?

Natural dyes derived from plant material avoid using the toxic chemicals and heavy metals used in synthetic colours. These won't be listed on a garment label, and you probably don't realise that you are being exposed to them. They can result in irritation of the skin and mucous membranes, and even cause organ damage with heavy exposure, especially in textile workers in developing countries, the source of our cheap clothes (and even many of the expensive ones).

Dyeing with plant materials is a satisfying craft that is always full of surprises, as you never quite know what colour you are going to get—it all depends on the freshness and concentration of the plant materials, the type of fabric you use, and the mordant (fixative) you use. The colours are softer and more subtle than chemical dyes, and when you wear clothes or robes coloured with them, they can help you feel like part of the landscape during ritual.

Do be prepared for the process to be time consuming, and do make sure you keep careful records so that you can reproduce your results as far as possible.

Equipment Needed

You will need some basic equipment, though you may already have these in your kitchen or be able to pick them up in secondhand shops.

- Large cooking pans (unchipped enamel and stainless steel ones are good, since iron, copper, and aluminium pots will alter the colour slightly)

- Thermometer for liquid

- Scales

- Stirring sticks or wooden spoons

- Tongs

- Sieves

- Rubber gloves

- Plastic bowls

- Labels and pen

- Glass jars

Safety First

Never use the same equipment that you use for dying for cooking. Some of the materials used may be toxic (though I have tried to use only fairly safe ones in this book), so keep them in a safe place, out of reach of children and animals. Make sure that you label everything clearly. Do not breathe the fumes when you are dying or mordanting, and do it in a well-ventilated space. Always wear rubber gloves throughout the process.

Obtaining the Plants

You can forage many plants that provide a wide range of colours. Different herbs, mosses, barks, berries, twigs, and leaves can be gathered at different times of the year, and this is rewarding in itself. Do bear in mind the rules of foraging, and never take too many plants from one spot or collect any rare species. Many lichens, for example, are on the edge of extinction, so please leave these alone. It's worth remembering that many of the plants we consider common weeds—such as nettles and dandelions—will provide a dye.

If you wish to, and have the space, it is easy to grow a wide range of traditional dye plants such as woad, alkanet, marigold, chamomile, madder, and goldenrod. If you don't have a garden or wild spaces nearby, you can even use kitchen waste such as avocado skins, beetroot, carrot peel and tops, and onion skins.

COLLECTING AND DRYING DYE PLANTS

Pick leaves and aerial plant parts on a dry, sunny day, but pick roots on a damp day. To dry the plants, tie them up and hang them upside down in a warm, dry place. For plants with flaky parts or seeds, you can put them in a paper bag before hanging them up.

A Note on Water

Some natural dyers will only use pure rainwater, as the acidity or alkalinity of the water used will affect the dye colour. While I would not worry too much about this in your early experiments, it is as well to be aware that soft water (more acidic) is best for practically all natural dyes. If you live in a hard water (more alkaline) area, add vinegar or lemon juice. Cream of tartar is often added as a pH buffer and softens the water for improved results. A few dyes, such as madder, weld, logwood, and brazilwood, develop better in hard water containing calcium and magnesium salts. If you live in a soft water area, you can add calcium carbonate in the form of finely ground chalk or household ammonia. If your tap water contains iron, the colours will be "saddened" and turn out darker and more muted than they otherwise would.

Stage 1: Prepare the Fabric

Natural dyes will only colour natural fabrics. (The exception is rayon, which is the only manmade fibre that will successfully take them.) Natural fabrics or fibres can be divided into two categories: those obtained from animal sources, such as wool, silk, and mohair, and those obtained from plant sources, such as cotton, linen, and hemp. Fibres from animal sources are much easier to colour, as they bond more readily with the dyes and take less time to mordant properly. Plant-based yarns and fabrics usually need premordanting to achieve successful results.

It is much easier to dye yarns than woven fabric or made-up garments, which can be tricky to achieve even coverage on. Remember that if the stitching uses synthetic fibres, it will not take the colour.

Dirt and grease will reject the mordant and the dye, so all yarn or fabric should be washed. If necessary, soak it overnight. Give it a final rinse in warm water to which a tablespoon of white vinegar has been added.

Wool is the easiest of all to dye, and whether in the form of fleece or skeins of yarn, it should be soaked in water for several hours. Never bring wool to the boil in the dye pot or mordant, as it will begin to felt (mat together). For the same reason, do not stir or agitate it.

Cotton and linen should be prepared by being brought to a boil with a spoonful of washing soda and soaking for 24 hours.

Stage 2: Mordant the Fabric

After washing and rinsing the fabric or yarn, the next stage is to mordant it, which prepares the fabric for dying. Derived from the Latin word *mordere*, meaning "to bite," a mordant is a chemical compound that helps the dye stick to the fibre of the fabric and set the colour permanently. Colours from natural dyes will vary depending on which mordant is used.

Some hobby dyers use chromium and tin as mordants, but both are known to be dangerous to health even in tiny amounts. Although these metallic salts work well to fix the dyes, they are an environmental hazard, producing toxic waste that requires special disposal. Safer mineral alternatives include alum (which can be used with most plant dyes), copper, and iron. Such mordants can be bought from pharmacies and specialist craft and dye suppliers.

There are greener alternatives from natural or household chemical sources, and though these do not create a completely permanent dye, they do greatly reduce fading. They include household chemicals like vinegar, cream of tartar, and bicarbonate of soda (baking soda). Ancient dyers used urine. Some plant materials provide natural mordants too, but they may also add a pale colour tint. However, some plants, such as onion skins, acorns, and walnut shells, need no mordants at all and have qualities that will bind with the fibre and are colour-fast all on their own. This can eliminate the mordanting step in the dyeing process.

Here are some of the safer mordants:

WOOD ASH

This takes a lot of ash and the results can be a bit unpredictable, but the outcome can be worth it. If you have pure wood fires or barbecues, save the ash—the whiter the better (birch wood is best). Use 50 percent weight of wood ash to the weight of dry fabric to be dyed. To prepare the ash as a mordant, put the ash in a large jar and cover with enough water to fill it. Put on the lid and shake. Leave for one week until the water clears. Strain it off carefully and retain as the mordant. To use, fill a large pan with water and add the wood ash liquid. Add the fabric and simmer for an hour. Remove from the heat and leave to soak overnight. Rinse and proceed to the dye stage.

PLANT MORDANTS

Some plant materials provide natural mordants but may also add a pale colour tint, such as rhubarb leaves (pale green—**note:** poisonous), rhubarb stems (yellow), lemon skins (no colour), privet leaves (greenish tint), sumac leaves (no colour), and nettles (browny-green). You will need about 25 percent of plant material to the weight of the fabric.

Pour boiling water over the plant stems, leaves, or peels, simmer for one hour, and strain. Pour the liquid into the mordant pan and heat to 80°C (176°F) and add the material to be dyed. Simmer for 50 minutes, remove from the heat, and soak for 24 hours. Wring out the fabric (do not rinse) and proceed to the dye stage.

OAK GALLS
(ALSO CALLED GALL NUTS OR OAK APPLES)

Found on oak trees, oak galls[43] are the home of gall wasps and are very rich in tannin, containing up to 70 percent. Used since ancient times in dying, ink making, and leather tanning, they are collected and ground. You will need about 20 percent of gall nuts to the weight of the fabric or yarn to be dyed. Grind the nuts to a powder, cover with water, and leave overnight, then boil for 90 minutes and strain. Take the resulting liquid and pour it

---

43   Oak apple galls are brown balls found hanging like fruit from oak twigs in the autumn, varying in size from half an inch to two inches in diameter. They are caused when the gall wasp lays its eggs in developing leaf buds in early summer. The larva inside eat their way out and emerge a few weeks later. The dried, empty galls are gathered in the autumn.

into the mordant pan, add the fabric to be dyed, and raise the temperature to 80°C (176°F) for one hour. Turn off the heat and soak for 4 hours. Wring out the fabric (do not rinse) and proceed to the dye stage.

ALUM
(ALUMINIUM POTASSIUM CHLORIDE/ POTASSIUM ALUMINIUM SULPHATE)

This is one of the cheapest and safest chemical mordants to use. Whereas other mordants may add colour to fabric, alum just makes shades brighter and clearer. True alums are double salts of aluminium such as potassium aluminium sulphate, but aluminium sulphate is also used and called alum. You can buy food-grade alum in the grocery store. Try using 1 ounce for every pound of dry fabric weight, and add 1 ounce cream of tartar (not suitable for addition if using linen and cotton). Dissolve, add 2 gallons water, bring slowly to a boil, reduce the heat, add the damp fabric, and simmer for 1 hour. Remove the fabric. Do not rinse but drip fairly dry. Continue to the dye stage.

IRON
(FERROUS SULPHATE, ALSO CALLED COPPERAS)

The ancients obtained this from bogs and iron ore. It makes colours more muted or "saddened," to use the correct term. It is usually used *after* the fabric has been dyed, rather than before. You can make it by soaking iron nails or horseshoes in four parts water to one part of white vinegar for a week. Strain through muslin before use. To use, fill a pan with water and the iron liquid, put in the damp fabric, and simmer at 60°C (140°F) for 40 minutes. Remove the fabric and rinse well.

COPPER SULPHATE
(ALSO CALLED BLUE VITRIOL OR VERDIGRIS)

This is used to bring out blue-greens in a dye and works best with natural wool yarn, rather than fabric. Use ½ ounce with ½ pint of white vinegar for every pound of dry yarn weight. Fill a pan with hot water and dissolve the copper sulphate. Put in the yarn and simmer for 40–60 minutes. Remove from the heat and soak for no more than an hour. Rinse the yarn well and proceed to the dye stage. You can make your own copper solution by putting a copper bracelet, copper pipe, or some pure copper coins in a small amount of white vinegar and enough water to cover. Leave three or four days until the water turns bluish, then use this liquid as per the above instructions.

Note: Poisonous. Handle with care!

Stage 3: Dye the Fabric

Generally speaking, use approximately 2 ounces of the plant material for every ounce of fabric. The plant should be chopped up (roots and barks ground), just covered in water and simmered to extract the dye; the longer and slower the simmer, the better the result, as most dye plants don't react well to temperatures over 40°C (104°F), though a few need to be boiled. Remove from the heat and let the mixture stand for 24 hours. You can then strain it and use it immediately or put the resulting decoction in a jar, label it, and store in a dark place until you need it.

Add the fabric and simmer, stirring, until the fabric takes on a good colour. You can then turn off the heat and leave the fabric to soak in the dye overnight.

Wearing rubber gloves, rinse the fabric several times, gradually decreasing the temperature of the rinsing water.

Hang up the fabric to dry naturally. Always dry out of direct sunlight, and do not put the article in a tumble dryer.

You can repeat the dyeing process two or three times to deepen the colour.

Dye Plants to Use

Many plants will produce some kind of dye, but *tinctorum* or *tinctoria* in their botanical name indicates a plant that is long established as a dyestuff. Various parts may be used—bark, berries, flowers, juice, leaves, shoots, or roots, depending on the particular plant.

ONION SKINS–YELLOW

Onion skins need no mordant, and they are readily available—whenever you peel an onion, just save the skin. To dye, put them in a pan with just enough water to cover them and boil until the water turns a deep brownish-yellow. Strain and return the liquid to the pan. Wet the material you want to dye and add it to the pan. Simmer gently until you have the depth of colour you require. Rinse the fabric well and dry.

WELD (*RESEDA LUTEOLA*) ALSO CALLED DYER'S WELD OR DYER'S WEED–YELLOW

Mordant the fabric with alum for bright yellow or with copper for a greeny-yellow. Use 50 percent weld to dry weight of fabric (so if you have 100 grams of fabric, use 50 grams of weld). Put the plant material into a pan and pour on enough boiling water to cover. Stand overnight. Add more water and bring the pot to a simmer at no more than 70°C (158°F). Strain off the dye into the dye pan. Add the damp fabric and simmer below 70°C (158°F) for an hour. Weld develops best in slightly hard water, so add some calcium carbonate to soft water.

DYER'S GREENWEED (*GENISTA TINCTORIA*)–YELLOW OR GREEN

Use an alum mordant for yellow or copper for greens. The flowers, tender twigs, or leaves are used for dying. Use 60 percent weight of the plant to dry weight of fabric. Steep the plant in cold water for 30 minutes. Add some white vinegar and bring to a boil. Strain off the liquid into a jar, and also reserve the plant material. Add more fresh water to the plant material, steep for 30 minutes, add a dash of white vinegar, and boil. Strain and discard the plant material. Put all the liquid into a dye pan along with the damp mordanted fabric. Heat to 70°C (158°F) for 15 minutes, longer if you want a darker yellow. Turn off the heat and allow the pan to cool. Remove the fabric and rinse.

MADDER (*RUBIA TINCTORIA*)–PINK AND RED

Historically, madder was one of the most important dyes; remains of the plant have been found at the Viking excavations in York. The colour is contained in the root, beneath the woody root-bark, and is best extracted from two-year-old plants. The roots should be washed and dried out for a few days, then ground to a powder. To dye your fabric, you will need about 25 percent of madder root to dry weight of fabric.

The fabric or yarn should be mordanted with alum for red or copper for a brownish-pink. Put the madder root in a pan of water and heat very slowly to no more than 60°C (140°F) for a couple of hours. Strain out the dye and add the fabric, heat to no more than 60°C (140°F) for one hour, turn off the heat, and leave to cool. Remove the fabric and rinse well. The water left in the dye bath will dye another load or two in ever paler shades.

This dye reacts to different levels of acidity and alkalinity in the water. You can change the shade by adding a teaspoon or two of lemon juice for orange shades or washing soda for a pinker colour. Madder develops to its deepest and richest reds in hard water, so if the water is soft, add calcium carbonate.

ALKANET (*ALKANNA TINCTORIA*)–VIOLET

Mordant with alum for wool and silk or with oak galls for cotton. The colourant from alkanet is not soluble in water, so the root shavings must be soaked in alcohol for several days; use methylated spirits or vodka. When the liquid has developed a strong colour, strain it off into the dye pan and add water. Heat gently to no more than 60°C (140°F) until all the colour has been taken up.

CHAMOMILE (*ANTHEMIS TINCTORIA*)–YELLOW

Use an alum mordant on the fabric to be dyed. Soak the chamomile in hot water for one hour, add the fabric, and slowly bring the temperature up to about 82°C (180°F) for about an hour.

HENNA (*LAWSONIA INERMIS*)–REDDISH-BROWN

Mordant the fabric with alum. Add henna powder at about 50 percent to the dry fabric weight to the dye pan and simmer for two hours or until the desired colour is obtained.

MARIGOLD (*CALENDULA OFFICINALIS*)–ORANGE

Use alum mordant on the fabric. Put the fresh flower petals in a pan, cover with water, and leave to steep for 40 minutes. Turn on the heat and simmer for 50 minutes at 40°C (104°F). Strain the liquid and return to the dye pan. Add the fabric and simmer at 70°C (158°F) until the desired shade is achieved. Remove from the heat and rinse immediately or the colour will dull.

SAFFLOWER (*CARTHAMUS TINCTORIA*)–YELLOW, PINK & RED

Both a red and a yellow dye can be extracted from safflower petals. When using safflower, use at least equal weights of dyestuff and fibres, more if you want a stronger colour.

The yellow dye can be applied to wool, cotton, linen, and silk. You don't have to use a mordant, though using an alum mordant will improve fastness. Extract the yellow dye from the petals by tying them in muslin and soaking them in a bucket of cold water for a few hours. Wearing rubber gloves, squeeze the bag of petals to extract the yellow colour. Keep doing this until the yellow colour stops coming out of the petals and the water in the bucket is strongly yellow. Remove the bag and put the yellow liquid into a dye bath, add your fabric, and heat to simmering point. (At this point you can reserve the bag of petals to make a red dye—see below.) Simmer for 45 minutes and remove from heat. Allow the fabric to cool in the liquid before removing and rinsing.

Extracting a red dye is more complicated. It is not necessary to add a mordant, but it will fade over time. Use for cotton, linen, and silk; it will not work on wool. Using the petals from which you have already extracted the yellow dye, put them in a bucket with enough cold water for your dye bath to which 1 tablespoon of washing soda has been added per gallon of water. Leave for an hour or two, squeeze the petals well, and strain off the liquid. Add enough clear vinegar or lemon juice to the strained-off liquid to turn it bright red. Add the fibres and leave them to soak overnight. Rinse well and dry away from direct sunlight.

DYER'S BUCKTHORN (*RHAMNUS TINCTORIA*)–YELLOW

A warm yellow colour comes from the unripe berries. Soak the berries in water, bring to a boil, and simmer until the colour is extracted. Strain, return to the dye pan, and simmer at about 80°C (176°F) as the colour develops. Add the fabric (premordanted with alum and cream of tartar) and turn off the heat. Leave to soak for 24 hours. Rinse.

GOLDENROD (*SOLIDAGO CANADENSIS*)–YELLOW

Mordant the fabric with alum or rhubarb. Simmer the flowering tops of the plant in water, strain, and return the liquid to the dye pan. Add the fabric and simmer at 70°C (158°F) for 60 minutes. Turn off the heat and allow to cool, then rinse.

MORE DYE PLANTS

PLANT	COLOUR	MORDANT
AGRIMONY	YELLOW	ALUM
ALDER BARK	RED-BROWN	ALUM
ALDER FLOWERS	GREEN	ALUM
ALDER TWIGS	BROWN	IRON
ALKANET	BEIGE	ALUM
APPLE BARK	GREEN	IRON
APPLE BARK	RED-YELLOW	ALUM
ASH INNER BARK	YELLOW	ALUM

PLANT	COLOUR	MORDANT
BAYBERRY LEAVES	YELLOW-BROWN	ALUM
BEDSTRAW ROOTS	RED	ALUM AND TARTAR
BILBERRIES	BLUE	IRON
BILBERRIES	PURPLE	ALUM
BIRCH	YELLOW	ALUM
BIRCH BARK	PURPLE	IRON
BIRCH LEAVES	GREEN-YELLOW	ALUM
BLACKBERRIES	LIGHT GREY	ALUM
BLACKBERRY SHOOTS	BLACK	IRON
BLACKTHORN	ORANGE	ALUM
BOG MYRTLE	YELLOW	ALUM
BRACKEN	YELLOW	ALUM
BROOM	YELLOW	ALUM
CRAB APPLE BARK	YELLOW	ALUM

PLANT	COLOUR	MORDANT
DOCK	BEIGE	ALUM
ELDER BARK	BLACK	IRON
ELDER BERRIES	PINK-PURPLE	ALUM
ELDER LEAVES	YELLOW	ALUM
FLAG IRIS	BLUE	IRON
GOLDEN ROD	YELLOW	ALUM
GORSE	YELLOW	ALUM
HEATHER	BEIGE	ALUM
HORSETAIL	GREEN	ALUM
ICELAND MOSS	LIGHT BROWN	NONE
INDIGO	BLUE	NONE NEEDED
LICHEN	YELLOW TO PURPLE	NONE NEEDED
LILY OF THE VALLEY LEAVES	GREEN-YELLOW	ALUM
MADDER	DARK RED	ALUM AND TARTAR

PLANT	COLOUR	MORDANT
MADDER ROOT	ORANGE-RED	ALUM OR IRON
MARIGOLD	BROWN	ALUM
MARSH MARIGOLD	YELLOW	ALUM
MEADOWSWEET	YELLOW	ALUM
NETTLE	YELLOW	ALUM
OAK BARK	BLACK	IRON
OAK BARK	BROWN	ALUM
ONION SKINS	YELLOW	ALUM
PARSLEY	GREEN-YELLOW	ALUM
PINE	RED-YELLOW	ALUM
PINE CONES	BEIGE	ALUM
PRIVET LEAVES	BLUE	ALUM AND SALT
SLOES	PURPLE	ALUM
SORREL LEAVES	YELLOW	ALUM

VEGETABLE DYES

PLANT	COLOUR	MORDANT
SORREL ROOT	RED	ALUM
ST. JOHN'S WORT FLOWERS	PURPLE	NONE
SUNFLOWER PETALS	YELLOW	ALUM
WALNUT LEAVES	BROWN	ALUM
WALNUT SHELLS	BROWN	ALUM
WOAD	GREEN-BLUE	NONE NEEDED

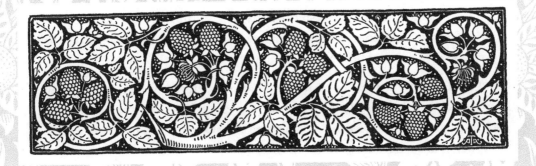

Colour Correspondences

BLACK: Banishing, repelling, death, endings, destruction, winding down, the elderly, ancestor contact, the void or womb, receptivity, reincarnation, rejection of ego, possibilities waiting to be realised, Samhain, crone goddesses, death deities, the planet Saturn, Scorpio, Capricorn

BLUE: Tranquillity, peace, calm, harmony, protection, healing, spiritual development, teaching, luck, autumn equinox, spiritual protection, throat chakra, moon, water spirits, the planet Jupiter, the element of water, Virgo, Aquarius

BROWN: Grounding, stability, earthiness, sexuality, practicality, environmental awareness, the planet Earth, autumn equinox, Mother Earth, nature deities

GOLD: Happiness, rejuvenation, spiritual strength, spiritual zest, service to others, friendship, healing, energy, spiritual energy, strength, life force, solar plexus chakra, sun and corn deities, Midsummer, the sun

GREEN: Fertility, growth, prosperity, wealth, money, creativity, love, attraction, art, music, change, balance, Beltane, Yule, earth magic, compassion, heart chakra, Mother Earth, fairies, dryads, vegetation deities, the planet Venus, the element of earth, Venus, Cancer, Capricorn

GREY: Communication, study, teaching, divination, the planet Mercury

INDIGO: Perceptiveness, vision, intuition, insight, third eye chakra, Taurus

MAGENTA: Vision, creativity, insight, inspiration, creative vitality, root chakra

ORANGE: Optimism, success, courage, bravery, energy, ambition, luck, career, legal matters, self-esteem, spleen chakra, Samhain, Lughnasa, the sun, Leo

PINK: Love, romance, friendship, happiness, harmony, peace, compassion, handfastings, beauty, heart chakra, love goddesses, Libra

PURPLE: Strength, mastery, power, occult power, protection, Pisces, crone goddesses

RED: Life, vitality, energy, sex drive, passion, lust, conflict, competition, courage, strength, health, root chakra, Yule, Midsummer, fire spirits, mother goddesses, warrior gods, the planet Mars, the element of fire

SILVER: Intuition, truth, enlightenment, agriculture, the home, medicine, psychic ability, removes negativity, communication, personal enlightenment, moon rituals, moon goddesses

TURQUOISE: Inventiveness, conception, philosophy, creativity, communication, throat chakra

VIOLET: Spiritual healing, mastery, ceremony, spirituality, self-respect, spiritual growth, spiritual fulfilment, self-esteem, third eye chakra, crown chakra, Sagittarius

WHITE: Peace, cleansing, defensive magic, protection, purity, harmony, spirit, psychic development, the dispelling of negativity, purification, tranquillity, Imbolc, maiden goddesses, waxing moon, crown chakra

YELLOW: Intellectual development, strength of mind, learning, study, eloquence, joy, air spirits, vision, solar plexus chakra, the planet Mercury, the element of air, Ostara, Leo

• • • • •

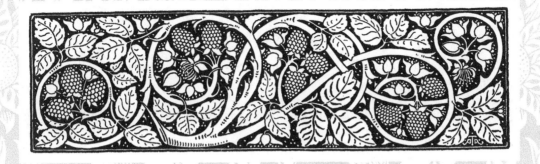

Planetary Influences

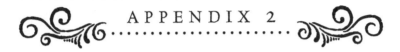

JUPITER: Rituals and spells to do with material things, money, property, and luck.

MARS: Rituals and spells to do with conflict, competition, debates, courage, and lust.

MERCURY: Rituals and spells to do with study, teaching, divination, and communications.

MOON: Rituals and spells to do with agriculture, psychic ability, the home, and medicine.

NEPTUNE: Rituals and workings of intuition, sensitivity, empathy, compassion, adaptability, imagination, harnessing spiritual energy, altered states of awareness, dance, music, creativity, poetry, writing, theatre, beauty, and glamour.

PLUTO: Rituals and workings linked to rebirth, transformation, destiny, the subconscious, releasing the old and embracing the new.

SATURN: Rituals and spells to do with the elderly, death, reincarnation, wills, destruction, and endings.

SUN: Rituals and spells to do with employers, friendship, healing, and work.

URANUS: Rituals and workings concerned with invention, innovation, new technologies, freedom, creativity, and altruistic and humanitarian pursuits.

VENUS: Rituals and spells to do with love, art, music, incense, and perfume making.

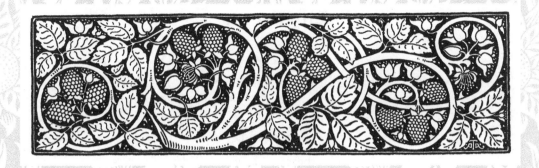

Magical Herbal Correspondences

Life Events

• • • •

BIRTH

Ash   Birch   Birthwort   Caraway   Nettle   Rosemary

• • • • • • •

FUNERALS

Aconite   Ash   Blackberry   Caraway   Cedar   Cypress
Forget-Me-Not   Iris   Marjoram   Myrrh   Nettle   Parsley
Rosemary   Rowan   Smallage   Tansy   Willow

• • • • • • • •

HANDFASTING

Anise   Apple   Broom   Cardamom   Cinnamon   Clove
Coriander   Dill   Lavender   Mallow   Marjoram   Meadowsweet
Myrtle   Patchouli   Rose   Rosemary   Rue   Saffron   Skullcap
Sorrel   Strawberry   Violet

Moon Phases

DARK MOON

Forget-Me-Not   Garlic   Parsley   Willow

FULL MOON

Alecost   Avens   Bindweed   Birch   Blackberry   Buckwheat
Chervil   Cinquefoil   Clover   Cornflower   Dandelion   Fir
Frankincense   Hawthorn   Jasmine   Lady's Mantle
Marshmallow   Mugwort   Periwinkle   Poppy   Red Rose
Strawberry   Sweet Cicely   Vine   Woodruff

NEW MOON

Aloe   Birch   Blackberry   Camphor   Clover   Daisy   Gorse
Ground Ivy   Jasmine   Lily   Mulberry   Ox-Eye Daisy   White Rose
Wormwood

WANING MOON

Aspen   Blackberry   Clover   Elder   Garlic   Henbane   Myrrh
Parsley   Willow   Yew

WAXING MOON

Aloe   Camphor   Cinquefoil   Lily   Mugwort
Ox-Eye Daisy   Poppy   White Rose

Sabbats

· · · · · · · · · · · ·

Autumn Equinox

Acorn Alder Apple Ash Basil Bean Benzoin
Blackberry Buckwheat Calendula Cedar Chicory Corn
Cornflower Cypress Daisy Dog Rose Elder Frankincense
Hawthorn Hazel Ivy Myrrh Parsley Poppy Rose Yew

· · · · · ·

Beltane

Apple Belladonna Birch Celandine Cinquefoil Clover
Cuckoo Pint Daisy Dandelion Dill Dog Rose Elder Fir
Hawthorn Honeysuckle Horse Chestnut Lily of the Valley
Mallow Oak Primrose Rose Sorrel Sweet Cicely Willow Woodruff

· · · · · ·

Imbolc

Alder Alfalfa Benzoin Birch
Chickweed Elm Fir Heather Hop Lily of the Valley
Periwinkle Rowan Snowdrop Tansy Willow Woad Wormwood

· · · · · · ·

Lughnasa

Alder Apple Basil Benzoin Borage Chicory Daisy Fennel
Fenugreek Frankincense Gorse Honeysuckle Ivy Marshmallow
Mugwort Nasturtium Oak Pine Poppy Sunflower Vine Woad

· · · · · · · ·

Midsummer

Alexanders Angelica Apples Ash Bay Calendula Chamomile
Celandine Daisy Dill Dog Rose Elder Elecampane
Fennel Fern Feverfew Fir Frankincense Heather Honeysuckle
Lavender Marjoram Mint Mistletoe Oak St. John's Wort
Strawberry Sunflower Sweet Cicely Violet Yarrow

· · · · ·

OSTARA

Acacia Alder Apple Ash Benzoin Birch Bistort Blackthorn
Bluebell Calendula Caraway Celandine Cleavers Coltsfoot Daisy
Forget-Me-Not Frankincense Gorse Ground Ivy Lemon Verbena
Mugwort Nettle Pine Tansy Violet

SAMHAIN

Aconite Alder Apple Aspen Belladonna Blackthorn Calamus
Catnip Chervil Cypress Damiana Dittany of Crete Elder
Fumitory Galangal Hellebore Hemlock Henbane
Honeysuckle Hop Ivy Juniper Mullein Myrrh Parsley
Pumpkin Rowan Thistle Valerian Wormwood Yew

YULE

Apple Ash Bayberry Blackthorn Calendula
Cinnamon Cypress Fern Frankincense Holly Hop Ivy
Juniper Mistletoe Oak Violet

Elements

· · · · · · · · · ·

AIR ELEMENT

Acacia   Agrimony   Alecost   Almond   Anise   Aspen   Bean
Benzoin   Bergamot   Caraway   Cedar   Celery   Chervil   Chicory
Clary Sage   Clover   Comfrey   Dandelion   Dill   Dock   Elecampane
Fenugreek   Fern   Hazel   Hop   Horehound   Houseleek   Lavender
Lemon Verbena   Lily of the valley   Marjoram   Mint   Mistletoe
Mulberry   Niaouli   Nutmeg   Parsley   Pine   Sage   Sandalwood
Sweet Cicely   Sweet Pea   Wormwood

· · · · · · · · · ·

EARTH ELEMENT

Alfalfa   Barley   Bayberry   Bistort   Blackthorn   Briony
Buckwheat   Clover   Cypress   Elm   Fir   Fumitory   Hollyhock
Honeysuckle   Lilac   Mimosa   Oakmoss   Patchouli   Pine   Primrose
Rhubarb   Sage   Soapwort   Sorrel   Strawberry   Tansy   Tonka   Tulip
Vervain   Vetiver

· · · · · · · · · ·

FIRE ELEMENT

Alder   Alexanders   Angelica   Asafoetida
Ash   Aspen   Avens   Basil   Bay   Betony   Cedar   Celandine
Centaury   Cinnamon   Cinquefoil   Clove   Clover   Cuckoo Pint
Coriander   Dill   Dragon's Blood   Fennel   Flax   Frankincense
Galangal   Garlic   Gorse   Holly   Horse Chestnut   Horseradish
Hyssop   Juniper   Lily of the Valley   Lovage   Madder   Mandrake
Mustard   Nasturtium   Nettle   Oak   Olive   Orange   Peony
Rosemary   Rue   Saffron   Sassafras   Smallage   Sneezewort
St. John's Wort   Sunflower   Tarragon   Vine   Walnut   Woodruff

· · · · ·

WATER ELEMENT

Aconite   Alder   Aloe   Apple   Ash   Balm of Gilead   Belladonna
Bindweed   Birch   Birthwort   Blackberry   Burdock   Camphor
Cardamom   Catnip   Cereus   Chamomile   Chervil   Cleavers   Clover
Coltsfoot   Columbine   Cornflower   Daisy   Damiana   Dog Rose
Feverfew   Forget-Me-Not   Foxglove   Freesia   Gardenia   Geranium
Hellebore   Hemlock   Hemp   Henbane   Herb Robert   Hyacinth
Indigo   Ivy   Jasmine   Lady's Mantle   Lemon Balm   Lily   Mallow
Marshmallow   Meadowsweet   Melon   Mugwort   Mullein   Myrrh   Myrtle
Narcissus   Opium   Orris (Iris)   Ox-Eye Daisy   Palmorosa   Periwinkle
Plumaria   Poppy (Red)   Purslane   Rose   Rowan   Skullcap   Snowdrop
Spider Lily   Stephanotis   Thyme   Valerian   Vanilla   Violet   Water Lily
Willow   Woad   Wood Aloe   Yarrow   Yew   Ylang-Ylang

Planets

· · · · ·
EARTH

Acorns   Amaranth   Barley   Buckthorn   Clary Sage
Comfrey   Cypress   Field Poppy   Horehound   Liquorice
Maize   Millet   Mugwort   Patchouli   Oak   Oak Moss
Oat   Rice   Rye   Sage   Spruce   Vervain   Vetiver   Wheat

· · · · · ·
JUPITER

Agrimony   Alexanders   Avens   Balm of Gilead   Betony   Borage
Chervil   Chicory   Cinquefoil   Clove   Dandelion   Datura   Dock
Hemp Agrimony   Honeysuckle   Horse Chestnut   Houseleek   Hyssop
Lemon Balm   Mace   Meadowsweet   Mistletoe   Nutmeg   Oak
Oakmoss   Red Rose   Sage   Sassafras   Star Anise   Sweet Cicely   Tonka

· · · · ·
MARS

Allspice   Anemone   Asafoetida   Basil   Bearberry   Beech   Black Pepper
Bryony   Broom   Coffee   Coriander   Cuckoo Pint   Deerstongue
Dragon's Blood   Fern   Galangal   Garlic   Ginger   Hawthorn
Holly   Hop   Horseradish   Juniper   Madder   Mustard   Nasturtium
Nettle   Onion   Pennyroyal   Pine   Rue   Sneezewort   Tarragon
Thistle   Woodruff   Wormwood

· · · · · ·
MERCURY

Almond   Anise   Aspen   Bayberry   Bean   Benzoin   Bergamot   Caraway
Cedar   Celery   Clary Sage   Clover   Dill   Elecampane   Eucalyptus   Fennel
Fenugreek   Fern   Flax   Hazel   Horehound   Lavender   Lemon Verbena
Lemongrass   Lily of the Valley   Liquorice   Mandrake   Marjoram   Mulberry
Niaouli   Parsley   Peppermint   Smallage   Spearmint   Sweet Pea   Valerian

· · · · ·

. . . . .

MOON

Alecost Aloe Camphor Cereus Clary Sage Cleavers Dog Rose
Fir Gardenia Honesty Jasmine Lemon Lemon Balm
Lily Lotus Marshmallow Melon Mugwort Myrrh Opium
Ox-Eye Daisy Peony Poppy Purslane Rowan Snowdrop
Stephanotis Water Lily White Rose White Sandalwood Willow

. . . .

NEPTUNE

Not one of the seven known ancient planets, but modern attributions include:
Hemp Lemon Lobelia Lotus Mugwort Opium Poppy Orange
Orange Blossom Passionflower Pine Reed
Wild Lettuce Willow Wisteria

. . . .

PLUTO

Not one of the seven known ancient planets, but modern attributions include:
Acacia Aquilegia Damiana Eucalyptus Hop Larkspur
Male Fern Patchouli Pine Wormwood

. . . . .

SATURN

Aconite Asafoetida Belladonna Bindweed Bistort Blackthorn
Comfrey Cornflower Cypress Datura Elm Fern Fumitory
Hellebore Hemlock Hemp Henbane Holly Indigo Ivy Mimosa
Mullein Myrrh Patchouli Skullcap Woad Yew

. . . . .

• • •

SUN

Acacia Angelica Arnica Ash Aspen Bay Benzoin Burnet
Butterbur Calendula Carnation Caraway Cedar Celandine Centaury
Chamomile Cinnamon Citron Clove Copal Eyebright Frankincense
Goldenseal Gorse Juniper Lovage Mastic Mistletoe Nasturtium
Neroli Olive Orange Peony Petitgrain Reed Rosemary Rue Saffron
Sandalwood (Red) St. John's Wort Sunflower Vine Walnut Witch Hazel

• • • • •

URANUS

Not one of the seven known ancient planets, but modern attributions include:
Bryony Cinnamon Clove Coffee Guarana
Kava-Kava Nutmeg Pokeweed

• • • •

VENUS

Alder Alfalfa Apple Balm of Gilead Birch Birthwort Blackberry
Buckwheat Bugle Burdock Cardamom Catnip Cherry Chickweed
Coltsfoot Columbine Cowslip Daffodil Daisy Dog Rose Elder
Feverfew Forget-Me-Not Foxglove Freesia Gardenia Geranium
Golden Rod Ground Ivy Heather Herb Robert Hollyhock Hyacinth
Iris Lady's Mantle Larkspur Lemon Verbena Lilac Magnolia Mallow
Marshmallow Meadowsweet Mint Mugwort Myrtle Narcissus
Orris (Iris) Palmorosa Patchouli Periwinkle Plumeria Primrose
Rose (Damask) Soapwort Sorrel Spider Lily Strawberry Sweetpea
Tansy Thyme Tuberose Tulip Vanilla Vetiver Violet Wood Aloe
Yarrow Ylang-Ylang

Rituals

. . . .

AURA CLEANSING

Agrimony   Angelica   Bean   Betony   Cinquefoil   Fumitory
Horehound   Jasmine   Rosemary   Sage

. . . .

CLEANSING AND PURIFICATION

Agrimony   Angelica   Agrimony   Avens   Basil   Bay   Bean   Beech
Benzoin   Birch   Broom   Burdock   Camphor   Caraway   Cinquefoil
Clove   Comfrey   Dill   Dragon's Blood   Eucalyptus   Fennel
Frankincense   Gorse   Garlic   Horehound, White   Hyssop   Juniper
Lavender   Lemon Balm   Lovage   Nettle   Oak   Pine   Primrose
Rosemary   Rue   Sage   Soapwort   St. John's Wort   Tansy   Thyme   Vervain

. . . .

CONSECRATION

Bay   Bayberry   Belladonna   Bindweed   Borage   Calendula   Caraway
Chicory   Clover   Dragon's Blood   Frankincense   Fumitory   Hemlock
Horehound   Hyssop   Mint   Nettle   Olive   Rue   Sunflower

. . . .

DIVINATION

Aloe   Anise   Bay   Belladonna   Bistort   Calendula
Camphor   Chicory   Cinnamon   Clary   Cleavers   Damiana
Dandelion   Fern   Hazel   Hemp   Honeysuckle   Mace   Mugwort
Nutmeg   Rowan   Sandalwood   Vervain   Wormwood   Yarrow

. . . .

EXORCISM

Asafoetida   Avens   Basil   Beans   Birch   Garlic   Hellebore
Horseradish   Juniper   Marshmallow   Rue   St. John's Wort

. . . . .

HEALING

Allspice   Angelica   Apple   Bay   Chamomile   Cinnamon   Comfrey
Dock   Elder   Eucalyptus   Garlic   Hollyhock   Juniper   Lavender
Lemon Balm   Rosemary   Sage   Sassafras

MEDITATION AND RELAXATION

Acacia   Acacia   Benzoin   Bergamot   Chamomile   Feverfew
Frankincense   Hollyhock   Horse Chestnut   Lavender   Lemon Balm
Patchouli   Rose   Sandalwood   Skullcap

PROTECTION

Acacia   Agrimony   Aloe   Angelica   Asafoetida   Avens   Basil   Bay
Betony   Birch   Bryony   Burdock   Cactus   Chamomile   Caraway   Celandine
Cinnamon   Cinquefoil   Clove   Clover   Comfrey   Coriander   Dandelion
Dill   Dragon's Blood   Elecampane   Fennel   Feverfew   Frankincense
Fumitory   Garlic   Geranium   Heather   Holly   Hollyhock   Houseleek
Hyssop   Iris   Ivy   Jasmine   Lavender   Mandrake   Marigold (Calendula)
Marjoram   Marshmallow   Mistletoe   Mugwort   Mullein   Nettle   Onion
Pennyroyal   Peony   Purslane   Poplar   Primrose   Rosemary   Rowan
Rue   Solomon's Seal   St. John's Wort   Thistle   Thyme   Vervain   Yarrow

PSYCHIC AWARENESS

Aloe   Angelica   Anise   Bay   Bearberry   Benzoin   Borage
Dandelion   Eyebright   Henbane   Myrrh   Smallage

Zodiac

· · · · · · ·
AQUARIUS

Acacia Almond Benzoin Citron Costmary Cypress Hops
Lavender Lemon Verbena Mace Mastic Mimosa Mint Parsley
Patchouli Pine Star Anise Sweet Pea

· · · ·
ARIES

Allspice Betony Black Pepper Blackberry Carnation Cedar Cinnamon
Clove Copal Coriander Cumin Fennel Frankincense Galangal Ginger
Juniper Marjoram Mustard Neroli Pennyroyal Peppermint Petitgrain
Pine Rosemary Thyme Woodruff

· · · · ·
CANCER

Agrimony Calamus Cardamom Chamomile Daisy Eucalyptus
Gardenia Honeysuckle Hyssop Jasmine Lemon Lemon Balm
Lilac Lily Myrrh Palmarosa Plumeria Sandalwood
Violet White Rose Yarrow

· · · · · · ·
CAPRICORN

Comfrey Cypress Honeysuckle Lilac Magnolia
Mimosa Moss Myrrh Patchouli Tonka Tulip Vetiver Vervain

· · · · ·
GEMINI

Almond Anise Benzoin Bergamot Caraway Citron Clover
Dill Horehound Lavender Lemongrass Lily Mace Mastic
Meadowsweet Mint Parsley Peppermint Sweet Pea

· · · · ·

• • •
LEO

Acacia Angelica Bay Basil Benzoin Borage Calendula Cinnamon
Copal Eyebright Frankincense Ginger Juniper Lime Mastic
Nasturtium Neroli Nutmeg Orange Peony Petitgrain
Rosemary Rue Rue Saffron Red Sandalwood Sunflower

• • • •
LIBRA

Apple Catnip Chamomile Daffodil Dill Eucalyptus Fennel
Geranium Lilac Magnolia Marjoram Mugwort Orchid Palmarosa
Peppermint Pine Rose Spearmint Sweetpea Thyme Vanilla
Vervain Violet

• • • •
PISCES

Alder Anise Apple Calamus Camphor Cardamom
Catnip Clove Eucalyptus Gardenia Honeysuckle Hyacinth
Jasmine Lemon Lily Mimosa Mugwort Myrrh Nutmeg
Orris (Iris) Palmarosa Sage Sarsaparilla Sweetpea
Vanilla White Sandalwood Ylang-Ylang

• • • • • • • •
SAGITTARIUS

Anise Bergamot (Citrus) Calendula Carnation
Cedar Clove Copal Dandelion Dragon's Blood Fir Frankincense
Ginger Honeysuckle Hyssop Juniper Lemon Balm Mace
Mallow Marshmallow Nutmeg Oakmoss Orange Rose Rosemary
Saffron Sage Sassafras Ylang-Ylang

• • • • • • •
SCORPIO

Allspice Basil Black Pepper Cardamom Coffee Clove Cumin
Galangal Gardenia Ginger Hyacinth Hops Myrrh
Pennyroyal Pine Thyme Tuberose Vanilla Violet Woodruff

TAURUS

Apple Cardamom Daisy Honeysuckle Lilac Lovage Magnolia
Moss Mugwort Oakmoss Orchid Patchouli Periwinkle
Plumeria Rose Thyme Tonka Vanilla Violet Ylang-Ylang

VIRGO

Almond Bergamot Caraway Cedar Clary Sage Costmary
Cypress Dill Fennel Honeysuckle Lavender Lemon Balm
Lily Mace Mint Moss Oakmoss Patchouli Valerian

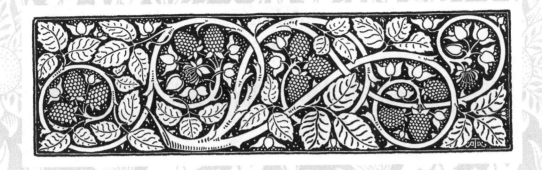

Weights & Measures

Volume
(Liquid Measures)

IMPERIAL	METRIC	US CUPS
½ FLUID OUNCE	15 MILLILITRES	1 TABLESPOON
1 FLUID OUNCE	30 MILLILITRES	2 TABLESPOONS
2 FLUID OUNCES	60 MILLILITRES	¼ CUP
2½ FLUID OUNCES	75 MILLILITRES	⅓ CUP
4 FLUID OUNCES	120 MILLILITRES	½ CUP
5 FLUID OUNCES	150 MILLILITRES	⅔ CUP
6 FLUID OUNCES	180 MILLILITRES	¾ CUP
8 FLUID OUNCES	250 MILLILITRES	1 CUP
10 FLUID OUNCES (½ PINT)	310 MILLILITRES	1¼ CUPS
20 FLUID OUNCES (1 PINT)	620 MILLILITRES	2½ CUPS

Weights
(Rough Equivalents)

IMPERIAL	METRIC
½ OUNCE	15 GRAMS
1 OUNCES	30 GRAMS
2 OUNCES	60 GRAMS
3 OUNCES	90 GRAMS
4 OUNCES	110 GRAMS
5 OUNCES	140 GRAMS
6 OUNCES	170 GRAMS
7 OUNCES	200 GRAMS
8 OUNCES	225 GRAMS
9 OUNCES	255 GRAMS
10 OUNCES	280 GRAMS
11 OUNCES	310 GRAMS
12 OUNCES	340 GRAMS
13 OUNCES	370 GRAMS
14 OUNCES	400 GRAMS
15 OUNCES	425 GRAMS
16 OUNCES (1 POUND)	450 GRAMS

Ingredient Weights
(Rough Equivalents)

ITEM	US CUPS	IMPERIAL	METRIC
BUTTER	1	8 OUNCES	225 GRAMS
OATMEAL	1	3 OUNCES	85 GRAMS
SUGAR, GRANULATED	1	7 OUNCES	200 GRAMS
SUGAR, SOFT BROWN	1	8 OUNCES	220 GRAMS
SUGAR, POWDERED	1	4 OUNCES	110 GRAMS
FLOUR	1	4½ OUNCES	125 GRAMS
APPLES, SLICED	1	4 OUNCES	223 GRAMS
CHEESE, GRATED	1	4 OUNCES	110 GRAMS
CORNFLOUR (CORNSTARCH)	1	4 OUNCES	110 GRAMS
MAYONNAISE	1	8 OUNCES	225 GRAMS

Temperatures

FAHRENHEIT	CELSIUS
32°F	0°C (FREEZING POINT)
70°F	21°C (AVERAGE ROOM TEMPERATURE/ LUKEWARM)
212°F	100°C (BOILING POINT OF WATER

Oven Temperatures

CELSIUS	FAHRENHEIT	GAS MARK	DESCRIPTION
110	225	¼	VERY COOL/SLOW
130	250	½	
140	275	1	COOL
150	300	2	
170	325	3	
180	350	4	MODERATE
190	375	5	
200	400	6	
220	425	7	HOT
230	450	8	
245	475	9	VERY HOT

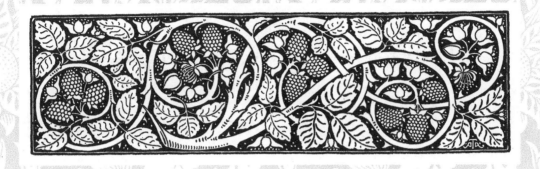

Your Recipes

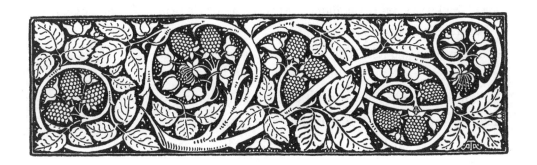

Select Bibliography

Arnold, James. *Country Crafts*. London: John Baker Ltd., 1968.

Baker, Margaret. *Folklore and Customs of Rural England*. David and Charles, 1974.

Beyerl, Paul. *The Master Book of Herbalism*. Washington: Phoenix Publishing, 1984.

Boxer, Arabella, and Philippa Back. *The Herb Book*. London: Octopus Books, 1980.

Brown, Deni. *Encyclopedia of Herbs and Their Uses*. New York: Dorling Kindersley, 1995.

Buhner, Stephen Harrod. *Sacred and Herbal Healing Beers*. Boulder: Siris Books, 1998.

Castleman, Michael. *The Healing Herbs*. Emmaus: Rodale Press, 1991.

Chevalier, Andrew. *The Encyclopaedia of Medicinal Plants*. London: Dorling Kindersley, 1996.

Culpeper's Complete Herbal. W. Foulsham & Co. Ltd, n/d.

De Menezes, Patricia. *Crafts from the Countryside*. London: Hamlyn, 1981.

Down, Deni. *The Royal Horticultural Society Encyclopaedia of Herbs and Their Uses.* London: Dorling Kindersley, 1997.

Elkington, John, and Julia Hailes. *The Green Consumer Guide.* London: Victor Gollancz Ltd, 1988.

Franklin, Anna, and Sue Lavender. *Herb Craft.* Chieveley: Capall Bann, 1995.

Franklin, Anna. *Hearth Witch.* Earl Shilton: Lear Books, 2004.

Genders, Roy. *Natural Beauty.* Lucerne: EMB Services, 1992.

Gerard's Herbal. London: Senate, 1994.

Gordon, Lesley. *A Country Herbal.* London: Peerage Books, 1980.

Green, James. *The Herbal Medicine Maker's Handbook.* Berkeley: Crossing Press, 2002.

Green, M. *Gods of the Celts.* Gloucester: Allan Sutton, 1986.

Grieve, Mrs. M. *A Modern Herbal.* New York: Dover Publications, 1981.

Griggs, Barbara. *Green Pharmacy: A History of Herbal Medicine.* New York: Viking Press, 1982.

Guyton, Anita. *The Book of Natural Beauty.* London: Stanley Paul & Co. Ltd., 1981.

Hemphill, Rosemary. *Herbs for All Seasons.* London: Penguin, 1975.

Hoffman, David. *The Holistic Herbal.* Shaftsbury: Element Books, 1986.

Holmes, Peter. *The Energetics of Western Herbs.* Boulder: Artemis Press, 1989.

Lawless, Julia. *The Illustrated Encyclopaedia of Essential Oils.* Shaftsbury: Element, 1995.

Little, Kitty. *Kitty Little's Book of Herbal Beauty.* Harmondsworth: Penguin Books, 1981.

Lust, John. *The Herb Book.* Bantam Books, 1974.

Mabey, Richard. *Flora Britannica.* London: Sinclair-Stevenson, 1996.

———. *Food for Free.* Glasgow: William Collins, 1972.

———. *Plants with a Purpose.* London: Fontana, 1979.

Newdick, Jane. *Sloe Gin and Beeswax.* London: Charles Letts & Co. Ltd., 1993.

Ody, Penelope. *The Complete Medicinal Herbal.* London: Dorling Kindersley, 1993.

Passebecq, Andre. *Aromatherapy.* Wellingborough: Thorsons, 1979.

Pennick, Nigel. *Secrets of East Anglian Magic.* Milverton: Capall Bann, 2004.

Price, Shirley. *Practical Aromatherapy.* Wellingborough: Thorsons, 1983.

Raven, J. E. *Plants and Plant Lore in Ancient Greece.* Oxford: Leopard's Head Press, 2000.

Seymour, John, and Sally Seymour. *Self Sufficiency.* London: Faber and Faber, 1973.

Stapley, Christina. *Herbcraft Naturally*. Chichester: Heartsease Books, 1994.

Steel, Susannah, ed. *Neal's Yard Remedies*. London: Dorling Kindersley, 2011.

Strauss, Rachelle. *Household Cleaning*. London: New Holland Publishers, 2009.

Tisserand, Robert B. *The Art of Aromatherapy*. Rochester: Healing Arts Press, 1977.

Vickery, Roy. *Oxford Dictionary of Plant Lore*. Oxford University Press, 1995.

Walsh, Penny. *Spinning, Dyeing and Weaving*. London: New Holland Publishers, 2009.

Watts, D. C. *Elsevier's Dictionary of Plant Lore*. San Diego: Elsevier, 2007.

Wong, James. *Grow Your Own Drugs*. London: Collins, 2009.

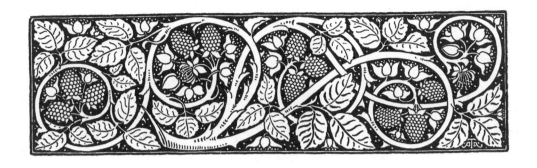

Index

RECIPE INDEX

• • • • •